Diagnosis and Treatment of Bone and Joint Disorders

Diagnosis and Treatment of Bone and Joint Disorders

Edited by Vincent Brooks

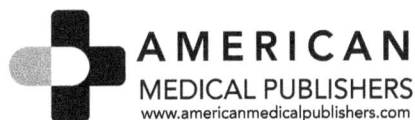

AMERICAN
MEDICAL PUBLISHERS
www.americanmedicalpublishers.com

American Medical Publishers,
41 Flatbush Avenue,
1st Floor, New York,
NY 11217, USA

Visit us on the World Wide Web at:
www.americanmedicalpublishers.com

ISBN: 978-1-63927-393-5

Cataloging-in-Publication Data

Diagnosis and treatment of bone and joint disorders / edited by Vincent Brooks.
    p. cm.
Includes bibliographical references and index.
ISBN 978-1-63927-393-5
1. Bones--Diseases. 2. Joints--Diseases. 3. Musculoskeletal system--Diseases. I. Brooks, Vincent.
RC930 .B66 2022
616.71--dc23

Table of Contents

Preface

This book has been an outcome of determined endeavour from a group of educationists in the field. The primary objective was to involve a broad spectrum of professionals from diverse cultural background involved in the field for developing new researches. The book not only targets students but also scholars pursuing higher research for further enhancement of the theoretical and practical applications of the subject.

The adult human skeletal system comprising of 206 bones provides support and protection to internal organs, and facilitates movement. The joints between bones can maintain heavy loads, withstand compression and execute smooth and precise movements. The bones are affected by a number of diseases, among which are fractures, infections, arthritis, osteoporosis and tumors. Fractures occur on exposure to a significant force or repeated trauma over time. It may also occur when a bone is considerably weakened with osteoporosis, cancer or affected with Paget's disease. Metastases in bones are generally secondary cancers but bones are a common site for the spread of lung cancer, breast cancer, thyroid cancer, kidney cancer and prostate cancer. These secondary cancers can destroy or create bone. Cancers of the bone marrow can affect the bone tissue. In osteoporosis, there is a reduction of bone mineral density thereby increasing the likelihood of fractures. When one or more joints are inflamed, the condition is called arthritis. It can be of different forms- osteoarthritis, septic arthritis, gouty arthritis, psoriatic arthritis, etc. The joints of the mandible may be affected by temporomandibular joint syndrome that inhibits jaw movement and cause facial pain. Bones and joints disorders are diagnosed with ultrasound, CT scan, MRI scan and X-ray. This book is compiled in such a manner, that it will provide in-depth knowledge about bone and joint disorders. It includes contributions of experts and scientists which will provide innovative insights into these disorders. For all those who are interested in orthopedics, this book can prove to be an essential guide.

It was an honour to edit such a profound book and also a challenging task to compile and examine all the relevant data for accuracy and originality. I wish to acknowledge the efforts of the contributors for submitting such brilliant and diverse chapters in the field and for endlessly working for the completion of the book. Last, but not the least; I thank my family for being a constant source of support in all my research endeavours.

Editor

Knee dGEMRIC at 7 T: comparison against 1.5 T and evaluation of T_1-mapping methods

Pernilla Peterson[1,2]* (ID), Carl Johan Tiderius[3], Emma Olsson[1], Björn Lundin[4], Lars E. Olsson[1,2] and Jonas Svensson[1,4]

Abstract

Background: dGEMRIC (delayed Gadolinium Enhanced Magnetic Resonance Image of Cartilage) is a well-established technique for cartilage quality assessment in osteoarthritis at clinical field strengths. The method is robust, but requires injection of contrast agent and a cumbersome examination procedure. New non-contrast-agent-based techniques for cartilage quality assessment are currently being developed at 7 T. However, dGEMRIC remains an important reference technique during this development. The aim of this work was to compare T_1 mapping for dGEMRIC at 7 T and 1.5 T, and to evaluate three T_1-mapping methods at 7 T.

Methods: The knee of 10 healthy volunteers and 9 patients with early signs of cartilage degradation were examined at 1.5 T and 7 T after a single (one) contrast agent injection ($Gd\text{-}(DTPA)^{2-}$). Inversion recovery (IR) sequences were acquired at both field strengths, and at 7 T variable flip angle (VFA) and Look-Locker (LL) sequences were additionally acquired. T_1 maps were calculated and average T_1 values were estimated within superficial and deep regions-of-interest (ROIs) in the lateral and medial condyles, respectively.

Results: T_1 values were 1.8 (1.4–2.3) times longer at 7 T. A strong correlation was detected between 1.5 T and 7 T T_1 values ($r = 0.80$). For IR, an additional inversion time was required to avoid underestimation (bias±limits of agreement -127 ± 234 ms) due to the longer T_1 values at 7 T. Out of the two 3D sequences tested, LL resulted in more accurate and precise T_1 estimation compared to VFA (average bias±limits of agreement LL: 12 ± 202 ms compared to VFA: 25 ± 622 ms). For both, B_1 correction improved agreement to IR.

Conclusion: With an adapted sampling scheme, dGEMRIC T_1 mapping is feasible at 7 T and correlates well to 1.5 T. If 3D is to be used for T_1 mapping of the knee at 7 T, LL is preferred and VFA is not recommended. For VFA and LL, B_1 correction is necessary for accurate T_1 estimation.

Keywords: dGEMRIC, Cartilage, 7 T, Inversion recovery, Variable flip angle, Look-locker

Background

Osteoarthritis is a common, painful, and disabling condition characterized by degradation and loss of cartilage. Although the disease progresses slowly, early detection is critical for development of treatment strategies which may prevent or slow down degradation before the cartilage is irreversibly lost.

The delayed Gadolinium Enhanced Magnetic Resonance Imaging of Cartilage (dGEMRIC) technique is a well-established method for early assessment of cartilage quality in osteoarthritis [1]. Using this technique, the distribution of $Gd\text{-}(DTPA)^{2-}$ contrast agent in cartilage after intravenous injection is assessed with quantitative T_1 mapping. The estimated T_1 is assumed to be indirectly related to the content of glycosaminoglycan (GAG) which is known to decrease early in osteoarthritis. The method is robust and has proved to sensitively detect early degenerative cartilage processes [2, 3] and loss of cartilage quality [4]. However, the technique requires injection of contrast agent, which in addition to a cumbersome

* Correspondence: pernilla.peterson@med.lu.se
[1]Medical Radiation Physics, Department of Translational Medicine, Lund University, Inga Marie Nilssons gata 49, SE-205 02 Malmö, Sweden
[2]Department of Oncology and Radiation Physics, Skåne University Hospital, Inga Marie Nilssons gata 49, SE-205 02 Malmö, Sweden
Full list of author information is available at the end of the article

examination procedure may also lead to long-term gadolinium deposits [5]. Thus, current development of magnetic resonance imaging (MRI) methods for assessment of cartilage quality is focused on methods that do not require contrast agent injection (e.g. GAG Chemical Exchange Saturation Transfer (gagCEST), ^{23}Na imaging, T_2 mapping, and $T_{1\rho}$ mapping [6]). In the development process of these new techniques there is still a real need for an established method for cartilage quality evaluation to use as a reference. For this purpose dGEMRIC may still be the most suitable choice.

gagCEST and ^{23}Na imaging benefit from the use of an ultra-high field strength, such as 7 T [7, 8]. Most dGEMRIC studies have so far been conducted at clinical field strengths. To enable the use of dGEMRIC as a reference tool during the development of the new techniques, there is a need to first validate dGEMRIC also at 7 T.

Translating the dGEMRIC technique to an ultra-high field strength may have some advantages but there are also several challenges. Increasing the field strength increases the signal-to-noise ratio (SNR), which may be used to improve either the measurement precision or imaging resolution. However, a higher field strength also increases the expected T_1 values [9] and decreases the relaxivity of Gd-(DTPA)$^{2-}$ [10]. These effects may require an altered dGEMRIC protocol and could reduce the sensitivity of the dGEMRIC experiment.

T_1 mapping is a core component of the dGEMRIC technique and several methods have been suggested in the literature. The gold standard approach is the 2D inversion recovery (IR) technique, but also 3D approaches such as the variable flip angle (VFA) [11] and Look-Locker (LL) techniques have been increasingly used over the last years [12–14]. Several challenges for accurate T_1 measurements are expected when moving to a higher field strength. First, the longer T_1 values likely require longer inversion and repetition times which increases the acquisition time. Second, the B_1 field is likely more inhomogeneous at ultra-high field strengths compared to clinical field strengths. This may affect the quality of the inversion pulse for the IR and LL experiments, but may also make B_1 correction approaches necessary for the VFA and LL techniques [14, 15]. For dGEMRIC at 7 T, IR [16] and VFA [17, 18] have previously been used for T_1 mapping, but as no quantitative comparison between the methods has been performed, further investigation is needed to find the optimal T_1-mapping approach at ultra-high field strength.

The aim of this study was to evaluate the feasibility of T1 mapping for knee dGEMRIC at 7 T by comparison against 1.5 T in human subjects in vivo. In order to identify a preferred choice of T_1-mapping approach at the ultra-high field strength, we additionally aim to compare and evaluate three T_1-mapping techniques – IR, VFA, and LL.

Methods
Human subjects
The study was approved by the regional ethical review board and all human subjects gave their written informed consent. To increase the expected range of T_1 values, both healthy volunteers ($N = 10$; 6 males, 4 females; median (range) age = 33.5 (23–56) years; body mass index (BMI) = 23.6 (20.7–26.3) kg/m^2) and patients with early degenerative changes in the knee cartilage ($N = 9$; 6 males, 3 females; median (range) age = 42.9 (36–48) years; BMI = 30.1 (23.8–33.3) kg/m^2) were included in the study. The inclusion criterion for the healthy volunteers was: No previous history of pain or other problem with the knee to be examined. Inclusion criteria for the patients were: superficial degenerative cartilage changes on the medial femoral condyle but no significant cartilage loss or fissuring deeper than 50% of the cartilage thickness as verified by arthroscopy conducted no more than 5 years before the MRI. The median time between arthroscopy and and imaging for the included subjects was 2.4 years (min 1.0 and max 2.8 years). Exclusion criteria for all subjects were: Kidney disease and implants which were not MRI compatible or risked induce artifacts.

Experiment procedure
Upon arrival at the hospital, an intravenous injection of a double dose (0.2 mmol/kg body weight) of Gd-(DTPA)$^{2-}$ (Magnevist®, Bayer Schering Pharma AG, Berlin, Germany) was administered. The subjects were then asked to walk at an easy pace along a specified path during 10 min to help distribution of the contrast agent in the cartilage [19].

Either the left or right knee of all subjects were imaged using both 1.5 T and 7 T MRI scanners (Philips Achieva dStream and Philips Achieva AS, Best, the Netherlands). Both examinations were conducted during one session after the same contrast agent injection. Half of the healthy subjects were examined at 1.5 T first and half at 7 T first. The order of the patient examinations was determined by practical scheduling considerations. Start of the first imaging session was planned such that the first IR sequence (see details below) was initiated 120 min after the contrast agent injection. The order of the sequences in the scan protocols was planned to ensure a minimum delay between the acquisitions of the IR sequences at the two field strengths. The subjects were transported between the two scanner rooms sitting in a wheel chair to minimize redistribution of the contrast agent in the knee joint between the examinations.

MRI examination

During the examinations, the knee was immobilized slightly bent in dedicated knee coils (1.5 T: receive only dStream Knee 15ch Coil, 7 T: transmit and receive QED Knee Coil 1TX / 28RX) using pads. A series of IR sequences with different inversion times (TI) were acquired at both 1.5 T and at 7 T. 2D slices were centered over the medial and lateral condyle, respectively, and imaged in separate sequences (single slice). At 1.5 T, 6 TIs were acquired (TI = 50 ms, 100 ms, 200 ms, 400 ms, 800 ms, and 1600 ms). Other parameters were: repetition time (TR) = 2000 ms, echo time (TE) = 7 ms, field of view (FOV) = 120x120x3 mm^3, bandwidth = 402 Hz/pixel, echo train length = 11, matrix size = 256 × 256, and acquisition time (TA)/IR sequence = 46 s. The corresponding parameters for the 7 IR acquisitions at 7 T were TI = 50 ms, 100 ms, 200 ms, 400 ms, 800 ms, 1600 ms, and 3800 ms, TR = 4000 ms, TE = 7 ms, FOV = 120x120x3 mm^3, bandwidth = 338 Hz/pixel, echo train length = 11, matrix size = 256 × 256, and TA/IR sequence = 1 min and 36 s. At 1.5 T a short diagnostic protocol was also executed in addition to the IR acquisition for all subjects. This was later used to exclude unexpected pathology and to aid in determining that the cartilage had adequate thickness for ROI evaluation.

At 7 T two different 3D T$_1$ methods were additionally evaluated: VFA and LL. For VFA, two 3D gradient echo sequences covering the knee joint were acquired with a non-selective excitation pulse and flip angles = 7° and 39°, TR = 30 ms, TE = 2.7 ms, FOV = 120 × 120 mm^2, slice thickness = 3 mm, pixel bandwidth = 338 Hz, matrix size = 256 × 256, and TA/ sequence = 4–6 min depending on number of slices. The flip angles were optimized expecting a T$_1$ of 700 ms [20]. For LL, a 3D gradient echo sequence was acquired with flip angle = 6°, TR = 5000 ms, time between each excitation pulse 5.5 ms, TE = 2.7 ms, FOV = 140x140x3 mm^3, pixel bandwidth = 338 Hz, echo train length = 15, matrix size = 256 × 256, and TA = 13–15 min depending on number of slices. 24 inversion times were acquired ranging from 16 ms – 3466 ms.

Finally, a Dual Refocusing Echo Acquisition Mode (DREAM) method for B$_1$ mapping [21] was acquired at 7 T with: flip angle = 15°, TR = 5.7 ms, TE = 2.9 ms, FOV = 120 × 120 mm^2, slice thickness = 3 mm, pixel bandwidth = 1695 Hz, matrix size = 120 × 110, and TA = 2–3 min depending on number of slices.

The acquisition of the IR sequences were prioritized and were acquired in all subjects. In some cases the 7 T examinations were limited by time,

and for this reason both 3D sequences where not acquired in all subjects. VFA was acquired in 10 subjects (5 patients and 5 healthy subjects) and LL in 14 subjects (5 patients and 9 healthy subjects). The total scan time for each volunteer was approximately 20 min at 1.5 T and 50 min at 7 T.

Estimation of T$_1$ maps

Voxel-based T$_1$ maps were created using the data from the three different methods (IR, VFA, and LL) in home-written Matlab scripts (v. R2013b, Mathworks, Nattick, USA). When necessary, affine image registration using the imregister Matlab function was conducted between the various image sequences before further T$_1$ estimation. The T1 calculations in the scripts were validated with phantom experiments using Ni-doped agarores gel phantoms with known T1 relaxation times before the start of this study (data not shown). The following calculations were performed:

B$_1$ error estimation

The relative B$_1$ error (c), expressed as a fraction of the nominal flip angle, was mapped using the DREAM sequence as described above [21]. An average value (c_{ROI}) within the investigated region-of-interest (ROI) (see below) was estimated and used for correction of VFA and LL data.

IR

T$_1$ was estimated with a 3-parameter fit to Eq. (1) using a Levenberg-Marquardt non-linear-least-squares algorithm:

$$S_{TI} = S_0 \left(1 - ke^{-\frac{TI}{T_1}} + e^{-\frac{TR}{T_1}} \right) \qquad (1)$$

S_{TI} is the signal acquired at inversion time TI, S_0 is the estimated signal at $TI = 0$, and k is the quality of the inversion pulse. A perfect inversion pulse corresponds to $k = 2$.

For estimation of T$_1$ at 1.5 T, all six acquired S_{TI} were used. For 7 T, T$_1$ was estimated both from the first six S_{TI} and from all seven S_{TI}s to investigate the importance of the additional longer TI at 7 T.

LL

From LL data (S_{TI}) the apparent T$_1$ (T$_1$*), M_A, and M_B were estimated in a 3-parameter fit to the following equation using a Levenberg-Marquardt non-linear-least-squares algorithm [22]:

$$S_{TI} = M_A - M_B e^{-\frac{TI}{T_{1*}}} \qquad (2)$$

For estimation of the actual T$_1$ the following equation was used:

$$T_1 = \frac{1}{\dfrac{1}{T_1*} + \dfrac{\ln(\cos(c\alpha))}{TR}} \tag{3}$$

The nominal flip angle is represented by α, and the relative error of the flip angle is given by the factor c. Both B_1-uncorrected ($c = 1$) and B_1-corrected ($c = c_{ROI}$, see above) T_1 values were estimated for comparison.

VFA

The T_1 was estimated from the signals S_1 and S_2 acquired at the two flip angles α_1 and α_2 according to [23]:

$$T_1 = \frac{TR}{\log\left(\dfrac{\sin(c\alpha_1)\cos(c\alpha_2) - \dfrac{S_1}{S_2}\sin(c\alpha_2)\cos(c\alpha_1)}{\sin(c\alpha_1) - \dfrac{S_1}{S_2}\sin(c\alpha_2)}\right)} \tag{4}$$

A B_1-uncorrected T_1 was obtained by setting $c = 1$, whereas $c = c_{ROI}$ was used for a B_1-corrected T_1.

Data analysis

Data analysis and ROI definition was performed in Matlab (v. R2013b, Mathworks, Nattick, USA). Two ROIs (one superficial and one deep) were drawn in each of the load-bearing lateral and medial femoral condyles for each field strength and method, respectively. Each ROI covered half the depth of the femoral cartilage from the center of the tibial plateau to the posterior boundary of the posterior meniscus. All ROIs were drawn by two readers to evaluate the variance in ROI definition. IR ROIs were drawn by Reader 1 and Reader 2 with 19 and 2 years of experience, respectively. VFA and LL ROIs were drawn by Reader 2 and Reader 3 (1 year of experience). For the 3D sequences, care was taken to choose the slice that best matched the position of the IR slice. In addition, the adjacent two slices were also evaluated for both 3D approaches to investigate the uncertainty introduced by non-identical slice positioning. To exclude any possible extreme values, all values above 1300 ms (1.5 T) and 2600 ms (7 T) were disregarded when estimating the average T_1 within each ROI. In addition, the average k factor was calculated within IR ROIs to investigate adiabatic pulse quality.

All estimated average T_1 values within an ROI were corrected for BMI differences between subjects with a reference BMI set to the mean value of all healthy subjects (BMI = 23.4 kg/m^2) [24].

Statistical analysis

Statistical analysis was conducted in Matlab (v. R2013b, Mathworks, Nattick, USA) and for all statistical testing,

$P < 0.05$ was considered a significant result. Median and range were used for descriptive statistics.

To investigate a potential difference between starting at 1.5 T or 7 T, the relative T_1 increase at 7 T was compared between the groups starting at 1.5 T and 7 T using a Mann-Whitney U test. The Pearson correlation coefficient was used to estimate the correlation between T_1 values at 1.5 T and 7 T. The coefficient of variation, defined as the ratio of the range and median T_1 values in the healthy and patient subject groups, was used as a measure of variability. The differences in T1 values between healthy subjects and patients were tested for the various ROIs using a Mann-Whitney U test at both 1.5 T and 7 T. The quality of the fit for IR T_1 calculations was estimated as the standard error of the estimate (SEE) defined as the root of the averaged squared distance from the data points to the fitted line. The SEE was normalized to the estimated S_0 and compared between using 6 and 7 TIs using a Wilcoxon signed rank test. A Wilcoxon signed rank test was also used to compare the average IR k factors between 1.5 T and 7 T.

The measured T1 relaxation times are expected to be longer at 7 T than at 1.5 T. To be able to compare the average T_1 relaxation times from each ROI compartment between field strengths, the T_1 values were normalized to the median value of all ROIs in healthy volunteers for the corresponding field strength. The resulting normalized T_1 values were compared between 1.5 T and 7 T for each ROI using a Wilcoxon signed rank test.

Method agreement between VFA, LL, and IR were estimated using linear regression and Bland-Altman analysis. Slope, intercept, average bias, and limits of agreement were presented as measures of agreement. Inter-reader and inter-slice variability were measured as average bias and limits of agreement.

Results

The cartilage in all included subjects were deemed of adequate thickness for ROI evaluation in deep as well as superficial regions, based on the images from the diagnostic acquisition and also directly from the images used for T1 evaluation. No cases of unexpected pathology was found.

Visually, the T_1 values within ROIs of T_1 maps obtained with the IR sequence were regarded precise and homogenous, both from 1.5 T and 7 T (Fig. 1). In contrast, T_1 varied considerably within the ROI for the 3D sequences (VFA and LL) in the healthy subject as well as the patient image examples.

The median T_1 values obtained with IR at 1.5 T and 7 T for the various ROI and subject groups are presented in Table 1. As expected, longer T_1 values were estimated at 7 T with an average factor of 1.8 (1.4–2.3)

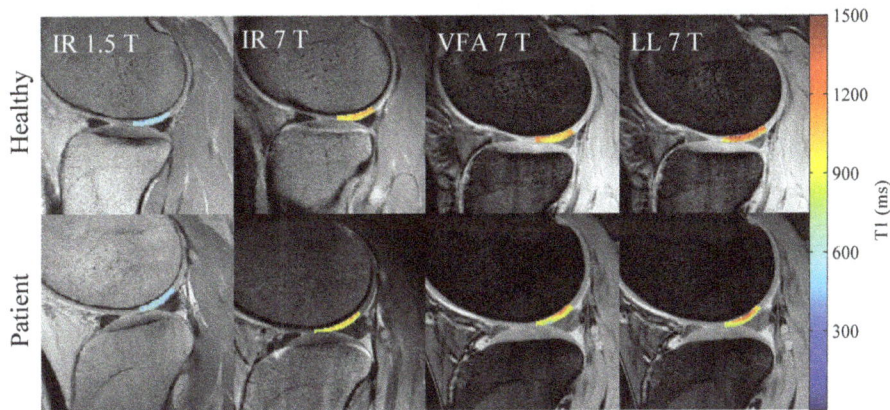

Fig. 1 Example post-contrast T_1 maps overlaid on raw images acquired at 1.5 T and 7 T from a healthy volunteer (top row) and a patient (bottom row). As, expected longer T_1 values were measured at 7 T compared to 1.5 T. IR resulted in homogenous and precise T_1 maps, whereas more variation was seen for the VFA and LL T_1 maps

times longer 7 T T_1 s compared to those at 1.5 T. The same overall patterns were observed at both field strengths with shorter T_1 values in superficial compared to deep cartilage, and shorter T_1 in the medial compared to the lateral condyle for both patients and healthy subjects. At both field strengths, patient T_1 values were slightly shorter and with a larger spread of values compared to healthy subjects. The difference between patient T1 values and healthy subjects T1 values were however not statistically significant. In the superficial medial region the difference was close to significant both at 1.5 T ($P = 0.11$) and at 7 T ($P = 0.09$), whereas for all other ROI's the test resulted in higher P-values ($P > 0.25$).

To be able to compare the T_1 values at the two field strengths, they were normalized to the median T_1 in healthy subjects at each field strength (Fig. 2). The differences in normalized T_1 values between 1.5 T and 7 T for the various ROIs were all small, with a largest relative difference of 10% in the superficial lateral region in patients.

Table 1 Estimated T_1 values in the femoral condyles of study subjects at the two field strengths

		$T1_{IR}$ at 1.5 T (ms)	$T1_{IR}$ at 7 T (ms)
Healthy ($N = 10$)			
Medial	Superficial	497 (361–562)	871 (695–1081)
	Deep	534 (459–587)	967 (854–1229)
Lateral	Superficial	530 (436–599)	944 (796–1080)
	Deep	556 (488–635)	1042 (921–1209)
Patients ($N = 9$)			
Medial	Superficial	463 (336–522)	799 (469–1031)
	Deep	507 (333–589)	984 (626–1261)
Lateral	Superficial	541 (343–624)	890 (473–1068)
	Deep	546 (364–622)	1029 (632–1193)

Values represent median (range) of the estimated T_1

The normalized T_1 values were not statistically different in most ROIs in neither patient (medial deep: $P = 0.36$, medial superficial: $P = 0.16$, lateral superficial: $P = 0.13$) nor healthy subjects (medial deep: $P = 0.77$, medial superficial: $P = 0.70$, lateral superficial: P = 0.70). The only exception was the deep lateral ROI were the difference in normalized T_1 between field strengths was statistically significant in patients ($P = 0.04$) and had a low P value also in healthy subjects ($P = 0.06$).

The median (range) time between the medial IR sequences at the two field strengths was 40 (28–63) minutes for healthy subjects and 40 (28–49) minutes for patients. To determine if this time difference would have impact on the comparison of the dGEMRIC results between the field strengths, the ratio of T_1 at 7 T and 1.5 T was compared between healthy subjects first scanned at 1.5 T and at 7 T, respectively. The median (range) T_1 ratios when starting at 1.5 T / 7 T was 1.92 (1.51–2.05) / 1.67 (1.47–2.26) for the superficial ROIs and 1.82 (1.71–2.20) / 1.85 (1.72–1.99) for the deep ROIs. The difference was larger for superficial ROIs, but not statistically different for neither superficial ($P = 0.16$) nor deep ROIs ($P = 0.62$). For this reason, we do not discriminate between in which order the measurements at the two field strengths were performed in the results presented here.

A linear correlation was found between the T_1 values at 1.5 T and 7 T with a Pearson correlation coefficient of 0.80 (Fig. 3). The coefficient of variation at 1.5 T/7 T T_1 s was 0.50/0.54 for healthy subjects and 0.57/0.88 for patients, thus indicating a slightly larger spread of the 7 T T_1 values, especially for patients. The inter-reader variability of the IR T_1s was 5.71 ± 49.2 ms at 1.5 T and -4.25 ± 96.1 ms at 7 T. The adiabatic pulse quality observed at 7 T was significantly lower compared to at 1.5 T with median (range) k factors equal to 1.85 (1.75–1.93) and 1.71

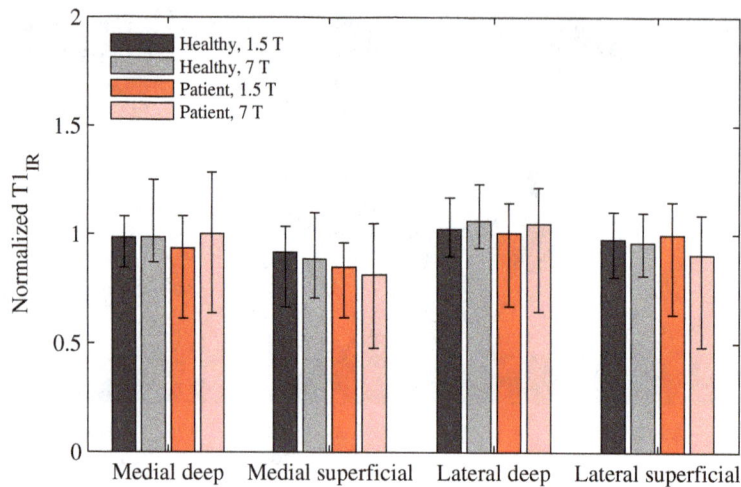

Fig. 2 Comparison of median normalized T_1 values at 1.5 T and 7 T in the various ROIs with error bars showing the range of values. The T_1 values were normalized to the median T_1 value of all healthy subject ROIs at 1.5 T and 7 T, respectively, to enable a comparison between the relaxation times at the two field strengths. Similar normalized T_1 values was seen at the two field strengths, and a significantly larger normalized T_1 at 7 T compared to 1.5 T was detected only in the deep lateral region in patients ($P = 0.04$)

(1.11–1.89) at 1.5 and 7 T, respectively ($P = 4 \cdot 10^{-13}$). Of the 38 acquired IR data sets at each field strength, three data sets at 7 T had too low SNR for a voxel-by-voxel T_1 estimation due to a poor quality adiabatic pulse. For these data sets, an ROI-based T_1 estimation was performed.

Using the same six TIs at 7 T as used at 1.5 T results in lower T_1 values (bias ± limits of agreement – 127 ± 234 ms) and a lower quality fit with significantly higher SEE (median

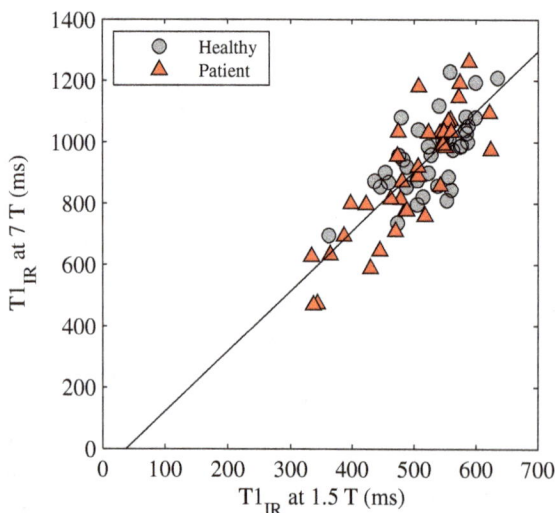

Fig. 3 A scatter plot of IR T_1s at 7 T against IR T_1 at 1.5 T for healthy (grey circles) and patient subjects (red triangles) demonstrating the strong correlation between dGEMRIC at the two field strengths (Pearson correlation coefficient = 0.80). The linear regression with slope = 1.95 (1.61–2.29) and intercept = – 71.9 (– 248–104) is shown in solid black

SEE = 138 (20.9–1180) compared to SEE = 77.0 (29.4–524), $P = 2 \cdot 10^{-6}$) compared to using an adapted sampling scheme with an additional longer TI at 7 T (Fig. 4). Thus, the presentation of 7 T T_1 results is based on the adapted sampling scheme.

A poor agreement was observed between the T_1 values measured with VFA and IR at 7 T (Fig. 5 and Table 2). With no B_1 correction the VFA technique severely underestimated T_1. Although the accuracy was improved using a B_1 correction, the precision worsened with wider limits of agreement. The inter-slice variability for the B_1-corrected case was – 2.55 ± 433 ms and the inter-reader variability was – 51.9 ± 327 ms. Both of these estimates of variability indicate a poor precision of the VFA method. Out of the 10 acquired VFA data sets, one was excluded due to technical difficulties during imaging.

The LL T_1 values agrees well with IR T_1 values at 7 T (Fig. 6 and Table 2). Compared to VFA, LL both with and without B_1 correction is more accurate and precise. The agreement also for LL is improved using B_1 correction, but the correction is not as vital as for VFA. For the B_1-corrected LL data, the inter-slice variability was 1.33 ± 172 ms and the inter-reader variability was 11.5 ± 63.7 ms, thus indicating a smaller variability of LL data compared to VFA. Out of the 14 acquired LL data sets, five were excluded due to insufficient B_0 shim causing a failed adiabatic inversion pulse, and two were excluded due to technical difficulties during imaging.

Discussion

This study compared dGEMRIC at 1.5 T and 7 T after a single (one) contrast-agent injection in both healthy

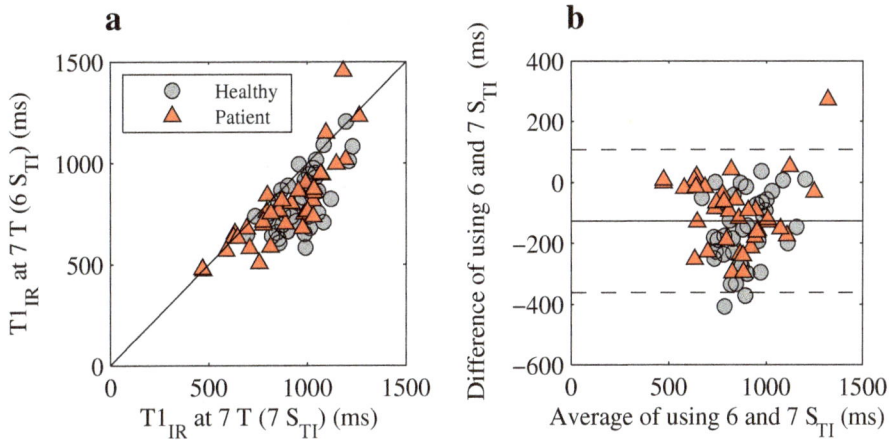

Fig. 4 Scatter (**a**) and Bland-Altman plot (**b**) comparing IR T_1 values at 7 T using an adapted TI sampling with an additional longer TI (7 TIs) and the IR TI sampling pattern with 6 TIs. In **a**) the line of identity is shown in solid black. In **b**) the average bias and limits of agreement are shown in solid and dashed black lines, respectively. The T_1 values using 6 TIs were underestimated compared to using 7 TIs

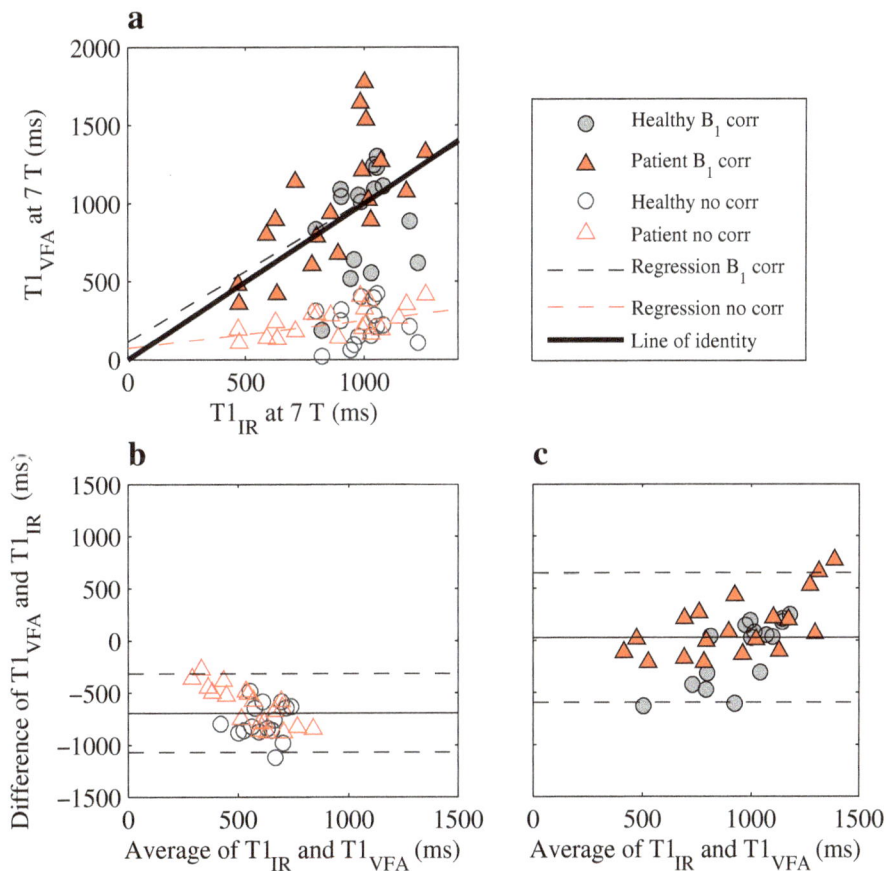

Fig. 5 Scatter (**a**) and Bland-Altman (**b**, **c**) plots comparing the VFA and IR techniques at 7 T for healthy (grey circles) and patient subjects (red triangles). The comparison was made both for B_1-corrected (**a**, **c**; filled markers) and B_1-uncorrected data (**a**, **b**; empty markers). In **b**) and **c**), the average bias and limits of agreement are shown as solid and dashed lines, respectively. A poor agreement was seen between the methods, especially without B_1 correction

Table 2 Measures of method agreement between IR and the VFA and LL techniques

	VFA		LL	
	B_1 correction	No correction	B_1 correction	No correction
Bias ± limits of agreement (ms)	39.6 ± 640	− 687 ± 389	12.2 ± 202	−239 ± 269
Slope ± 95% CI	0.90 ± 0.57	0.18 ± 0.18	0.88 ± 0.29	0.38 ± 0.29
Intercept ±95% CI (ms)	114 ± 537	74 ± 169	119 ± 265	326 ± 274

Regression and Bland-Altman analysis was used as measures of method agreement

subjects and patients. A randomized alternation of the 1.5 T and 7 T examinations of healthy subjects indicated that it was possible to obtain both measurements after a single contrast-agent administration without significant bias due to the difference in time delay after injection. Using an adapted sampling scheme with an additional longer TI, dGEMRIC based on T_1 measurements with IR is feasible at 7 T. The estimated T_1 values at the two field strengths were strongly correlated, although there was a slightly wider distribution of the 7 T T_1 s. Similar normalized T_1 values were found using the two field strengths with significant, yet small, difference between the two only for the deep lateral region. Out of the investigated 3D options at 7 T, LL showed a higher agreement to IR results compared to VFA. For both LL and VFA, B_1 correction is necessary at 7 T. Careful B_0 shimming is crucial, especially for the IR and LL methods.

The feasibility of dGEMRIC at 7 T has previously been studied for knee [16] and hip applications [17, 18]. Our estimated postcontrast femoral T_1 values are slightly longer than those presented by Welsh et al. in healthy volunteers [16]. In expectation of longer T_1 values at 7 T, we chose to use an additional longer TI, compared to what was used in the Welsh study. The results from our study indicate that this choice is necessary to avoid underestimation of T_1 at 7 T.

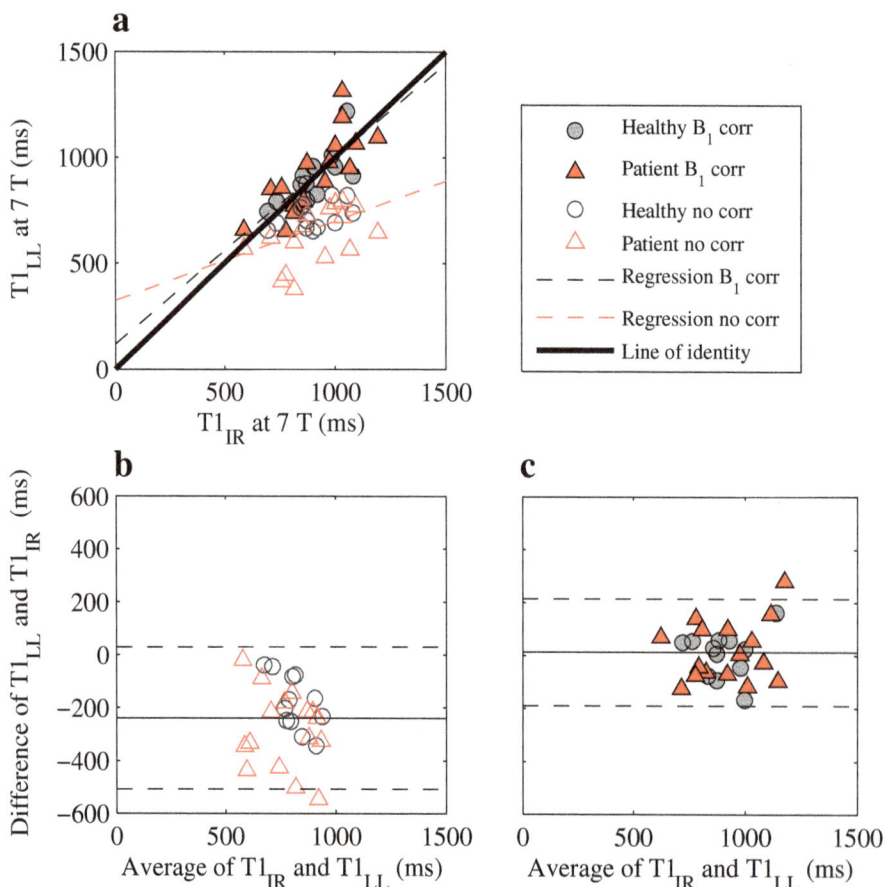

Fig. 6 Scatter (**a**) and Bland-Altman (**b**, **c**) plots comparing the LL and IR techniques at 7 T for healthy (grey circles) and patient subjects (red triangles). The comparison was made both for B_1-corrected (**a**, **c**; filled markers) and B_1-uncorrected data (**a**, **b**; empty markers). In **b**) and **c**), the average bias and limits of agreement are shown as solid and dashed lines, respectively. A strong agreement was seen between the two methods, especially with B_1 correction

dGEMRIC has previously been compared between 7 T and a clinical field strength in repaired cartilage tissue of the hip, where dGEMRIC at 7 T resulted in an unexpected T_1 decrease compared to dGEMRIC at 3 T [18]. Our study, however, resulted in the expected markedly longer T_1 values at 7 T compared to 1.5 T in native knee cartilage of both healthy volunteers and patients. In the previous study [18], the VFA technique was used, while we in contrast chose an IR T_1-mapping method for the field strength comparison. Based on the evaluation of these techniques at 7 T presented in our current study, we believe that this resulted in a more accurate comparison of T_1 values between field strengths.

VFA, LL, and IR have previously been compared at clinical field strengths [25]. Similarly to the results in this study, both the accuracy and precision of LL was superior to VFA also at 1.5 T. Previous studies using dGEMRIC at 7 T has used IR [16] and VFA [17, 18] for T_1 mapping. In a few healthy hips, these two techniques have also been semi-quantitatively compared at 7 T and their respective measures were considered comparable [17]. Success of the VFA technique is dependent on an optimal choice of flip angle pair and B_1-inhomogeneity correction at high field strengths [11, 15]. Thus, at 7 T VFA is expected to be especially challenging as B_1 inhomogeneity is likely high enough to also affect the optimal choice of flip angles. This issue may explain why VFA showed poor agreement with IR even after B_1 correction in our quantitative comparison.

The inversion pulses used in IR sequences were of better quality at 1.5 T compared to at 7 T in this study. This might be explained by the use of a transmit/receive coil at 7 T compared to a receive-only coil at 1.5 T. In addition, the adiabatic-type pulses rely on a successful B_0 shim which is more challenging at 7 T. Especially, this issue was apparent for the LL technique of which several data sets had to be excluded for this reason. However, also a few IR data sets suffered from poor SNR due to this problem. The B_0-shim procedure was improved during the course of the study, and after the volume-based first-order shim technique first used was replaced by use of the Shimtool [26] (an image-based second-order shim technique) the shim was sufficient in all the remaining LL data sets and the SNR of the remaining IR data sets were consistently high.

In our implementation, dGEMRIC using IR required a longer scan time at 7 T compared to at 1.5 T. The reason is that we, as we expected longer T_1s at the higher field strength, chose to increase the repetition time and add an extra acquisition with longer TI at 7 T. Our comparison of using six and seven TIs for the T_1 estimation demonstrates that this was necessary to achieve an accurate T_1 estimation at 7 T. However, we also noticed that the longer acquisition time made the sequences more sensitive to patient motion as motion correction was more frequently needed in the 7 T scans as compared to the shorter 1.5 T scans. In a practical case when designing a study protocol it is important to take both the benefits and the potential disadvantages of a longer scan time into consideration.

Focus of this work was on the T_1-mapping techniques used for the dGEMRIC method at 7 T, and patients were primarily recruited to increase the expected range of T_1 values. For this reason, a full comparison of dGEMRIC indices and diagnostic performance was beyond the scope of this study. However, although the difference in post-contrast T_1 values between patients and healthy volunteers was small (not statistically significant) in this study, it was similarly small at both 1.5 T and 7 T. At both field strengths it was the same region (superficial medial) that was closest to a significant difference, which is also the region were cartilage changes had been observed in the patients. The normalized T_1 values were also similar at the two field strengths. This hence implies that the methods perform similarly at the two field strengths. As possible explanation for the small differences found, we speculate that the difference in timing between the protocols starting at 1.5 T and 7 T may have increased the spread of the data making comparisons between groups more difficult.

dGEMRIC using $Gd-(DTPA)^{2-}$ (Magnevist) will probably be performed less frequently in the future given the fact that its use will be restricted based on the recent reports about long-term gadolinium deposits [5]. However, dGEMRIC could potentially also be used with other contrast agents such as gadoterate meglumine (Dotarem, Guerbet, Villepinte, France). To date almost all dGEMRIC studies have been performed using Magnevist, and future dGEMRIC studies with other contrast agents would of course first need careful and in depth validation studies. After such validation, the results from our evaluation of T1 mapping methods and field strength comparison would still be valuable for future studies with dGEMRIC at 7 T.

There were mainly two limitations of the study design of this work: the time difference between the examinations at the two field strengths and that no precontrast T_1 values were measured. Both for ethical and study design purposes, the examinations at the two field strengths were conducted after a single (one) contrast agent injection. Thus they could not be performed at identical post-injection time delays. Efforts were made to minimize the time delay between examinations and the subjects were moved in a wheel chair between the examination rooms to avoid loading the knee and thus redistributing the contrast agent between measurements. The achieved time delay between examinations are within the previously reported plateau of dGEMRIC values between 2 h and 3 h after injection [27]. Although no statistically significant difference in T_1 was found due to timing differences in healthy volunteers, they may have increased the spread of the data as mentioned in the paragraph above. Precontrast T_1 values were not measured neither at 1.5 T nor 7 T. This choice was made as the addition of these measurements would make the visit and scan time unbearably long for the study subjects. Instead, it was prioritized to make it feasible to perform the examinations at the two field strengths in a single visit and after a single contrast agent injection. Previous work indicates that the precontrast T_1 value contributes little additional information compared to postcontrast values at both 1.5 T and 3 T in native cartilage [3, 28]. In repaired cartilage tissue, measurements of precontrast T_1 may be more important [29]. The importance of a precontrast T_1 value may need to be investigated further also at 7 T.

Conclusions

In conclusion, T_1 mapping for use in the dGEMRIC method is feasible at 7 T with similar normalized T_1 values compared to at 1.5 T and with a strong correlation between T_1 values at 1.5 T and 7 T. However, the IR protocol at 7 T needs to be adapted to the longer T_1 values at this field strength. As a 3D alternative to IR at 7 T, LL is preferred and VFA is not recommended without further optimization of the method. For both 3D methods, B_1 correction is necessary for an accurate T_1 estimation. For LL and IR, careful B_0 shimming is crucial at 7 T.

Abbreviations

BMI: Body mass index; CEST: Chemical exchange saturation transfer; dGEMRIC: Delayed gadolinium enhanced magnetic resonance imaging of cartilage; DREAM: Dual refocusing echo acquisition mode; FOV: Field of view; GAG: Glycosaminoglycan; IR: Inversion recovery; LL: Look-locker; MRI: Magnetic resonance imaging; ROI: Region of interest; SEE: Standard error of the estimate; TE: Echo time; TI: Inversion time; TR: Repetition time; VFA: Variable flip angle

Acknowledgments

We would like to thank the staff at the Swedish National 7 T Facility, especially Boel Hansson, Johanna Arborelius, and Karin Markenroth Bloch, for their invaluable help.

Funding

This research was supported by the Swedish Research Council [grant number K2013-52X-22196-01-3] and Greta och Johan Kocks stiftelser.

Authors' contributions

The study was conceived and designed by PP, CJT, LEO, and JS. Data was acquired by PP and EO, and the acquired images were read and inspected by BL. Analysis of the data was conducted by PP, CJT, and EO. The manuscript was drafted by PP. All authors contributed to interpretation of the results and critical review of the manuscript. All authors have read and approved the manuscript.

Competing interests

The authors declare that they have no competing interests.

Author details

Medical Radiation Physics, Department of Translational Medicine, Lund University, Inga Marie Nilssons gata 49, SE-205 02 Malmö, Sweden. Department of Oncology and Radiation Physics, Skåne University Hospital, Inga Marie Nilssons gata 49, SE-205 02 Malmö, Sweden. [3]Orthopedics, Department of Clinical Sciences, Lund University, Skåne University Hospital, SE-221 85 Lund, Sweden. [4]Department of Medical Imaging and Physiology, Skåne University Hospital, SE-221 85 Lund, Sweden.

References

1. Bashir A, Gray ML, Burstein D. Gd-DTPA2- as a measure of cartilage degradation. Magn Reson Med. 1996;36(5):665–73.
2. Owman H, Tiderius CJ, Neuman P, Nyquist F, Dahlberg LE. Association between findings on delayed gadolinium-enhanced magnetic resonance imaging of cartilage and future knee osteoarthritis. Arthritis Rheum. 2008; 58(6):1727–30.
3. Tiderius CJ, Olsson LE, Leander P, Ekberg O, Dahlberg L. Delayed gadolinium-enhanced MRI of cartilage (dGEMRIC) in early knee osteoarthritis. Magn Reson Med. 2003;49(3):488–92.
4. Tiderius CJ, Svensson J, Leander P, Ola T, Dahlberg L. dGEMRIC (delayed gadolinium-enhanced MRI of cartilage) indicates adaptive capacity of human knee cartilage. Magn Reson Med. 2004;51(2):286–90.
5. Fraum TJ, Ludwig DR, Bashir MR, Fowler KJ. Gadolinium-based contrast agents: a comprehensive risk assessment. J Magn Reson Imaging. 2017; https://doi.org/10.1002/jmri.25625.
6. Trattnig S, Zbyn S, Schmitt B, Friedrich K, Juras V, Szomolanyi P, et al. Advanced MR methods at ultra-high field (7 tesla) for clinical musculoskeletal applications. Eur Radiol. 2012;22(11):2338–46.
7. Singh A, Haris M, Cai K, Kassey VB, Kogan F, Reddy D, et al. Chemical exchange saturation transfer magnetic resonance imaging of human knee cartilage at 3 T and 7 T. Magn Reson Med. 2012;68(2):588–94.
8. Staroswiecki E, Bangerter NK, Gurney PT, Grafendorfer T, Gold GE, Hargreaves BA. In vivo sodium imaging of human patellar cartilage with a 3D cones sequence at 3 T and 7 T. J Magn Reson Imaging. 2010;32(2):446–51.
9. McKenzie CA, Williams A, Prasad PV, Burstein D. Three-dimensional delayed gadolinium-enhanced MRI of cartilage (dGEMRIC) at 1.5T and 3.0T. J Magn Reson Imaging. 2006;24(4):928–33.
10. Rohrer M, Bauer H, Mintorovitch J, Requardt M, Weinmann HJ. Comparison of magnetic properties of MRI contrast media solutions at different magnetic field strengths. Investig Radiol. 2005;40(11):715–24.
11. Mamisch TC, Dudda M, Hughes T, Burstein D, Kim YJ. Comparison of delayed gadolinium enhanced MRI of cartilage (dGEMRIC) using inversion recovery and fast T1 mapping sequences. Magn Reson Med. 2008;60(4):768–73.
12. Kimelman T, Vu A, Storey P, McKenzie C, Burstein D, Prasad P. Three-dimensional T1 mapping for dGEMRIC at 3.0 T using the look locker method. Investig Radiol. 2006;41(2):198–203.
13. Li W, Scheidegger R, Wu Y, Vu A, Prasad PV. Accuracy of T1 measurement with 3-D look-locker technique for dGEMRIC. J Magn Reson Imaging. 2008; 27(3):678–82.
14. Siversson C, Tiderius CJ, Dahlberg L, Svensson J. Local flip angle correction for improved volume T1-quantification in three-dimensional dGEMRIC using the look-locker technique. J Magn Reson Imaging. 2009;30(4):834–41.
15. Siversson C, Chan J, Tiderius CJ, Mamisch TC, Jellus V, Svensson J, et al. Effects of B1 inhomogeneity correction for three-dimensional variable flip angle T1 measurements in hip dGEMRIC at 3 T and 1.5 T. Magn Reson Med. 2012;67(6):1776–81.
16. Welsch GH, Mamisch TC, Hughes T, Zilkens C, Quirbach S, Scheffler K, et al. In vivo biochemical 7.0 tesla magnetic resonance: preliminary results of dGEMRIC, zonal T2, and T2* mapping of articular cartilage. Investig Radiol. 2008;43(9):619–26.
17. Lazik A, Theysohn JM, Geis C, Johst S, Ladd ME, Quick HH, et al. 7 tesla quantitative hip MRI: T1, T2 and T2* mapping of hip cartilage in healthy volunteers. Eur Radiol. 2016;26(5):1245–53.
18. Lazik-Palm A, Kraff O, Johst S, Quick HH, Ladd ME, Geis C, et al.

Morphological and quantitative 7 T MRI of hip cartilage transplants in comparison to 3 T-initial experiences. Investig Radiol. 2016;51(9):552 9.

19. Burstein D, Velyvis J, Scott KT, Stock KW, Kim YJ, Jaramillo D, et al. Protocol issues for delayed Gd(DTPA)(2-)-enhanced MRI (dGEMRIC) for clinical evaluation of articular cartilage. Magn Reson Med. 2001;45(1):36–41.

20. Deoni SC, Rutt BK, Peters TM. Rapid combined T1 and T2 mapping using gradient recalled acquisition in the steady state. Magn Reson Med. 2003;49(3):515–26.

21. Nehrke K, Bornert P. DREAM–a novel approach for robust, ultrafast, multislice B(1) mapping. Magn Reson Med. 2012;68(5):1517–26.

22. Deichmann R, Haase A. Quantification of T1 values by snapshot-flash Nmr imaging. J Magn Reson. 1992;96(3):608–12.

23. Homer J, Beevers MS. Driven-equilibrium single-pulse observation of T1 relaxation - a reevaluation of a rapid new method for determining Nmr spin-lattice relaxation-times. J Magn Reson. 1985;63(2):287–97.

24. Tiderius C, Hori M, Williams A, Sharma L, Prasad PV, Finnell M, et al. dGEMRIC as a function of BMI. Osteoarthr Cartil. 2006;14(11):1091–7.

25. Siversson C, Tiderius CJ, Neuman P, Dahlberg L, Svensson J. Repeatability of T1-quantification in dGEMRIC for three different acquisition techniques: two-dimensional inversion recovery, three-dimensional look locker, and three-dimensional variable flip angle. J Magn Reson Imaging. 2010;31(5):1203–9.

26. Schar M, Kozerke S, Fischer SE, Boesiger P. Cardiac SSFP imaging at 3 tesla. Magn Reson Med. 2004;51(4):799–806.

27. Tiderius CJ, Olsson LE, de Verdier H, Leander P, Ekberg O, Dahlberg L. Gd-DTPA2- -enhanced MRI of femoral knee cartilage: a dose-response study in healthy volunteers. Magn Reson Med. 2001;46(6):1067–71.

28. Williams A, Mikulis B, Krishnan N, Gray M, McKenzie C, Burstein D. Suitability of T(1Gd) as the dGEMRIC index at 1.5T and 3.0T. Magn Reson Med. 2007;58(4):830–4.

29. Watanabe A, Wada Y, Obata T, Ueda T, Tamura M, Ikehira H, et al. Delayed gadolinium-enhanced MR to determine glycosaminoglycan concentration in reparative cartilage after autologous chondrocyte implantation: preliminary results. Radiology. 2006;239(1):201–8.

2

Is unilateral lower leg orthosis with a circular foot unit in the treatment of idiopathic clubfeet a reasonable bracing alternative in the Ponseti method? Five-year results of a supraregional paediatric-orthopaedic centre

N. Berger[1]* ⓘ, D. Lewens[2], M. Salzmann[1], A. Hapfelmeier[1,3], L. Döderlein[2] and P. M. Prodinger[1]

Abstract

Background: In the Ponseti treatment of idiopathic clubfoot, children are generally provided with a standard foot abduction orthosis (FAO). A significant proportion of these patients experience irresolvable problems with the FAO leading to therapeutic non-compliance and eventual relapse. Accordingly, these patients were equipped with a unilateral lower leg orthosis (LLO) developed in our institution. The goal of this retrospective study was to determine compliance with and the efficacy of the LLO as an alternative treatment measure. The minimum follow-up was 5 years.

Results: A total of 45 patients (75 ft) were retrospectively registered and included in the study. Compliance with the bracing protocol was 91% with the LLO and 46% with the FAO. The most common problems with the FAO were sleep disturbance (50%) and cutaneous problems (45%). Nine percent of patients experienced sleep disturbance, and no cutaneous problems occurred with the LLO. Thirteen percent of patients being treated with an FAO until the age of four (23 patients; 40 ft) underwent surgery because of relapse, defined by rigid recurrence of any of the components of a clubfoot. Fourteen percent of patients being treated with an LLO (22 patients; 35 ft), mostly following initial treatment with an FAO, experienced recurrence.

Conclusion: Changing from FAO to LLO at any point during treatment did not result in an increased rate of surgery and caused few problems.

Keywords: Clubfoot, Ponseti, Brace, Unilateral Orthosis, AFO, Pohlig Baise articulated lower leg Orthosis

Background

The Ponseti method [1] is universally accepted as the gold standard for correcting idiopathic clubfoot. It involves serial manipulation and casting of the feet, mostly combined with an Achilles tenotomy, followed by the use of a foot abduction orthosis (FAO) to maintain the correction. This orthosis, which holds the foot in external rotation and dorsiflexion, must be worn for 23 h a day for 3 months, and for at least 10 h per night for an additional 3–4 years [2, 3]. The most common models follow the design of Denis Browne [4, 5], employing a rigid middle bar, high-top shoes, and maintaining the affected foot in up to 70° external rotation (non-affected foot: 30–40°) and 10° dorsiflexion. If the protocol is correctly maintained, recurrences needing surgery are reported to be around 12% [6–8].

However, parental non-compliance with the use of FAO during the course of treatment is an often

* Correspondence: nina.berger@tum.de
[1]Klinikum rechts der Isar der Technischen Universität München, Munich, Germany
Full list of author information is available at the end of the article

reported problem [9–13]. Although it is well known that non-adherence to the bracing protocol results in elevated odds of recurrence (5- to 17-fold higher [6, 11, 14]), non-compliance is as high as 34–61% [3, 9, 11, 14–17].

To date, existing literature has identified low income and low educational levels as predicting factors for non-compliance [12, 16, 18]. Reasons given by parents for not using the brace are prolonged crying, disturbed sleep [10, 17, 19], and cutaneous problems such as skin irritation, blisters, and pressure sores [9, 18, 20].

In recent years, efforts have been made to develop more comfortable braces. Dynamic braces allowing a certain range of motion have shown promising results [9, 20, 21]. However, existing designs of ankle–foot orthoses have not yet provided an alternative to bracing because of the reported high recurrence rates (31% [22] and 83% [23]). George et al. [22] built an above knee orthosis, which consisted of three parts, shoe (sandal with laces), angled metal bar, and leg straps. The orthosis could be picked from the shelf and assembled as required. Janicki et al. [23] used a standard AFO consisting of a one piece plastic half-tube that was applied to the dorsal side of the leg and ended below the knee. Foot and shank were fixed with Velcro straps. The authors stated that their orthosis could not control abduction of the foot, which is required to stretch the medial soft tissues.

After completing Ponseti casting, our patients are generally provided with a standard FAO. If problems occur and cannot be solved, we provide the patient with a custom-made unilateral lower leg orthosis (LLO). In this retrospective study, we aimed to (1) evaluate compliance rates with FAO and LLO treatment, and (2) gain a first-hand impression of the efficacy of LLO in avoiding clubfoot recurrence.

Methods

Inclusion criteria for the present study were the diagnosis of idiopathic clubfoot, complete documentation, a minimum bracing period of 3 years after completion of casting (or less, if an operation was performed within the bracing period), and a minimum age at follow-up of 5 years.

After completing the Ponseti series of castings, children were routinely provided with a standard foot abduction orthosis according to Denis Browne. High-top leather sandals closed by Velcro straps could be attached separately to a rigid middle bar (Fig. 1).

At each visit, we asked the parents about difficulties in complying with the bracing protocol. If the brace or orthosis was not put on for 23 h during the first 3 months of life and for at least 10 h per night until the end of the third year of life, it was regarded as non-compliance, and the reasons given by the parents

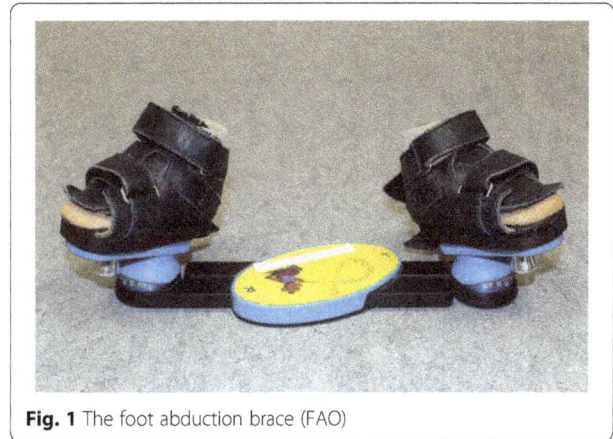

Fig. 1 The foot abduction brace (FAO)

were documented. The absence of signs of brace or orthosis use was also recorded.

Parents who reported problems with the FAO were specifically asked about the nature of the problem. Cutaneous problems were treated by adjusting the size and configuration of the standard shoes. If we detected a problem understanding the necessity for therapy, then the parents were advised thoroughly and encouraged to continue using the FAO. Parents who reported acceptance difficulties by the child, usually expressed by prolonged crying and problems sleeping through the night, were helped to implement a bed-time routine. If none of these measures were successful in re-establishing compliance with the bracing protocol, then we proposed an LLO. Some children were initially provided with the LLO if the treating doctor felt that the FAO might not be well tolerated.

Construction of the LLO

The unilateral LLOs were custom-made with resin and carbon and were built in three parts following Baise and Pohlig's 2005 design (Fig. 2a-c) [24]: a circular foot unit, a lower leg unit, and an inner liner made out of Tepefoam.

The foot unit follows the principles of the Calcaneus-Rotation-Ring type orthosis, described by Baise and Pohlig (2004) for the treatment of spastic clubfeet [25]. It fixes the subtalar joint in a valgus position. It does so by encasing the calcaneopedal unit [26], which is then everted in the subtalar joint line by a turning movement by the person who applies the orthosis. Once in place, the ring-like enclosure (completed by a heel cap) works like an external arthrodesis of the subtalar joint [25] (Fig. 2a-i). The resulting hindfoot valgus is 10–15°. In the beginning, we externally rotated the foot against the knee joint line 40° and more, but this resulted in overcorrection. Hence, we reduced the rotation and now seek for an external rotation of 20° (Fig. 3a-d).

The foot unit is fixed to the lower leg unit by screws and hinges and allows a range of motion of 0–5-20°

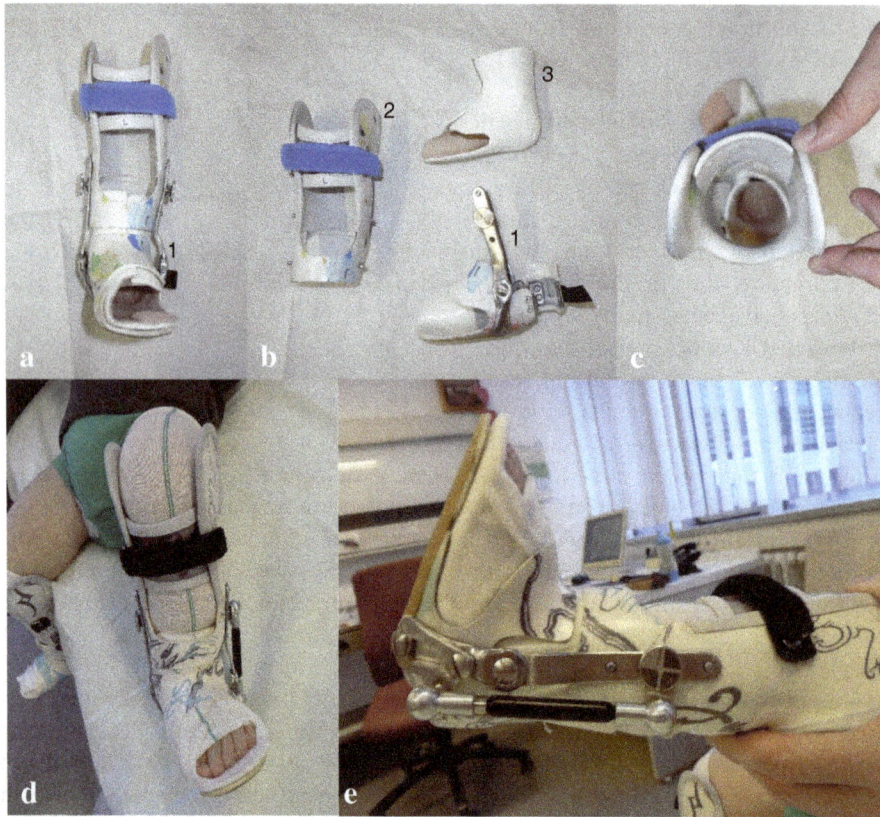

Fig. 2 a-e The Pohlig lower leg orthosis (LLO). **a** + **b** Note the circular foot unit (1) closed by a heel cap as seen in **b**), the lower leg unit (2) and the inner liner made out of Tepefoam (3). The calcaneo-pedis block is held in 20° external rotation (see **a** and **c**) and 20° dorsal extension (see **e**). A mounted gas pressure spring to push into dorsal extension that can be adjusted, if desired, is also shown

plantarflexion/dorsiflexion. Rotational stability of the orthosis in relation to the axis of the knee is mandatory to maintain the position and therefore the correctional capacity of the foot unit. This is achieved by mounting the lower leg unit with a combination of ear-shaped supports encompassing the femoral condyles at the proximal ending of the lower leg unit, working as a counter bearing against the rotational forces. The range of motion of the knee joint is not limited by those encompasses. Further stability is provided by a firm intake of the calf, realized by a Velcro-fixed resin cap above the tibial tuberosity that provides an intake working like a Sarmiento brace (Fig. 2a-e).

The inner liner or "Inliner" made out of Tepefoam works simultaneously as a pressure absorber and distributer of the correctional forces to the entire foot surface. Padding of Bisgaard's region in the Inliner further prevents slipping of the heel. Besides, the Inliner alleviates the process of slipping into the foot unit (see also our online Additional file 1: Video S1).

These principles of construction allowed us to meet the demands of a post-Ponseti-brace: (1) stretching of the structures of the posterior and medial ankle and tarsal ligaments and musculo-tendinous units [2]; (2) allowing free kicking (and even walking), and thereby stretching of the gastrosoleus complex [27].

We did not use the term 'ankle–foot orthosis', because the orthosis also encompasses parts of the knee. Instead, we chose to introduce the term 'lower leg orthosis'.

During follow-up, recurrence of the clubfoot position in one or more of its components (hindfoot varus, midfoot cavus, and forefoot adductus; defined on clinical basis) was documented and, if necessary, a second series of casting, re-tenotomy, or other invasive operative measures were performed.

Statistics

The distribution of quantitative data is described by mean and range. Qualitative data is presented by absolute and relative frequencies. Corresponding hypothesis testing on group differences was performed by t-tests and Pearson's chi-squared tests using exploratory two-sided 5% levels of significance. All statistical analyses were performed using R 3.4.2 (R Foundation for Statistical Computing, Vienna, Austria).

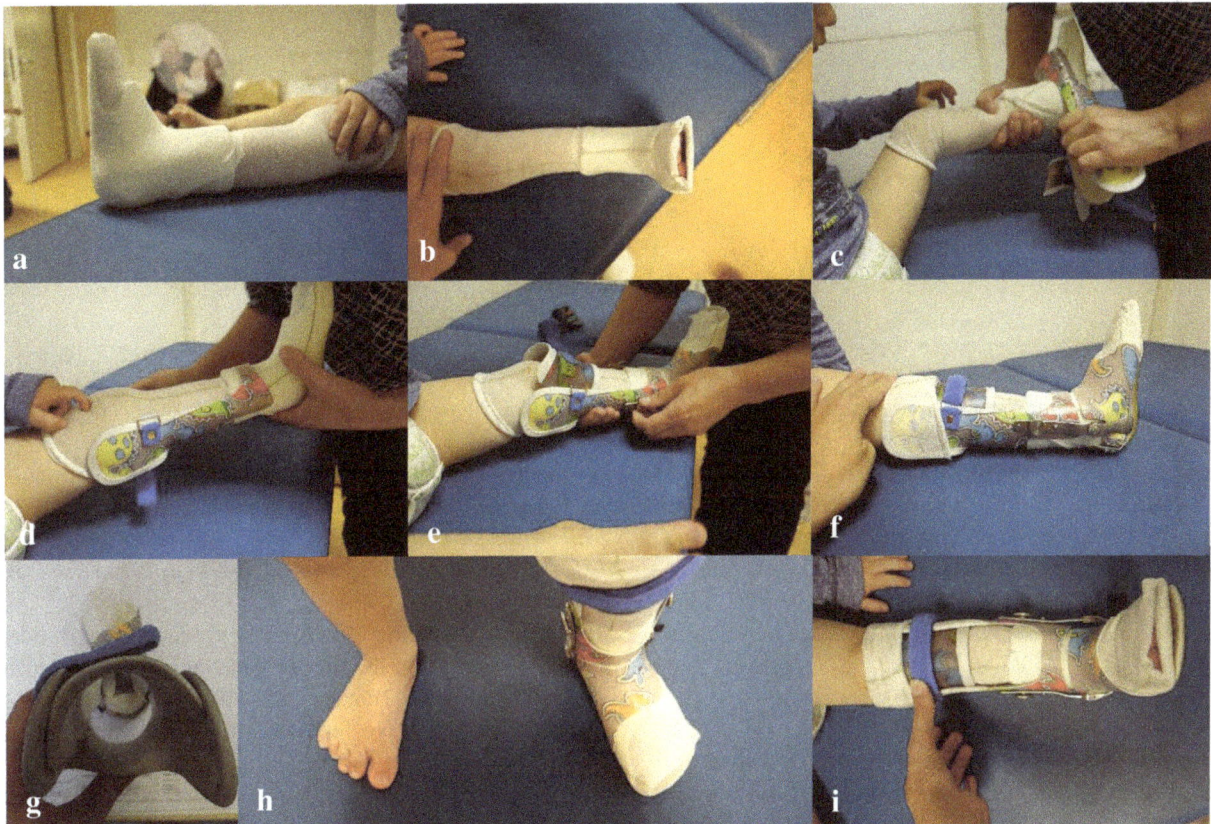

Fig. 3 a-i Putting-on of the Pohlig lower leg orthosis: (**a** + **b**) A stocking is put on the leg before the Inliner is applied, then the stocking is pulled over the Inliner (**c** + **d**) Now the lower leg unit is slipped over the foot and fixed to the shank (**e**) The foot unit is slipped over the foot and fixed to the lower leg unit by screws. (**f**, **h**, **i**) The mounted orthosis fixes the foot in neutral dorsiflexion and 20° of external rotation. Further 5–10° of dorsiflexion are allowed by hinges when walking in the orthosis (**g**) Top view of the orthosis, demonstrating external rotation of the foot unit versus the lower leg unit

Results

Between 2004 and 2011, we treated 177 children with clubfoot according to the Ponseti method. Forty-four patients were excluded from this study because of a non-idiopathic clubfoot. Ten patients had accompanying hip problems, so the Ponseti treatment had to be modified. Forty-nine patients were lost during follow-up and continued treatment with their local orthopaedic doctor. Of the remaining patients, 45 (75 ft) had a minimum follow-up of 5 years and were included in this study.

The mean age at follow-up was 8.2 years (range: 5.0–11.6 years). Fifty-three percent of the patients ($n = 24$) were pre-treated and referred to our clinic owing to persistence of the deformity. Children with pre-treated feet presented at our hospital at a mean age of 6.4 weeks. Fifteen children had unilateral clubfoot. The female to male ratio was 1:1.8. The mean initial Pirani score [28] at first presentation in our clinic was 4.9 (range: 1.0–6.0). A mean of seven casts (range: 1–12) were necessary. The foot with only one cast had an initial Pirani score of 1.5. Achilles tenotomy was performed in 88% of all feet.

Complete initial correction was observed in all patients at the mean age of 14.6 weeks (range: 7.9–45.9 weeks). There was no residual cavus or adduction deformity and the minimum dorsiflexion capacity of the foot (measured in extended knee position) was 15° and the minimum passive abduction was 40° of the foot against the fixed talus as described by Ponseti [2].

Compliance with the FAO and LLO

We registered problems with the FAO in 54% and with the LLO in 9% of treated patients (Table 1).

Forty-one children (70 ft) were initially treated with an FAO. Twenty-two children (54%) developed intermittent or lasting non-compliance with the bracing protocol. The most common problems were skin irritations/pressure sores (45%) and/or sleep problems (50%). Three out of ten patients suffering from serious cutaneous problems were successfully managed by changing to custom-made resin shoes, so the children could continue with FAO treatment.

Table 1 Characteristics of patients in terms of compliance

Characteristic	Value
Non-compliance with FAO total, patients (% of patients; feet)	22 (54%; 34)
Non-compliance with FAO because of skin problems, patients (% of non-compliant patients; feet)	10 (45%; 14)
Non-compliance with FAO because of sleep disturbance, patients (% of non-compliant patients; feet)	11 (50%; 18)
Non-compliance with FAO for other reasons, patients (% of non-compliant patients; feet)	1 (5%; 2)
Non-compliance with LLO total, patients (% of patients; feet)	2 (9%; 4)
Non-compliance with LLO because of skin problems, patients (feet)	0
Non-compliance with LLO because of sleep disturbance, patients (feet)	2 (9%; 4)
Non-compliance with LLO for other reasons, patients (feet)	0

Twenty-two children (35 ft) were treated with an LLO. Of those, 18 children (30 ft) were converted to LLO treatment as a consequence of discontent with the FAO at a mean age of 14.5 months (range: 2–34 months). Only two children (four feet; 11%) developed problems with the LLOs and showed prolonged crying and sleep disturbance (Table 1). No unresolvable pressure sores or complaints about the complexity of brace handling were noted with the LLOs.

Efficacy of the FAO and LLO

Two groups of patients were defined with respect to the treatments: patients who remained on FAO treatment throughout ('FAO only'; 23 patients, 40 ft) and patients who began treatment with LLO at any time-point during the treatment (LLO initially or following FAO treatment: 'FAO > LLO group'; 22 patients, 35 ft) (Fig. 4 and Table 2). There was similar age at the beginning of cast treatment between the 'FAO only' group (mean 3.7 weeks, range 0.3–22.7) and the FAO > LLO (mean 5.1 weeks, range 0.3–40.3) patients ($p = 0.527$; t-test). There was minor difference between the groups in the number of pre-treated feet (FAO only: 38%, FAO > LLO: 44%; $p = 0.6277$), Pirani-score (mean: FAO only: 4,9; FAO > LLO: 4,8; $p = 0.905$), or mean follow-up period (FAO only: 8.0 years; FAO > LLO: 8.4 years; $p = 0.597$).

Four patients (five feet) started bracing therapy directly with an LLO. At the beginning of the bracing treatment, these patients had a mean age of 26.1 weeks (range: 13–46 weeks). They were all pre-treated with a minimum of four casts for a period of 0.5–9 months. At the time of presentation to our institution, their Pirani scores were 3, 4.5, 2 × 5, and 6 (Fig. 5).

Eighteen children (30 ft) changed to LLO treatment at a mean age of 14.5 months (range: 2–34 months). The mean wearing time of FAO per foot before switching to LLO was 8.1 months (range: 0–27 months) (see also Additional file 2).

The mean wearing time of LLO per foot (of all children treated with LLO, initially or following FAO treatment) was 30.7 months (range: 13.9–80.5 months) (Table 2). Three children (three feet; 14%) required additional surgery. Two children had a peritalar release performed at age 4.9 and 6.5 years. They had started with FAO treatment at the age of 2.6 and 2.3 months, respectively, and switched to LLO treatment owing to sleeping issues at age 3.9 and 6.9 months, respectively. Another child had received 9 months of casting elsewhere before being referred to us. This child first received an additional four casts at our institution; subsequently, bracing treatment was initiated directly with an LLO. Anterior tibial tendon transfer and calcaneal osteotomy followed at the age of 7 years.

In patients treated exclusively with the FAO ($n = 23$), the mean wearing time until end of treatment or relapse was 41.6 months (range: 28–49 months) per foot. One patient required a second series of casting. Three patients (three feet; 13%) developed recurrence requiring re-tenotomy of Achilles tendon and additional dorsal capsulotomy in one case (one patient, at age 13 months) or had major surgery (peritalar release; [two patients, at age 3.8 and 8.5 years]).

Discussion

In this retrospective study, we investigated compliance with unilateral LLO or standard FAO. We also attempted to obtain some first impressions regarding the efficacy of the unilateral LLO. As this study took place at a specialized hospital, many patients were referred after pre-treatment at a relatively "old" age compared with patients normally seen at an outpatient clinic. Therefore, these patients may represent a negative selection regarding severity of the deformity or overall parental compliance.

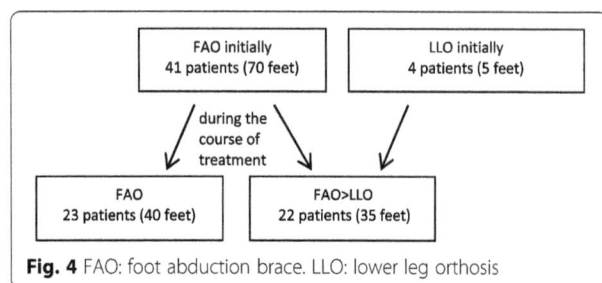

Fig. 4 FAO: foot abduction brace. LLO: lower leg orthosis

Table 2 Characteristics of patients treated with a foot abduction brace (FAO) either exclusively until the end of treatment or follow-up (FAO only), or who were began on or switched to a lower leg orthosis (FAO > LLO)

Characteristic	FAO only	FAO > LLO
No. patients (feet)	23 (40)	22 (35)
Sex, female/male	10/13	6/16
Unilateral/ bilateral affected patients	6/17	9/13
Age at beginning of cast treatment, weeks (range)	3.7 (0.3–22.7)	5.1 (0.3–40.3)
Pre-treated feet, n	15 (38%)	16 (44%)
Initial Pirani score (range)	4.9 (1–6)	4.8 (1.5–6)
Mean wearing time, months per foot: FAO/LLO	40.9/–	8.1/30.7
Follow-up period, years (range)	8.4 (5.0–11.6)	8.0 (5.0–11.3)
Second series of casting/second tenotomy Achilles tendon, patients (feet)	1 (1)	0
Surgery because of relapse (retenotomy of Achilles tendon, soft tissue and bony procedures), patients (feet)	3 (3)	3 (3)

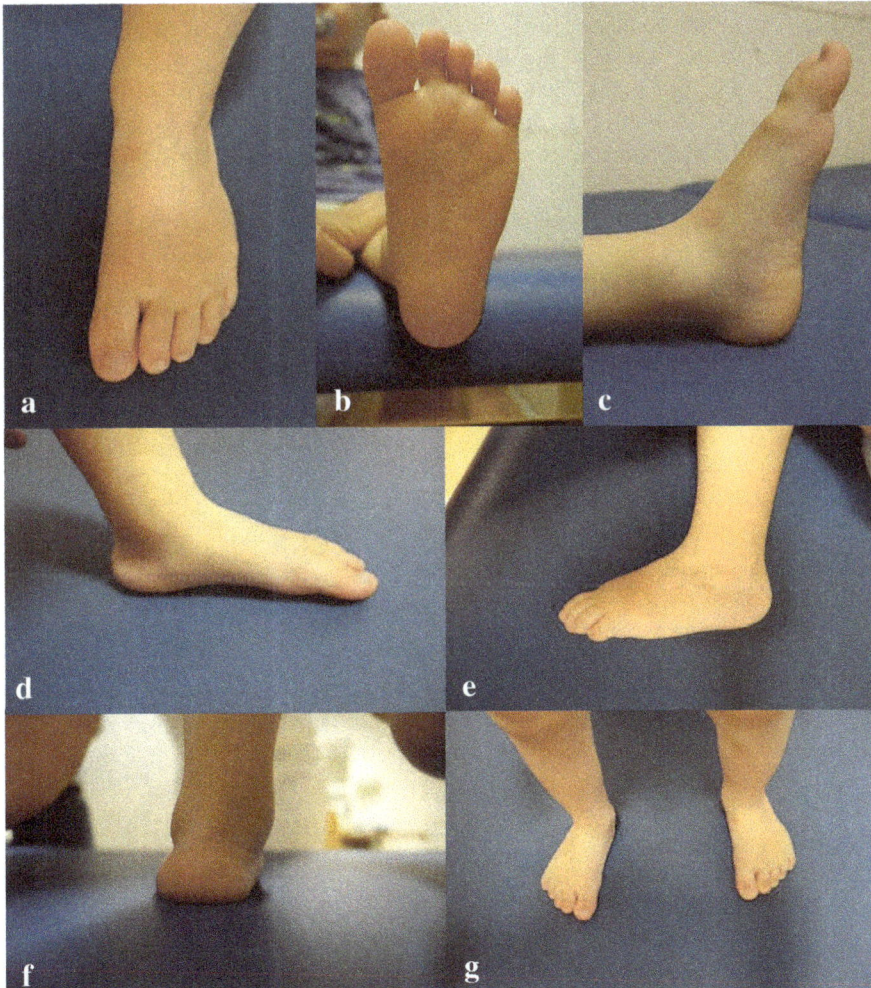

Fig. 5 a-g This otherwise healthy boy (same boy as in Fig. 2) presented at birth with a congenital vertical talus at the right foot and a congenital clubfoot at the left side (Pirani score 6, stiff-soft). His treatment with LLO started right after removing the last casts. At the time the photographs were taken, he was 2.5 years old. (**a** + **b**) There is only minimal adduction of the greater toe and neutral orientation of the left forefoot (**c**, **d**). The heel is in slight valgus position (**f**). Residual from his deformity is a pronounced internal rotation of the left tibia (**g**)

Difficulties in maintaining the bracing-protocol for standard FAOs is well known in literature [29], with cutaneous problems reported in up to 45% of patients [9, 18, 20] and non-compliance rates of 34–61% [3, 9, 11, 14–17]. Non-compliance is usually defined as the interruption or discontinuation of the recommended scheme (23 h of bracing for the first 3 months, then 10–12 h per day until the age of 3–4 years). In a recent study by Goksan et al. [29], compliance with the orthosis was defined as fulltime brace use for 3 months and during sleep for ≥9 months. In this study, difficulties with the brace were encountered in 80% of affected children [29]. Comparatively, dynamic orthoses seem to result in fewer cutaneous problems (0–3.6%) and less non-compliance (7–38%), probably by reducing the lever on the heel and allowing more active movement [9, 20, 21].

The rate of non-adherence with the bracing protocol in our study was 9% with the lower leg orthosis, and 54% in children treated with a foot abduction orthosis. The most important problems reported with the FAO were problems sleeping through the night (50%) and skin problems (45%). With the LLO, only sleep disturbance was observed. In our study, non-compliance meant that patients did not wear the brace full-time for the advised time of three whole months and at least 10 h during night-time until the age of 3–4 years. Of the 18 patients who did not accept the FAO and probably would have discontinued the bracing protocol, 16 patients successfully continued with the LLO.

At present, it is of doubt whether an 'ankle–foot orthosis' can guarantee foot abduction or external rotation [3, 22, 23] representing major columns in treating clubfeet. To our knowledge, the literature has so far reported only two studies of post-Ponseti bracing with a unilateral ankle–foot orthosis. Janicki et al. investigated the use of a classic AFO fixed with Velcro straps [23] (Fig. 6), while

George et al. presented a system consisting of a shoe fixed to a lateral bar spanning the knee at a 90° angle, fixed by straps at the shank [22] (Fig. 7). Although compliance was good (up to 85% [22]) with both versions, relapse was seen in 83% [23] and 31% [22] of feet, respectively, over follow-up periods of 60 (range: 50–72) [23] and 25 (range: 16–36) months [22]. Recurrence occurred after an average of 33.3 weeks (range: 4–76) [23]. To summarize, the results were not encouraging and both authors recommended not using the unilateral orthoses any further.

In the classic orthotic AFO design as used by Janicki et al. [23] the foot is fixed into a dorsally applied shell by Velcro straps (Fig. 6). To our experience, a foot can move in a plastic half-tube shell to a certain amount around its axis, and supination of the foot is quite easily performed. In our design of the articulated lower leg orthosis the foot is held in a full-contact custom-made circular encompassing, preventing any undesired movement of the foot once the heel cap is closed. The

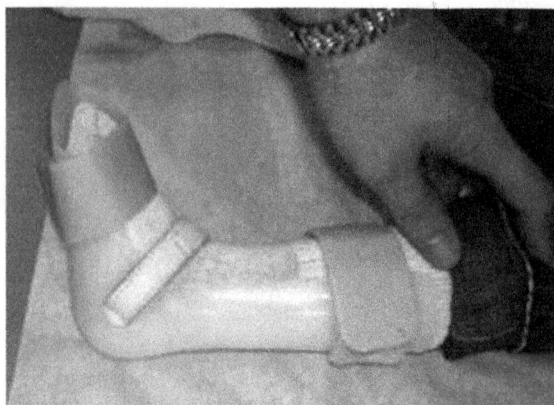

Fig. 6 The orthosis used by Janicki et al. 2011, following the classic AFO design [23]

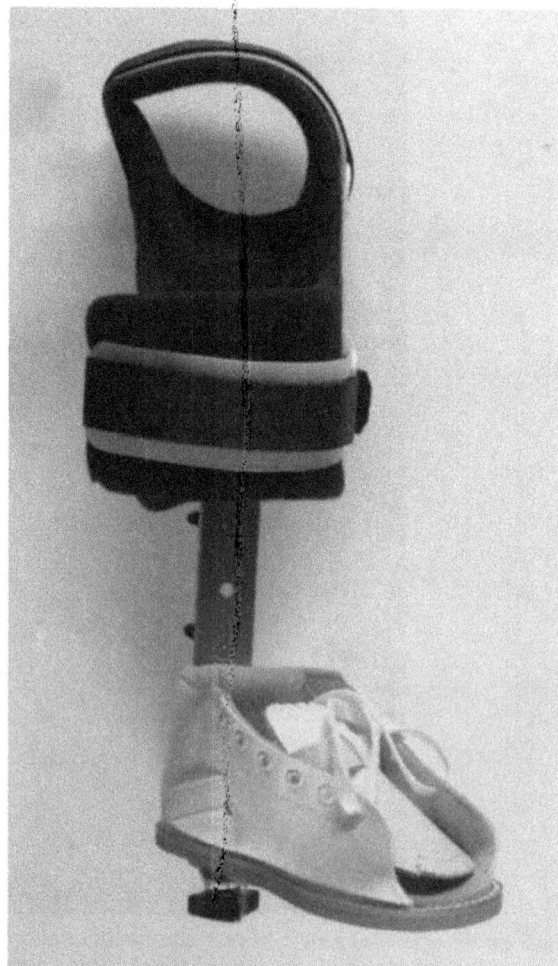

Fig. 7 The orthosis used by George et al. 2011, using a modular system [22]

pressure in this circular holding is applied on a large scale and thereby prevents pressure sores.

Another problem in the classic AFO design is to maintain external rotation of the foot to the knee joint line. The rotational forces have to be antagonised by sufficient friction and abutment.

In the classic AFO design a counter bearing is missing. The articulated LLO works with a lateral support at the femoral level via condylar encompasses that transmit the rotational forces to the femoral condyles, whether in knee flexion or extension. This follows the same principles as the toe-to-groin cast suggested by Ponseti [1].

The second pillar of rotational control, which is friction to the shaft, is realized by a firm intake of the lower leg by using a closing cap at the level of the tibial tuberosity. Thereby and by using a three-point support the LLO is applying sufficient pressure on the bone and soft tissue to create enough friction to prevent slipping and rotation. In the shell-like slick plastic shaft of the classic AFO there is only few friction created by the punctual pressure of one or two Velcro straps bandings.

The orthotic design used by George et al. [22] consists of a sandal which is fixed to a longitudinal bar in external rotation (Fig. 7). The bar in turn is fixed to the shank by straps, holding the knee in constant flexion. Though being an interesting approach, the rotational control and in consequence stretching of the medial tissues of the foot was difficult to achieve and the deformity reoccurred in 31% of feet [22]. The authors supposed that the failing of the orthosis was due to full time knee flexion at 90° preventing active contractions of gastrocnemius and assumed that this in turn might result in tightness and a higher relapse rate.

Another feature of our articulated lower leg orthosis is the possible dorsiflexion of up to 20°. The dorsiflexion can be attained by active movement, by either walking in the orthosis or adding gas pressure springs. Thereby, the possibility to stretch and exercise the gastrosoleus complex as suggested by Desai et al. [27] is another advantage of the LLO design.

The efficacy of the Pohlig LLO in preventing clubfoot recurrence is difficult to assess in our retrospective study. Almost all the patients in the LLO group were secondarily provided with LLOs after failed FAO treatment; therefore, the whole group represents negatively selected cases.

Four children (one with bilateral and three with unilateral involvement) were treated with a lower leg orthosis from the beginning. All of them were pretreated. One of these children had received 9 months of casting elsewhere before being referred to us (unilateral clubfoot, Pirani score 3 at presentation). The parents were strongly inclined towards LLO. This approach failed, and the child had to be re-operated at the age of 7 years.

The other three children (Pirani score, 4.5–6) were deliberately provided with LLO by the treating doctor who was at that time convinced that the LLO treatment was equally effective as the FAO. These three children showed no recurrence over a follow-up period of 8.1–9.5 years.

The children who were converted during treatment were treated with the LLO for a mean time of 31 months (subsequently to a mean treatment time of 8 months with a foot abduction brace), leaving a considerable amount of time for the LLO to 'fail'. We did not detect an elevated percentage of recurrence in this group after a mean follow-up of 8.4 years.

Although we are satisfied with the compliance and efficacy of the Pohlig LLO, this system does have certain disadvantages. The orthoses can in fact be adjusted one or two times in size (by grinding down the Inliner and displacing the hinges that fix the foot-unit to the lower leg-unit), but it is still rather time-consuming to adjust the orthosis to the child's growth. Another difficulty is that babies sometimes have a lot of soft tissue. This can limit the firm fitting and therefore reduces rotational stability and control of the foot. The orthosis cannot properly support itself to bony structures in these cases and instead 'swims' on soft tissue. Especially when a child has only a unilateral clubfoot, parents are often quite demanding to switch to a unilateral orthosis. If possible, we try to convince the parents to stick to the FAO until the age of at least one year before switching to an LLO. We feel that one year of age is likely the appropriate cut-off age for relevant technical problems. Nevertheless, if necessary, children below one year of age can be provided with an LLO, but it can be technically demanding and time consuming for the reasons noted above. In this age group, we now like to replace the lower leg unit by a thigh long L-shaped dorsal channelling with ventral cover in fixed 90° knee flexion. This unit is attached to the foot unit by screws in the same manner as in the LLO. The resulting construction strongly resembles the thigh long casting as performed in the Ponseti casting and provides – in our opinion - equivalent stability.

Limitations of the study

There are several limitations to our study. First, the study is retrospective. Second, since most patients included in the study have been treated with a standard foot abduction brace before converting to the LLO, a comparison of the two methods is not possible and the statistical analysis is limited. Furthermore, the diagnosis of recurrence was established on a clinical basis. Because there were no objective measures in this decision (e.g. degrees of hindfoot-varus), there might be a selection bias. Another limitation is that the original work of Baise and Pohlig is only available in German language, which limits visibility and dissemination of this treatment option. Finally, the costs and efforts to construct a LLO are higher than purchasing a standard FAO from the shelf.

Conclusion

Changing from FAO to LLO at any point during treatment did not result in an increased rate of surgery. The Pohlig LLO was associated with good compliance and efficacy in terms of recurrence of congenital talipes-equinovarus being treated with the Ponseti method. If treatment with a standard foot abduction brace cannot be continued, our results show that the LLO is an efficient alternative. This study is serving as a pilot for further investigations performed in a prospective and randomized manner.

Abbreviations
FAO: Foot abduction orthosis; LLO: Lower leg orthosis

Acknowledgements
We would like to thank Dr. Christel Schäfer from Behandlungszentrum Aschau im Chiemgau/Germany for her major contribution to this work in terms of performing the casting, bracing, and follow-up controls of all the patients. We also would like to thank Dr. Josien van Den Noort for her thorough and insightful help to improve the quality of this paper by reviewing it.

Funding
The study was performed in Behandlungszentrum Aschau im Chiemgau, Head Dr. L. Döderlein.

Authors' contributions
NB and LD drafted the study. NB, DL, MS and PMP took part in the design and conception of the study. NB, DL, and MS collected the clinical data. Analysis of the dataset was done by NB and AH. NB, MS, LD and PMP contributed to the interpretation of the results. The manuscript was written by NB and PMP. All authors revised the manuscript and approved the final version submitted for publication.

Consent for publication
Written consent was obtained from the practitioner performing in the Additional file 2: Video "Putting on LLO".

Competing interests
The authors declare that they have no competing interests.

Author details
[1]Klinikum rechts der Isar der Technischen Universität München, Munich, Germany. [2]Behandlungszentrum Aschau im Chiemgau, Aschau, Germany. [3]Institute of Medical Informatics, Statistics and Epidemiology, Technical University Munich, Munich, Germany.

References
1. Ponseti IV, Smoley EN. Congenital Club foot: the results of treatment. The Journal of Bone & Joint Surgery. 1963;45(2):261–344.
2. Ponseti IV: Congenital clubfoot: fundamentals of treatment: Oxford university press; 1996.
3. Zhao D, Liu J, Zhao L, Wu Z. Relapse of clubfoot after treatment with the Ponseti method and the function of the foot abduction orthosis. Clinics in orthopedic surgery. 2014;6(3):245–52.
4. Browne D. Modern methods of treatment of Club-foot. Br Med J. 1937; 2(4002):570–2.
5. Browne D. TALIPES EQUINO-VARUS. Lancet. 1934;224(5801):969–74.
6. Morcuende JA, Dolan LA, Dietz FR, Ponseti IV. Radical reduction in the rate of extensive corrective surgery for clubfoot using the Ponseti method. Pediatrics. 2004;113(2):376–80.
7. Shabtai L, Segev E, Yavor A, Wientroub S, Hemo Y. Prolonged use of foot abduction brace reduces the rate of surgery in Ponseti-treated idiopathic club feet. J Child Orthop. 2015;9(3):177–82.
8. Zionts LE, Zhao G, Hitchcock K, Maewal J, Ebramzadeh E. Has the rate of extensive surgery to treat idiopathic clubfoot declined in the United States? J Bone Joint Surg Am. 2010;92(4):882–9.
9. Garg S, Porter K. Improved bracing compliance in children with clubfeet using a dynamic orthosis. J Child Orthop. 2009;3(4):271–6.
10. Hemo Y, Segev E, Yavor A, Ovadia D, Wientroub S, Hayek S. The influence of brace type on the success rate of the Ponseti treatment protocol for idiopathic clubfoot. J Child Orthop. 2011;5(2):115–9.
11. Ramírez N, Flynn JM, Fernández S, Seda W, Macchiavelli RE: Orthosis Noncompliance After the Ponseti Method for the Treatment of Idiopathic Clubfeet: A Relevant Problem That Needs Reevaluation. J. Pediatr. Orthop.2011, 31(6):710–715 7https://doi.org/10.1097/BPO.1090b1013e318221eaa318221.
12. Zionts LE, Dietz FR. Bracing following correction of idiopathic clubfoot using the Ponseti method. J. Am. Acad. Orthop. Surg. 2010;18(8):486–93.
13. Zionts LE, Frost N, Kim R, Ebramzadeh E, Sangiorgio SN: Treatment of Idiopathic Clubfoot: Experience With the Mitchell-Ponseti Brace. J. Pediatr. Orthop 2012, 32(7):706–713 7https://doi.org/10.1097/BPO.1090b1013e3182694f3182694d.
14. Haft GF, Walker CG, Crawford HA. Early clubfoot recurrence after use of the Ponseti method in a New Zealand population. J Bone Joint Surg Am. 2007; 89(3):487–93.
15. Abdelgawad AA, Lehman WB, van Bosse HJ, Scher DM, Sala DA. Treatment of idiopathic clubfoot using the Ponseti method: minimum 2-year follow-up. J Pediatr Orthop B. 2007;16(2):98–105.
16. Dobbs MB, Rudzki JR, Purcell DB, Walton T, Porter KR, Gurnett CA. Factors predictive of outcome after use of the Ponseti method for the treatment of idiopathic clubfeet. J Bone Joint Surg Am. 2004;86-A(1):22–7.
17. Richards BS, Faulks S, Rathjen KE, Karol LA, Johnston CE, Jones SA. A comparison of two nonoperative methods of idiopathic clubfoot correction: the Ponseti method and the French functional (physiotherapy) method. J Bone Joint Surg Am. 2008;90(11):2313–21.
18. Boehm S, Sinclair M: Foot Abduction Brace in the Ponseti Method for Idiopathic Clubfoot Deformity: Torsional Deformities and Compliance. J. Pediatr. Orthop2007, 27(6):712–716 7https://doi.org/10.1097/BPO.1090b1013e3181425508.
19. Avilucea FR, Szalay EA, Bosch PP, Sweet KR, Schwend RM. Effect of cultural factors on outcome of Ponseti treatment of clubfeet in rural America. J Bone Joint Surg Am. 2009;91(3):530–40.
20. Chen RC, Gordon JE, Luhmann SJ, Schoenecker PL, Dobbs MB: A New Dynamic Foot Abduction Orthosis for Clubfoot Treatment. JPediatr. Orthop 2007, 27(5):522–528 5https://doi.org/10.1097/bpo.1090b1013e318070cc318019.
21. Kessler JI. A new flexible brace used in the Ponseti treatment of talipes equinovarus. J Pediatr Orthop B. 2008;17(5):247–50.
22. George HL, Unnikrishnan PN, Garg NK, Sampath J, Bruce CE. Unilateral foot abduction orthosis: is it a substitute for Denis Browne boots following Ponseti technique? J Pediatr Orthop B. 2011;20(1):22–5.
23. Janicki JA, Wright JG, Weir S, Narayanan UG. A comparison of ankle foot orthoses with foot abduction orthoses to prevent recurrence following correction of idiopathic clubfoot by the Ponseti method. J Bone Joint Surg Br. 2011;93(5):700–4.
24. Baise M, Pohlig K. Behandlung des reversiblen dynamischen Spitzfußes mittels Unterschenkelorthesen mit ringförmiger Fussfassung. Ergebnisse bei Kindern mit infantiler Zerebralparese Med Orth Techn. 2005;3:1–19.
25. Baise M K P: [A new concept in the treatment of spastic clubfoot with the calcaneus-rotation-ring type orthosis]. Med Orth Tech 2004, 124(5):61–68.

26. Seringe R, Wicart P. The talonavicular and subtalar joints: the "calcaneopedal unit" concept. Orthop Traumatol Surg Res. 2013;99(6 Suppl):S345–55.
27. Desai L, Oprescu F, DiMeo A, Morcuende JA. Bracing in the treatment of children with clubfoot: past, present, and future. The Iowa orthopaedic journal. 2010;30:15–23.
28. Pirani S, Outerbridge H, Moran M, Sawatsky B: A method of evaluating the virgin clubfoot with substantial inter-observer reliability. 1995.
29. Goksan SB, Bilgili F, Eren I, Bursali A, Koc E. Factors affecting adherence with foot abduction orthosis following Ponseti method. Acta Orthop Traumatol Turc. 2015;49(6):620–6.

3

Quality of internet-based decision aids for shoulder arthritis: what are patients reading?

Jeremy S. Somerson[1], Aaron J. Bois[2*], Jeffrey Jeng[3], Kamal I. Bohsali[4], John W. Hinchey[5] and Michael A. Wirth[5]

Abstract

Background: The objective of this study was to assess the source, quality, accuracy, and completeness of Internet-based information for shoulder arthritis.

Methods: A web search was performed using three common Internet search engines and the top 50 sites from each search were analyzed. Information sources were categorized into academic, commercial, non-profit, and physician sites. Information quality was measured using the Health On the Net (HON) Foundation principles, content accuracy by counting factual errors and completeness using a custom template.

Results: After removal of duplicates and sites that did not provide an overview of shoulder arthritis, 49 websites remained for analysis. The majority of sites were from commercial ($n = 16$, 33%) and physician ($n = 16$, 33%) sources. An additional 12 sites (24%) were from an academic institution and five sites (10%) were from a non-profit organization. Commercial sites had the highest number of errors, with a five-fold likelihood of containing an error compared to an academic site. Non-profit sites had the highest HON scores, with an average of 9.6 points on a 16-point scale. The completeness score was highest for academic sites, with an average score of 19.2 ± 6.7 (maximum score of 49 points); other information sources had lower scores (commercial, 15.2 ± 2.9; non-profit, 18.7 ± 6.8; physician, 16.6 ± 6.3).

Conclusions: Patient information on the Internet regarding shoulder arthritis is of mixed accuracy, quality, and completeness. Surgeons should actively direct patients to higher-quality Internet sources.

Keywords: Shoulder, Arthritis, Internet-based information

Background

Internet growth and popularity over the past two decades has required healthcare to evolve in many ways. Traditional methods of disseminating medical information (i.e., pamphlets from local healthcare providers) have been largely replaced by websites. This expansion of health information available on the Internet has continued at an accelerated pace. The search engine Google (www.google.com) yields over 21 million results when the search term "arthritis" is entered. The unregulated format of the Internet provides opportunity for any source to publish health-related information regardless of validity and veracity.

* Correspondence: ajmbois@gmail.com
[2]Sport Medicine Centre, University of Calgary, 2500 University Drive NW, Calgary, AB T2N 1N4, Canada
Full list of author information is available at the end of the article

Recent surveys have found that nearly 81% of U.S. adults use the Internet and, of those, 72% reported searching for health-related information online [1]. Many patients choose the Internet as their initial source for information to evaluate medical conditions before deciding whether or not to seek a physician [1–4]. Consequently, the quality and informational content on the Internet has the capacity to substantially impact patient health outcomes.

Over the past decade, the orthopaedic community has started to evaluate the quality and accuracy of informational websites for specific diagnoses. A 2005 study found that the Internet-based content on scoliosis primarily originates from academic sites, yet is of limited quality and poor accuracy [5]. More recently, the results of a study evaluating anterior cruciate ligament

Quality of internet-based decision aids for shoulder arthritis: what are patients...

23

reconstruction revealed progress in the quality of information compared to prior studies [6]; however, to the best of the authors' knowledge, similar studies on shoulder arthritis have not been published.

Shoulder pain is a common orthopaedic complaint with a prevalence as high as 50% in the elderly population [7]. Shoulder arthritis is an increasing problem in the aging population and surgical treatment is becoming more common. A recent study in the United States found that nearly 47,000 shoulder arthroplasties were performed as inpatient procedures in 2008, which represented a 2.5-fold increase when compared to only 19,000 shoulder arthroplasties in 1998 [8].

The primary objective of this study was to assess the source, quality, accuracy, and completeness of Internet-based information for glenohumeral joint arthritis by objectively analyzing the content with a predetermined set of criteria. We hypothesized that the websites available for glenohumeral joint arthritis would be lacking in quality and incomplete in content. To our knowledge, a comprehensive assessment of Internet-based information for glenohumeral joint arthritis has not been previously performed.

Methods

To evaluate the quality and content of Internet information, the search term "shoulder arthritis" was entered into three major search engines (www.google.com, www.yahoo.com, and www.bing.com). These were chosen in an attempt to simulate real-world usage as research has shown that these three search engines account for over 89% of all Internet searches in the United States [9]. The first 50 websites from each search engine were selected to be included in our study. Paid advertising links were excluded from this study. Duplicate websites within and between search engines were excluded from the final list to ensure each website was only evaluated once. Also, links that did not relate to shoulder arthritis and websites requiring paid subscription were removed from the final list to more accurately simulate patient usage. Of the 150 potentially eligible websites to be evaluated by each reviewer, the final number of sites included after all exclusion criteria were applied was 49 (Fig. 1). Three independent orthopaedic surgeons with shoulder and elbow fellowship training graded the websites selected for this study (A.J.B., K.I.B. and J.W.H.).

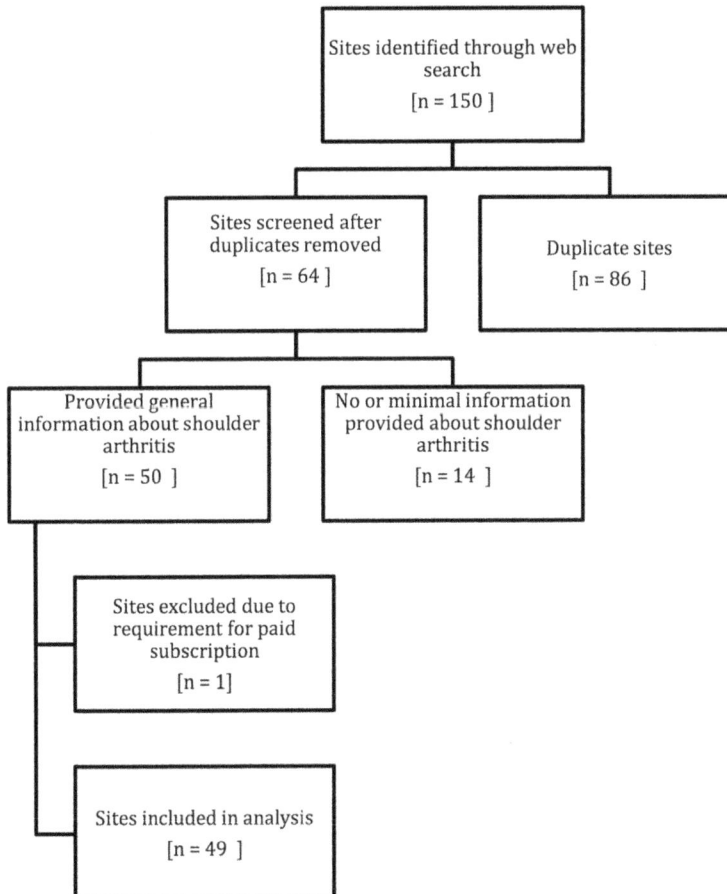

Fig. 1 Flowchart demonstrating number of websites included and excluded at each stage of the review

A grading template was developed to evaluate the source, quality, accuracy and completeness of each website. Source was divided into 1 of 4 categories: 1) *academic* included any university-affiliated physician group; 2) *commercial* if any websites received industry funding, displayed advertisements, or sold products for profit; 3) *nonprofit* included any organization that does not earn profits for its owners; and 4) *physician* encompassed any professional sites for an individual or group of physicians not affiliated with an academic institution. In cases of website categorization discrepancy amongst reviewers, the final category was assigned based on the agreement between the 3 reviewers; however, if all 3 reviewers were in disagreement, the site in question was presented and reviewed as a group to reach consensus for final categorization.

The second aspect of the grading template evaluated the quality of information being presented on each site. The Health On the Net (HON) Foundation is a non-governmental organization serving to monitor and encourage the dissemination of quality healthcare information throughout the Internet. The HON Foundation developed a certification system for websites that choose to follow the HONcode principles established by the organization. Certified sites are permitted to display a HONcode seal of approval to demonstrate their commitment to providing reliable health and medical information on the Internet. Following the methods used by Starman et al. [10], each website's quality of information was measured by a 16-point scale used to assess the compliance of websites according to the HON Foundation principles (HON Quality Score)(Table 1). If a site displayed a HONcode seal of approval, it was noted but still evaluated using the 16-point scale. A score of 0 indicated that none of the benchmarks for reliability and quality was met, while a score of 16 indicated that all benchmarks were met.

Accuracy of the source in question was calculated by counting the number of factual errors identified by each reviewer. When disagreements occurred, the average number of errors identified for each site from the three reviewers was recorded. Content completeness was graded on a custom 49-point scale (Table 2) developed by two orthopaedic surgeons (J.S.S. and M.A.W.) based on a previously-described algorithm [5]. Criteria were generated for 4 categories of information through a review of information in 4 shoulder textbooks [11–14]: 1) disease pathophysiology, pathoanatomy, and pathogenesis; 2) clinical evaluation; 3) treatment; 4) indications, outcomes, and complications. Disease-specific concepts were calculated based on frequency of appearance in each textbook. The final grading rubric excluded any inconsistent and/or low-yield information. For completeness, a board-certified orthopaedic surgeon with

Table 1 Health On the Net Foundation (HON) Quality Score (as described by Starman et al. [10])

Transparency and honesty

- Transparency of provider of site – including name (1), physical address or electronic address (1) of the person or organization responsible for the site (2 points).
- Transparency of purpose and objective (1) of the site (1 point).
- Target audience (1) clearly defined (further detail on purpose, multiple audiences could be defined at different levels)(1 point).
- Transparency of all sources of funding (1) for site (grants, sponsors, advertisers, nonprofit, voluntary assistance)(1 point).

Authority

- Clear statement of sources for all information (0 = none, 1 = some, and 2 = all) provided and date of publication (1) of source (3 points).
- Names and credentials of all human/institutional authors of information (0 = none, 1 = some, and 2 = all) put up on the site, including dates at which credentials were received (2 points).

Privacy and data protection

- Privacy (1) and data protection policy and system for the processing of personal data, including processing invisible to users (1 point).

Updating of information

- Clear and regular updating of the site, with date of update clearly displayed for each page and/or item as relevant (1 = listed). Regular checking of relevance of information (1 point).

Accountability

- Accountability—user feedback (1), and appropriate oversight responsibility (such as a named quality compliance officer (1) for each site) (2 points).
- Responsible partnering—all efforts should be made to ensure that partnering or linking to other web sites is undertaken only with trustworthy individuals and organizations who themselves comply with relevant codes of good practice
- Editorial policy—clear statement describing what procedure was used for selection of content (1 point).

Accessibility

- Accessibility—attention to guidelines on physical accessibility as well as general findability, searchability, readability (1 = clear organization of topics without embedded advertisements, etc.), and usability (1 point).

shoulder and elbow fellowship training reviewed all of the grading criteria. Each website was awarded 1 point for every disease-specific concept mentioned, for a maximum score of 49 points.

Statistical analysis

Descriptive statistics were generated based on average scores for content score, HON quality score, and number of errors reported from each reviewer. Mean and standard deviation were reported for these 3 outcome measures by website authorship. These measures were then compared by authorship group of websites (academic, commercial, non-profit, physician) to all other websites using a non-parametric 2-sample Wilcoxon rank sum test. Statistical significance was

Table 2 Shoulder Arthritis Content

Disease Pathophysiology, Pathoanatomy, and Pathogenesis

- - Mean score: 5.1±2.0 (maximum score 15)
- • Description of glenohumeral joint structures
- • Physical wear leading to articular cartilage failure and degeneration
- • Humeral head changes
- • Glenoid changes
- • Posterior humeral head subluxation
- • Anterior capsule contracture
- • Joint space narrowing
- • Age
- • Post-traumatic
- • Systemic factors (gender, smoking, diabetes, genetics)
- • History of previous surgery for glenohumeral instability
- • Increased load bearing
- • Cuff tear arthropathy
- • Avascular necrosis
- • Autoimmune disease

Clinical Evaluation

- - Mean score 5.1±2.1 (maximum score 12)
- • Complaint of pain
- • History of disease
- • Sleep difficulties
- • Progression of functional difficulties
- • Joint crepitation
- • Limited glenohumeral motion/loss of external rotation
- • Tenderness over posterior joint line
- • Muscle weakness/atrophy
- • Plain radiographs
- • CT scan
- • Arthrography
- • MRI

Treatment

- - Mean score 5.2±1.4 (maximum score 11)
- • Patient education
- • Rest/avoiding provocative activities (i.e., activity modification)
- • Physical therapy
- • Anti- inflammatory medications
- • Corticosteroid injection
- • Arthroscopy
- • Hemiarthroplasty
- • Total shoulder arthroplasty
- • Reverse total shoulder arthroplasty

Table 2 Shoulder Arthritis Content *(Continued)*

Indications, Outcomes, and Complications

- - Mean score: 1.5±1.8 (maximum score 11)
- • Pain/stiffness/weakness
- • Degree of dysfunction unacceptable to patient
- • Severe pain failing conservative (i.e., nonoperative) treatment
- • Expected outcomes and success rates of surgery
- • Rehabilitation protocols
- • Inherent surgical complications
- • Component loosening
- • Instability
- • Periprosthetic fractures
- • Rotator cuff tears
- • Neurologic injuries

established at $p \leq 0.05$. Consistency between the 3 graders was measured using Cronbach's alpha statistic for completeness and accuracy outcome measures.

Results

The distribution of sites by authorship was as follows: 12 (24%) were considered to be from an academic source, 16 (33%) were commercial, 5 (10%) were from non-profit organizations, and 16 (33%) were considered physician-based.

The HON Quality score was 5.8 ± 2.1 (mean ± SD) for academic sites, 6.4 ± 4.2 for commercial sites, 9.6 ± 3.6 for non-profit sites and 6.6 ± 2.7 for physician sites on a maximum 16-point scale (Fig. 2). We found only 3 out of 49 websites reviewed displayed the HONcode compliance seal of approval, but none of those websites received a full score using the 16-point scale. The top HON quality score of 14 points was attained by 4 websites (3 commercial and 1 non-profit website). The average number of mistakes (i.e., factual errors) per site was 0.2 (range: 0–1) for academic sites, 1.0 (range 0–3) for commercial sites, 0.5 (range 0–2) for non-profit sites and 0.4 (range: 0–2) for physician sites. These mistakes most commonly included unproven statements, such as the ability of shoulder injections or nutritional supplements to improve the health of articular cartilage. Non-profit sites had significantly higher HON quality scores than other types of sites ($P < 0.05$). Commercial sites had more errors than other types of sites ($P < 0.01$) while academic sites had fewer errors ($P = 0.02$). The content completeness score was 19.2 ± 6.7 (mean ± SD) for academic sites, 15.2 ± 2.9 for commercial sites, 18.7 ± 6.8 for non-profit sites and 16.6 ± 6.3 for physician sites on a maximum 49-point scale (Fig. 3). The 5 websites with the highest content completeness scores

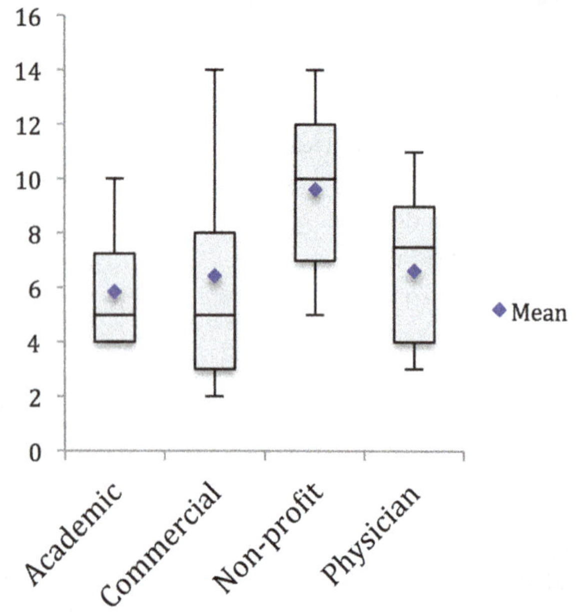

Fig. 2 Box plot depicting the HON Quality Score by authorship. Bars represent maximum and minimum data values

are presented in Table 3. We further analyzed each website's content completeness score and found consistently low scores for the subcategory of "Indications, Outcomes, and Complications"; the average score was 1.5 out of 11 possible subcategory points (13.6%) (Table 1).

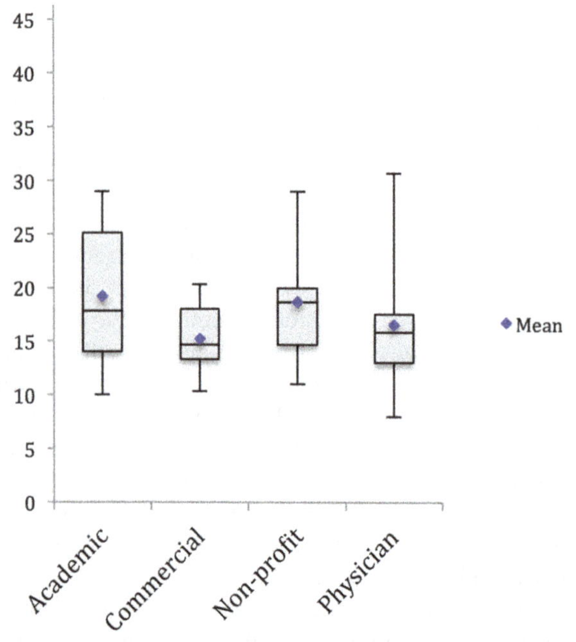

Fig. 3 Box plot depicting content completeness score by authorship. Bars represent maximum and minimum data values

Interobserver reliability

Total scores for content completeness points on a 49-point scale demonstrated excellent interobserver item reliability (Cronbach's alpha: 0.90). Subgroups for content completeness also revealed a high level of consistency (Disease Pathophysiology: 0.84, Clinical Evaluation: 0.89, Treatment: 0.86, Indications, Outcomes, and Complications: 0.86). The number of mistakes detected per website demonstrated good consistency (Cronbach's alpha: 0.67).

Discussion

Variability in the content that patients read on the Internet can present an obstacle to informed decision-making. This study reviewed Internet-based resources regarding shoulder arthritis and characterized the source, quality, accuracy and completeness of the information.

One of the first orthopaedic studies to look at Internet-based information evaluated the type, quality, and reliability of information regarding carpal tunnel syndrome [15]. The authors of this study found that only 23% of the 49 sites were created by a physician or an academic organization. Moreover, neither category scored above 40%, with an informational value score that ranged from 0 to 100. In 2005, Mathur et al. [5] conducted a similar study using 5 search engines and the key word "scoliosis," and found that the majority of websites for scoliosis were academic; however, they determined the content and accuracy of those sites to be poor. They found that 21 out of the 50 websites evaluated had an accuracy score of less than 25%.

In our study, academic websites had the highest average content completeness score of 19.2 out of 49 (39.2%), whereas commercial websites had the lowest average content completeness score of 15.2 (31%). However, we found that certain popular commercial sites, such as Medscape and WebMD, had content completeness scores above the category's average (47% and 41%, respectively). Physician authorship of individual content pages on these commercial sites may have contributed to this finding.

Regarding distribution of sources, we found commercial (33%) and physician-based (33%) websites were most common, followed closely by academic websites (24%) and lastly by non-profit websites (10%). There were no personal websites identified. Of the top 10 scores for content completeness, 5 were from academic organizations, 2 each from physician-based and non-profit groups, and only 1 from a commercial website. These results may reflect recent efforts by academic institutions and other healthcare organizations to provide patients with accurate and comprehensive healthcare information. Nevertheless, over 85% of all websites had content scores of less than 24 points, suggesting improvement is warranted. In particular, the low scores for the subcategory of "Indications, Outcomes, and

Table 3 Top-rated shoulder arthritis websites for content completeness

Site Name	Hyperlink	Content Score (49-point maximum)
The Steadman Clinic – Glenohumeral Arthritis	www.thesteadmanclinic.com/patient-education/shoulder/glenohumeral-arthritis	31 (Path: 9.7, Eval: 10.3, Tx: 6.0, I/O/C: 4.7)
Shoulder Arthritis and Rotator Cuff Tears: Causes of Shoulder Pain	shoulderarthritis.blogspot.com	30 (Path: 10.7, Eval: 6.7, Tx: 7.0, I/O/C: 6.0)
UCLA Health – Shoulder Arthritis	ortho.ucla.edu/body.cfm?id=181	29 (Path: 9.0, Eval: 6.7, Tx: 6.0, I/O/C: 7.3)
Arthritis of the Shoulder - OrthoInfo – AAOS	orthoinfo.aaos.org/en/diseases–conditions/arthritis-of-the-shoulder	29 (Path: 9.0, Eval: 7.3, Tx: 9.0, I/O/C: 3.7)
University of Washington - Shoulder Arthritis	http://www.orthop.washington.edu/?q=patient-care/shoulder-arthritis.html	29 (Path: 10.0, Eval: 9.3, Tx: 7.3, I/O/C: 2)

Path Pathology Content subscore, Eval Clinical Evaluation subscore, Tx Treatment subscore, I/O/C Indications/Outcomes/Complications subscore

Complications" is consistent with a previous orthopaedic study that found a lack of information on potential complications of various treatments [16].

The HON Foundation evaluates health-related sites and has established guidelines in an attempt to standardize the reliability and credibility of medical information on the Internet. Candidate websites are subjected to a thorough evaluation based upon HON ethical standards and, if certified, are permitted to display a HONcode seal of approval free of charge. The ethical aspects of the HONcode include the author's credentials, the date of the last modification with respect to clinical documents, confidentiality of data, source data reference, funding, and advertising [17]. However, over 83% of websites scored below 10 points (of a maximum of 16 points) to suggest that the majority of glenohumeral arthritis websites are of relatively low quality. This is consistent with recent studies that have found low quality Internet information for both shoulder- and elbow-related disorders, such as shoulder instability [18], and rotator cuff tears [19], and ulnar collateral ligament injuries [20], as well as shoulder-related surgery, such as total shoulder arthroplasty [21].

Ideally, a high-quality patient information website should be developed by a credible source and display accurate information regarding diagnostic tests, treatment options, outcomes, and possible complications. Information should also be at a reading level that is comprehensible to an average patient, as recent studies have shown patient materials on the Internet to be written at a much higher level than many patients can comprehend [18–20, 22]. The OrthoInfo site (www.orthoinfo.aaos.org), created by the American Academy of Orthopaedic Surgeons (AAOS), scored among the top five websites for HON score and content completeness. The OrthoInfo site received 14 out of 16 points for HON score and 29 (59%) out of 49 points for content completeness. Patients should be

actively directed to this and other high-scoring information sources.

There were a few limitations of this study that need to be considered. Although we used the 3 most popular Internet search engines, our method for selecting websites may not accurately reflect the way in which all patients locate a website for medical information (i.e., not all patients use Google, Yahoo, or Bing as their primary search engines). Second, selection of the top 50 websites may be affected by strategies for website optimization, as some sites may employ commercially available methods for improving their search engine ranking. Third, it was often unclear to what extent third parties were used to provide content for each website; this could have an impact on accuracy and completeness. Lastly, the subjective nature of the grading system created to evaluate each website is a potential source of bias; we did not engage patients or non-physician health care providers in the process to better understand what would constitute complete information from other perspectives. To limit the variability of the selected criteria, 2 orthopaedic surgeons developed the grading rubric through a systematic review of 4 primary shoulder textbooks. This resulted in a high level of interobserver reliability for total content completeness scores as well as subgroup scores.

Conclusions

The majority of information on the Internet regarding shoulder arthritis is of mixed quality and comprehensive sources are lacking. One-third of the top-ranked websites are commercial in nature and were more likely to contain factual errors. Academic sites were less likely to contain factual errors, and non-profit sites met a greater number of quality measures for information sources. We believe orthopaedic surgeons should be knowledgeable about where patients are likely to browse for medical information on the Internet and be responsible in directing them to optimal sources.

Abbreviations
AAOS: American Academy of Orthopaedic Surgeons; HON: Health On the Net

Acknowledgements
Not applicable.

Funding
Not applicable.

Authors' contributions
JSS participated in the design of the study, analyzed and interpreted data, major contributor to writing and editing the manuscript. AJB collected and interpreted data, major contributor to writing and editing the manuscript. JJ participated in the design of the study, major contributor to writing the manuscript. KIB collected and interpreted data, contributed to writing and editing the manuscript. JWH collected and interpreted data, contributed to writing and editing the manuscript. MAW participated in the design of the study, analyzed and interpreted data, contributed to writing and editing the manuscript. All authors read and approved the final manuscript.

Authors' information
Presented in poster format at the 13th Meeting of the Combined Orthopaedic Associations, Cape Town, South Africa, April 2016 (presenting author AJB).

Consent for publication
Not applicable.

Competing interests
The authors declare that they have no competing interests.

Author details
[1]University of Texas Medical Branch, 301 University Blvd, Galveston, TX 77555, USA. [2]Sport Medicine Centre, University of Calgary, 2500 University Drive NW, Calgary, AB T2N 1N4, Canada. [3]University of California Los Angeles, Los Angeles, USA. [4]Jacksonville Orthopaedic Institute-Beaches Division, 6100 Kennerly Road Suite 101, Jacksonville, FL 32216, USA. [5]Department of Orthopaedics, The University of Texas Health Science Center San Antonio, 7703 Floyd Curl Drive – MC 7774, San Antonio, TX 78229, USA.

References
1. Fox S, Duggan M. Health Online 2013. Pew Internet and American Life Project. 2013. http://www.pewinternet.org/~/media//Files/Reports/PIP_HealthOnline.pdf. Accessed 2 Feb 2014.
2. Benigeri M, Pluye P. Shortcomings of health information on the internet. Health Promot Int. 2003;18:381–6.
3. Diaz JA, Griffith RA, Ng JJ, Reinert SE, Friedmann PD, Moulton AW. Patients' use of the internet for medical information. J Gen Intern Med. 2002;17:180–5.
4. Hesse BW, Nelson DE, Kreps GL, Croyle RT, Arora NK, Rimer BK, et al. Trust and sources of health information. Arch Intern Med. 2005;165:2618–24.
5. Mathur S, Shanti N, Brkaric M, Sood V, Kubeck J, Paulino C, Merola A. Surfing for scoliosis: the quality of information available on the internet. Spine. 2005;30:2695–700.
6. Duncan IC, Kane PW, Lawson KA, Cohen SB, Ciccotti MG, Dodson CC. Evaluation of information available on the internet regarding anterior cruciate ligament reconstruction. Arthroscopy. 2013;29:1095–100.
7. Wofford JL, Mansfield RJ, Watkins RS. Patient characteristics and clinical management of patients with shoulder pain in U.S. primary care settings: secondary data analysis of the National Ambulatory Medical Care Survey. BMC Musculoskelet Disord. 2005;6:4.
8. Kim SH, Wise BL, Zhang Y, Szabo RM. Increasing incidence of shoulder arthroplasty in the United States. J Bone Joint Surg Am. 2011;93:2249–54.
9. Purcell K, Brenner J, Rainie L. Search Engine Use 2012. Pew Internet and American Life Project. 2012. https://www.eff.org/files/Pew%202012_0.pdf. Accessed 3 Feb 2014.
10. Starman JS, Gettys FK, Capo JA, Fleischli JE, Norton HJ, Karunakar MA. Quality and content of internet-based information for ten common Orthopaedic sports medicine diagnoses. J Bone Joint Surg Am. 2010;92:1612–8.
11. Gartsman GM. Shoulder arthroscopy. 2nd ed: W.B. Saunders Company; 2009.
12. Iannotti JP, Williams GR, Miniaci A, Zuckerman JD. Disorders of the shoulder, reconstruction. 3rd ed: Lippincott Williams & Wilkins; 2013.
13. Rockwood CA Jr, Matsen FA, Wirth MA, Lippitt SB, Fehringer EV, Sperling JW. The shoulder. 4th ed: Elsevier Health Sciences; 2009.
14. Williams GR Jr, Yamaguchi K, Ramsey ML, Galatz LM. Shoulder and elbow arthroplasty. 1st ed: Lippincott Williams & Wilkins; 2004.
15. Beredjiklian PK, Bozentka DJ, Steinberg DR, Bernstein J. Evaluating the source and content of Orthopaedic information on the internet: the case of carpal tunnel syndrome. J Bone Joint Surg Am. 2000;82:1540.
16. Lutsky K, Bernstein J, Beredjiklian PK. Quality of information on the internet about carpal tunnel syndrome: an update. Orthopedics. 2013;36:e1038–41.
17. Boyer C, Selby M, Scherrer JR, Appel RD. The health on the net code of conduct for medical and health websites. Comput Biol Med. 1998;28:603–10.
18. Garcia GH, Taylor SA, Dy CJ, Christ A, Patel RM, Dines JS. Online resources for shoulder instability: what are patients reading? J Bone Joint Surg Am. 2014;96(20):e177.
19. Dalton DM, Kelly EG, Molony DC. Availability of accessible and high-quality information on the internet for patients regarding the diagnosis and management of rotator cuff tears. J Shoulder Elb Surg. 2015;24(5):e135–40.
20. Johnson CC, Garcia GH, Liu JN, Stepan JG, Patel RM, Dines JS. Internet resources for Tommy John injuries: what are patients reading? J Shoulder Elb Surg. 2016;25(12):e386–93.
21. Matthews JR, Harrison CM, Hughes TM, Dezfuli B, Sheppard J. Web page content and quality assessed for shoulder replacement. Am J Orthop (Belle Mead NJ). 2016;45(1):e20–6.
22. Shah AK, Yi PH, Stein A. Readability of Orthopaedic oncology-related patient education materials available on the internet. J Am Acad Orthop Surg. 2015; 23(12):783–8.

4

Associations between circulating adipokines and bone mineral density in patients with knee osteoarthritis

Juan Wu[1] , Jianhua Xu[1], Kang Wang[1,2], Qicui Zhu[1], Jingyu Cai[1], Jiale Ren[1], Shuang Zheng[2] and Changhai Ding[1,2,3]*

Abstract

Background: Associations between adipokines and bone mineral density (BMD) in knee osteoarthritis (OA) remain indistinct. The aim of this study was to investigate the cross-sectional associations between serum levels of adipokines and BMD in patients with knee OA.

Methods: This study included 164 patients with symptomatic knee OA from the Anhui Osteoarthritis study. Serum levels of leptin, adiponectin, and resistin were measured using an enzyme-linked immunosorbent assay (ELISA). BMD at total body, spine, hip, and femur were measured by dual-energy X-ray absorptiometry (DXA).

Results: In multivariable analyses, serum levels of leptin were significantly associated with reduced BMD at total body, hip, total femur, femoral neck, and femoral shaft ($\beta = -0.019$, 95% CI -0.034 to -0.005; $\beta = -0.018$, 95% CI -0.034 to -0.003; $\beta = -0.018$, 95% CI -0.034 to -0.002; $\beta = -0.016$, 95% CI -0.032 to 0.000; $\beta = -0.026$, 95% CI -0.046 to -0.006; respectively). Serum levels of adiponectin were significantly and negatively associated with BMD at total femur and femoral shaft ($\beta = -0.007$, 95% CI -0.013 to 0.000; $\beta = -0.011$, 95% CI -0.018 to -0.003; respectively). However, no significant associations were found between serum levels of resistin and BMD at any site measured.

Conclusions: Serum levels of leptin and adiponectin were significantly and negatively associated with BMD, suggesting potentially detrimental effects of leptin and adiponectin on BMD in knee OA patients.

Keywords: Adiponectin, Bone mineral density, Leptin, Osteoarthritis, Resistin

Background

Osteoarthritis (OA) is the most prevalent joint disease worldwide, characterized by gradual loss of articular cartilage, synovial inflammation, osteophyte formation, and other structural changes. OA affected approximately 18% of women and 10% of men aged over 60 years according to the WHO's report [1].

Obesity is a well-recognized risk factor for OA, particularly in the weight-bearing joints. However, obesity-increased joint loading could not account for the associations between OA and non-weight-bearing joints such as hand and shoulder joints. Recent studies considered that obesity-related metabolic inflammation might contribute to OA [2, 3].

Adipokines, including leptin, adiponectin, and resistin which are mostly studied, are secreted by white adipose tissue, and have been found in synovial fluid and cartilage tissues obtained from OA patients [4, 5]. Leptin had been shown to be positively associated with the severity of OA [6, 7]; however, leptin was significantly associated with increased knee cartilage volume in patients with radiographic OA [8]. Another study [9] reported that leptin was not significantly associated with cartilage damage in OA patients. The role of adiponectin in OA

* Correspondence: changhai.ding@utas.edu.au
[1]Department of Rheumatology and Immunology, Arthritis Research Institute, the First Affiliated Hospital of Anhui Medical University, 218 Jixi Street, Hefei, China
[2]Menzies Institute for Medical Research, University of Tasmania, Private Bag 23, Hobart, TAS 7000, Australia
Full list of author information is available at the end of the article

remains inconclusive. Some studies suggested a protective effect of adiponectin in OA [8, 10, 11], while others found no association [12, 13] or even a positive association between serum adiponectin and disease severity in knee OA [14]. Studies regarding correlations between resistin and OA are sparse and have been controversial [15, 16].

The relationship between OA and bone mineral density (BMD) has been reported in various cross-sectional and longitudinal studies, but remains controversial. Previous studies revealed that higher BMD was associated with an increased risk of incident OA defined by osteophyte or Kellgren-Lawrence (KL) grade, suggesting that increased BMD was a risk factor for OA [17–19], but a recent study using MRI reported a positive association between systemic and subchondral BMD and cartilage thickness in patients with radiographic OA, indicating that BMD may play a protective role in OA [20].

Given that both adipokines and BMD might be involved in the etiology of OA, they would have a close relationship; however, associations between adipokines and BMD in OA are rarely reported though numerous studies reported the associations between adipokines and BMD in healthy human which remains controversial. One study was conducted in 60 postmenopausal women with hip or knee OA and reported no correlation between leptin and BMD [21]. Another study found that whole body BMD was positively correlated with the serum leptin level in 50 postmenopausal women with knee OA, but the correlation disappeared after adjustment for covariates [22]. To the best of our knowledge, there were no studies reporting the associations between adiponectin, resistin and BMD in OA patients so far. The aim of this study, therefore, was to investigate the

cross-sectional associations between serum adipokines levels and BMD in patients with knee OA.

Methods

Subjects

This study was part of the Anhui Osteoarthritis (AHOA) Study, a clinical study of 205 patients aged 34-74 years, aimed to identify the environmental and biochemical factors associated with the progression of knee OA. Patients with clinical knee OA, diagnosed using American College of Rheumatology criteria [23], were consecutively recruited from the Department of Rheumatology and Immunology in the First Affiliated Hospital of Anhui Medical University, from January 2012 to November 2013. We excluded institutionalized patients, patients with rheumatoid arthritis or other inflammatory diseases, patients with severe OA planning to have knee arthroplasty in 2 years, patients who did not have blood samples so the adipokines were not able to be measured, and patients who didn't have BMD measured due to personal reasons. Forty-one patients fulfilled the exclusion criteria and therefore were excluded from this study, leaving 164 patients. The study was approved by the First Affiliated Hospital Anhui Medical University ethics committee (the ethics approval number: H1000589), and written informed consent was obtained from all participants according to the Declaration of Helsinki.

Anthropometrics

Weight was measured to the nearest 0.1 kg (with shoes, socks and bulky clothing removed) by using a single pair of electronic scales that were calibrated using a known weight at the beginning. Height was measured to the

Table 1 Characteristics of participants (split by median level of leptin)

	Total (n = 164)	Leptin ≤ median (n = 82)	Leptin > median (n = 82)	p value
Age, yrs[a]	55.42(8.57)	54.57(8.94)	56.27(8.14)	0.206
Females, %[b]	88.4	81.7	95.1	**0.015**
Height, cm[a]	158.64(6.83)	158.62(7.70)	158.66(5.90)	0.971
Weight, kg[a]	65.07(10.29)	63.00(9.57)	67.08(10.61)	**0.012**
BMI, kg/m^{2a}	25.84(3.75)	24.98(2.83)	26.68(4.32)	**0.004**
BMD, kg/m^2				
Total body[a]	10,55(1.22)	10.64(1.41)	10.46(1.02)	0.361
Spine[a]	10.03(1.34)	10.09(1.66)	9.99(1.08)	0.709
Hip[a]	8.65(1.23)	8.90(1.42)	8.47(1.06)	0.060
Total femur[a]	9.31(1.30)	9.43(1.37)	9.21(1.24)	0.283
Knee ROA, %[b]	71.95	78.05	65.85	0.082
Adiponectin, ug/ml[c]	27.09(6.80,60.88)	11.73(3.56,35.25)	49.70(20.62,74.10)	**< 0.001**
Resistin, ng/ml[c]	2.22(1.40,4.55)	2.06(1.17,4.39)	2.27(1.48,4.63)	0.327

Leptin median level: 5.92 ng/ml
Data in bold denote statistically significant results
BMI body mass index, *BMD* bone mineral density, *BMC* bone mineral content, *ROA* radiographic osteoarthritis
[a]t tests were used for mean (standard deviation), [b]x^2 tests for the proportions, [c]Mann-Whitney U tests for median (interquartile range)

nearest 0.1 cm (with shoes, socks and headgear removed) by using a stadiometer. Body mass index (BMI) was calculated [weight (kg)/height (m)^2].

Serum adipokines measurements

Fasting blood was obtained from all patients in the morning. Serum was separated and aliquotted into plastic storage tubes. Aliquots were stored at − 80 °C till analysis. Serum levels of leptin, adiponectin, and resistin were measured by using enzyme-linked immunosorbent assay (ELISA; eBioscience, USA) kits, according to the manufacturer's instructions. The intra- and inter-assay coefficient of variations for leptin, adiponectin, and resistin were 5.7 and 6.9%, 4.2 and 3.1%, 5.1 and 8.1%, respectively.

BMD measurement

BMD of the total body, spine, hip and total femur, including femoral neck, Wards triangle, greater trochanter, and femoral shaft were measured using dual-energy x-ray absorptiometry (DXA) (Lunar Prodigy DF + 310,504, GE Healthcare, USA). BMD was calculated from the bone area (cm^2) and bone mineral content (g) and expressed in g/cm^2 [24]. The unit of BMD was converted to kg/m^2 to keep the levels of adipokines and BMD at the similar magnitudes.

Knee radiographic assessment

A standing anteroposterior semiflexed view of the diseased knee (the severer one if both were affected) with 15° of fixed knee flexion, was performed in all participants. KL grading system (grades 0-4) was used to assess the radiographic severity of OA [25]. Radiographic OA (ROA) was defined as KL grade of ≥2.

Statistical analysis

Student's t tests, Mann-Whitney U tests or chi-squared tests were used to compare means, median or proportions, respectively. Univariable and multivariable linear

regression analyses were used to examine the associations between adipokines and BMD before and after adjustment for age, sex, BMI and ROA. Scatter plots were also used to depict the associations between adipokines and BMD after adjustment for the above-mentioned covariates. Standard diagnostic checks of model fit and residuals were routinely made, and data points with large residuals and/or high influence were investigated for data errors. A p value < 0.05 (two-tailed) or a 95% confidence interval (CI) not including the null point was regarded as statistically significant. All statistical analyses were performed using SPSS 13.0 for Windows (SPSS, Chicago, IL, USA).

Results

A total of 164 subjects between 34 and 74 years of age (mean, 55.4 yrs) participated in our study. Of these, all subjects measured the BMD of total body and total femur, however, only 133 subjects measured the BMD of spine and hip. There were no significant differences in demographic factors (age, sex, and BMI) between these participants and those excluded ($n = 41$; data not shown). Characteristics of the participants are presented in Table 1. The mean BMI was 25.84 kg/m^2. The median levels of leptin, adiponectin, and resistin were 5.92 ng/ml, 27.09 μg/ml, and 2.22 ng/ml, respectively. Subjects with higher and lower levels of leptin (split at the median level) were similar in age, height, BMD at all sites measured, prevalence of ROA and levels of resistin; however, subjects with higher leptin levels had greater proportion of females, higher weight, higher BMI and higher adiponectin levels.

There were no interactions between serum levels of adipokines and sex on the BMD (data not shown). Therefore, males and females were combined for analyses in our study.

Associations between leptin and BMD were shown in Table 2. In univariable analyses, we did not find any significant associations between serum levels of leptin and BMD at any site measured. However, after

Table 2 Associations between leptin and BMD in various regions

	Univariable		Multivariable[a]	
	β(95% CI)	p value	β(95% CI)	p value
Total body BMD	−0.011(− 0.026,0.004)	0.155	**− 0.019(− 0.034,-0.005)**	**0.009**
Spine BMD	0.004(− 0.013,0.021)	0.653	− 0.010(− 0.028,0.007)	0.248
Hip BMD	− 0.010(− 0.025,0.006)	0.213	**− 0.018(− 0.034,-0.003)**	**0.018**
Total femur BMD	− 0.007(− 0.023,0.008)	0.352	**− 0.018(− 0.034,-0.002)**	**0.024**
Femoral neck	−0.010(− 0.025,0.006)	0.218	**−0.016(− 0.032,0.000)**	**0.048**
Wards triangle	−0.007(− 0.025,0.011)	0.462	−0.012(− 0.029,0.006)	0.194
Greater trochanter	−0.004(− 0.018,0.009)	0.538	−0.013(− 0.026,0.001)	0.074
Femoral shaft	−0.008(− 0.028,0.011)	0.386	**−0.026(− 0.046,-0.006)**	**0.012**

Dependent variable: BMD in respective compartment
Independent variable: leptin
Data in bold denote statistically significant results
BMD bone mineral density, *BMI* body mass index, *ROA* radiographic osteoarthritis
[a]Adjusted for age, sex, BMI and ROA

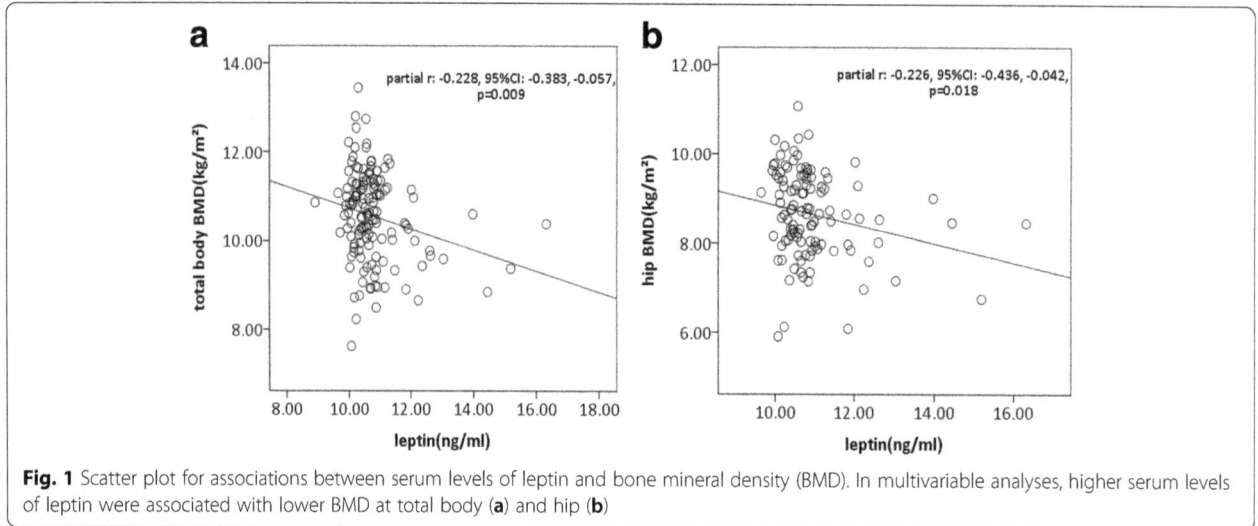

Fig. 1 Scatter plot for associations between serum levels of leptin and bone mineral density (BMD). In multivariable analyses, higher serum levels of leptin were associated with lower BMD at total body (**a**) and hip (**b**)

adjustment for age, sex, BMI and ROA, serum levels of leptin were significantly associated with reduced BMD at total body, hip, femoral neck, femoral shaft, and total femur (Table 2, Fig. 1).

Serum adiponectin was significantly and negatively associated with BMD at femoral shaft and total femur in univariable analyses. These negative associations remained unchanged after adjustment for the covariates mentioned above (Table 3, Fig. 2). We did not find any significant associations between serum adiponectin and BMD at total body, spine, and hip. The association between adiponectin and femoral neck BMD was also negative but of borderline statistical significance (Table 3).

The associations between serum resistin and BMD at any site did not reach statistical significance before and after adjustment for age, sex, BMI and ROA (Table 4).

Discussion

The present study investigated the cross-sectional associations between adipokines (including leptin, adiponectin, and resistin) and BMD in patients with knee OA. We found that the serum leptin levels were negatively associated with total body, hip and total femur (including femoral neck and femoral shaft) BMD. Serum adiponectin was also significantly associated with reduced BMD at total femur and femoral shaft. In contrast, no association was found between serum resistin and BMD.

Leptin, a protein encoded by the ob gene, was found to regulate bone metabolism. Various studies have demonstrated the association between leptin and BMD. Ducy et al. [26] found that intracerebroventricular infusion of leptin induced bone loss in both leptin-deficient and wild-type mice, suggesting that leptin could inhibit bone formation acting through the hypothalamus.

Table 3 Associations between adiponectin and BMD in various regions

	Univariable		Multivariable[a]	
	β(95% CI)	p value	β(95% CI)	p value
Total body BMD	−0.005(− 0.010,0.000)	0.072	−0.002(− 0.007,0.003)	0.432
Spine BMD	−0.006(− 0.013,0.002)	0.123	−0.002(− 0.010,0.005)	0.518
Hip BMD	−0.006(− 0.012,0.001)	0.100	−0.002(− 0.009,0.004)	0.456
Total femur BMD	**−0.006(− 0.012,0.000)**	**0.034**	**−0.007(− 0.013,0.000)**	**0.030**
Femoral neck	−0.006(− 0.011,0.000)	0.061	−0.005(− 0.011,0.001)	0.088
Wards triangle	−0.005(− 0.012,0.002)	0.137	−0.004(− 0.010,0.003)	0.234
Greater trochanter	−0.004(− 0.009,0.001)	0.116	−0.002(− 0.007,0.003)	0.436
Femoral shaft	**−0.008(− 0.015,-0.001)**	**0.025**	**−0.011(− 0.018,-0.003)**	**0.006**

Dependent variable: BMD in respective compartment
Independent variable: adiponectin
Data in bold denote statistically significant results
BMD bone mineral density, BMI body mass index, ROA radiographic osteoarthritis
[a]Adjusted for age, sex, BMI and ROA

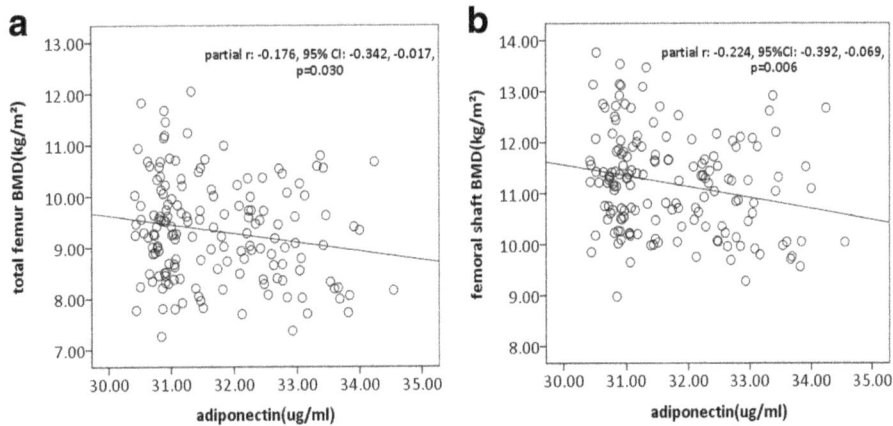

Fig. 2 Scatter plot for associations between serum levels of adiponectin and bone mineral density (BMD). In multivariable analyses, higher serum levels of adiponectin were associated with lower BMD at total femur (**a**) and femoral shaft (**b**)

Epidemiological studies reported that serum leptin concentrations were inversely associated with calcaneal BMD after adjustment for body weight in 221 healthy adult men [27], and leptin had a negative correlation with lumbar spine BMD in perimenopausal healthy women [28]. On the contrary, some studies reported a positive association between leptin and BMD. Martin et al. [29] demonstrated that peripheral administration of leptin could prevent disuse-induced bone loss through inhibiting the increase in bone resorption mediated by the RANKL/OPG and preventing the decrease in bone formation in tail-suspended female rats. Blain et al. [30] found that leptin was positively associated with whole body and femoral neck BMD in 155 postmenopausal women. Weiss et al. [31] reported that leptin predicted an increase in BMD in postmenopausal women but not older men after adjustment for age, BMI, and other bone related factors. In addition, several clinical studies reported no association between leptin and BMD or BMD

change [32, 33]. It was noteworthy that these studies mentioned above were conducted in healthy persons. Only two clinical studies investigated the association between leptin and BMD in OA [21, 22] and reported inconsistent results. Our study found that serum leptin was significantly associated with reduced BMD in patients with knee OA, independent of age, sex, BMI, and ROA. This suggests that leptin may play a potentially detrimental effect on BMD in knee OA.

Adiponectin was considered to have a negative effect on bone metabolism. Adiponectin levels were negatively associated with femoral neck and total body BMD in postmenopausal women after adjustment for potential confounders [32], and highest tertile of adiponectin had significantly greater hip BMD loss than the lowest tertile of adiponectin in women [33]. A meta-analysis indicated that adiponectin was the mostly relevant adipokine that was negatively associated with BMD in healthy subjects, regardless of menopausal status and gender [34].

Table 4 Associations between resistin and BMD in various regions

	Univariable		Multivariable[a]	
	β(95% CI)	p value	β(95% CI)	p value
Total body BMD	0.005(−0.042,0.053)	0.825	0.005(−0.037,0.048)	0.801
Spine BMD	−0.022(−0.117,0.072)	0.639	−0.024(−0.120,0.071)	0.612
Hip BMD	−0.005(−0.093,0.083)	0.913	0.012(−0.072,0.096)	0.777
Total femur BMD	−0.010(−0.061,0.042)	0.712	−0.007(−0.056,0.043)	0.792
Femoral neck	−0.023(−0.075,0.029)	0.376	−0.023(−0.073,0.027)	0.358
Wards triangle	−0.030(−0.090,0.030)	0.327	−0.031(−0.086,0.023)	0.257
Greater trochanter	−0.014(−0.059,0.031)	0.528	−0.012(−0.054,0.030)	0.568
Femoral shaft	0.002(−0.062,0.066)	0.951	0.003(−0.061,0.067)	0.918

Dependent variable: BMD in respective compartment
Independent variable: resistin
BMD bone mineral density, *BMI* body mass index, *ROA* radiographic osteoarthritis
[a]Adjusted for age, sex, BMI and ROA

Oshima et al. [35] reported that adiponectin supplement increased bone mass in trabecular bone via inhibiting osteoclast and activating osteoblast. In contrast, Kontogianni et al. [28] found no associations between adiponectin and lumber spine BMD in perimenopausal women, and Barbour et al. [33] found adiponectin levels were not correlated with whole-body areal BMD or trabecular lumbar spine volumetric BMD loss in older women and men. Our current study is the first to investigate the association between adiponectin and BMD in patients with knee OA, indicating a potentially detrimental effect of adiponectin on BMD in knee OA.

Serum leptin levels are positively correlated with BMI, while serum adiponectin levels are negatively correlated with BMI [36]. However, we found that both serum levels of leptin and adiponectin were negatively associated with BMD in OA. The potential mechanism is unclear, and it needs to be further investigated.

So far, there are a few studies reporting the association between resistin and BMD. Serum resistin was not associated with BMD of total body, lumbar spine, and total hip before and after adjustment for age and fat mass in 232 Chinese men [37], and was not an independent predictor of BMD in 336 healthy postmenopausal Chinese women aged 41-81 years [38]. One study reported that serum resistin levels were significantly and negatively associated with lumbar spine BMD in 80 middle-aged men [39]. In our current study, we didn't find any significant association between serum resistin and BMD in patients with knee OA.

There are several limitations in our study. First, due to the cross-sectional nature, the causality between adipokines and BMD is not able to be determined. Further longitudinal studies are needed to verify our findings. Second, the sample size was modest. This may be the reason why we did not find significant association between resistin and BMD. Third, 41 patients were excluded from this study which may cause selection bias; however, there were no significant differences in age, sex, and BMI between patients who were included and excluded. Last, there would be variations in muscle and fat mass which may affect the associations; however, the results remained largely unchanged after the adjustment for muscle or fat mass.

Conclusions
Serum leptin and adiponectin levels were significantly and negatively associated with BMD, suggesting potentially detrimental effects of leptin and adiponectin on BMD in knee OA patients.

Abbreviations
BMD: Bone mineral density; BMI: Body mass index; CI: Confidence interval; DXA: Dual-energy X-ray absorptiometry; ELISA: Enzyme-linked immunosorbent assay; KL: Kellgren-Lawrence; OA: Osteoarthritis; ROA: Radiographic OA

Acknowledgments
We would like to thank the participants who made this study possible, and thank the staff and volunteers who collected the data.

Funding
This study was supported by the National Natural Science Foundation of China (81172865).

Authors' contributions
Study conception and design: CD and JX. Acquisition of data: JW, KW, QZ, JC, JR and SZ. Analysis and interpretation of data: JW and CD. Drafting of the article: JW and CD. Revising and final approval of the article: All authors.

Consent for publication
Not applicable.

Competing interests
The authors declare that they have no competing interests. Changhai Ding is a Deputy Section Editor of BMC Musculoskeletal Disorders.

Author details
[1]Department of Rheumatology and Immunology, Arthritis Research Institute, the First Affiliated Hospital of Anhui Medical University, 218 Jixi Street, Hefei, China. [2]Menzies Institute for Medical Research, University of Tasmania, Private Bag 23, Hobart, TAS 7000, Australia. [3]Institute of Bone & Joint Translational Research, Southern Medical University, Guangzhou, Guangdong, China.

References
1. Woolf AD, Pfleger B. Burden of major musculoskeletal conditions. Bull World Health Organ. 2003;81:646–56.
2. Sowers MR, Karvonen-Gutierrez CA. The evolving role of obesity in knee osteoarthritis. Curr Opin Rheumatol. 2010;22:533–7.
3. Wang X, Hunter D, Xu J, Ding C. Metabolic triggered inflammation in osteoarthritis. Osteoarthr Cartil. 2015;23:22–30.
4. Presle N, Pottie P, Dumond H, Guillaume C, Lapicque F, Pallu S, et al. Differential distribution of adipokines between serum and synovial fluid in patients with osteoarthritis. Contribution of joint tissues to their articular production. Osteoarthr Cartil. 2006;14:690–5.
5. Francin PJ, Abot A, Guillaume C, Moulin D, Bianchi A, Gegout-Pottie P, et al. Association between adiponectin and cartilage degradation in human osteoarthritis. Osteoarthr Cartil. 2014;22:519–26.
6. Stannus OP, Jones G, Quinn SJ, Cicuttini FM, Dore D, Ding C. The association between leptin, interleukin-6, and hip radiographic osteoarthritis in older people: a cross-sectional study. Arthritis Res Ther. 2010;12:R95.
7. Staikos C, Ververidis A, Drosos G, Manolopoulos VG, Verettas DA, Tavridou A. The association of adipokine levels in plasma and synovial fluid with the severity of knee osteoarthritis. Rheumatology (Oxford). 2013;52:1077–83.
8. Zheng S, Xu J, Xu S, Zhang M, Huang S, He F, et al. Association between circulating adipokines, radiographic changes, and knee cartilage volume in patients with knee osteoarthritis. Scand J Rheumatol. 2016;45:224–9.
9. de Boer TN, van Spil WE, Huisman AM, Polak AA, Bijlsma JW, Lafeber FP, et al. Serum adipokines in osteoarthritis; comparison with controls and relationship with local parameters of synovial inflammation and cartilage damage. Osteoarthr Cartil. 2012;20:846–53.
10. Honsawek S, Chayanupatkul M. Correlation of plasma and synovial fluid adiponectin with knee osteoarthritis severity. Arch Med Res. 2010;41:593–8.
11. Yusuf E, Ioan-Facsinay A, Bijsterbosch J, Klein-Wieringa I, Kwekkeboom J, Slagboom PE, et al. Association between leptin, adiponectin and resistin and long-term progression of hand osteoarthritis. Ann Rheum Dis. 2011; 70:1282–4.
12. Berry PA, Jones SW, Cicuttini FM, Wluka AE, Maciewicz RA. Temporal relationship between serum adipokines, biomarkers of bone and cartilage turnover, and cartilage volume loss in a population with clinical knee osteoarthritis. Arthritis Rheum. 2011;63:700–7.
13. Massengale M, Lu B, Pan JJ, Katz JN, Solomon DH. Adipokine hormones and hand osteoarthritis: radiographic severity and pain. PLoS One. 2012; 7:e47860.

14. Cuzdan Coskun N, Ay S, Evcik FD, Oztuna D. Adiponectin: is it a biomarker for assessing the disease severity in knee osteoarthritis patients? Int J Rheum Dis. 2015;6 [Epub ahead of print]

15. Koskinen A, Vuolteenaho K, Moilanen T, Moilanen E. Resistin as a factor in osteoarthritis: synovial fluid resistin concentrations correlate positively with interleukin 6 and matrix metalloproteinases MMP-1 and MMP-3. Scand J Rheumatol. 2014;43:249-53.

16. Martel-Pelletier J, Raynauld JP, Dorais M, Abram F, Pelletier JP. The levels of the adipokines adipsin and leptin are associated with knee osteoarthritis progression as assessed by MRI and incidence of total knee replacement in symptomatic osteoarthritis patients: a post hoc analysis. Rheumatology (Oxford). 2016;55:680-8.

17. Zhang Y, Hannan MT, Chaisson CE, McAlindon TE, Evans SR, Aliabadi P, et al. Bone mineral density and risk of incident and progressive radiographic knee osteoarthritis in women: the Framingham study. J Rheumatol. 2000;27:1032-7.

18. Hochberg MC, Lethbridge-Cejku M, Tobin JD. Bone mineral density and osteoarthritis: data from the Baltimore longitudinal study of aging. Osteoarthr Cartil. 2004;12(Suppl A):S45-8.

19. Hart DJ, Cronin C, Daniels M, Worthy T, Doyle DV, Spector TD. The relationship of bone density and fracture to incident and progressive radiographic osteoarthritis of the knee: the Chingford study. Arthritis Rheum. 2002;46:92-9.

20. Cao Y, Stannus OP, Aitken D, Cicuttini F, Antony B, Jones G, et al. Cross-sectional and longitudinal associations between systemic, subchondral bone mineral density and knee cartilage thickness in older adults with or without radiographic osteoarthritis. Ann Rheum Dis. 2014;73:2003-9.

21. Jiang LS, Zhang ZM, Jiang SD, Chen WH, Dai LY. Differential bone metabolism between postmenopausal women with osteoarthritis and osteoporosis. J Bone Miner Res. 2008;23:475-83.

22. Iwamoto J, Takeda T, Sato Y, Matsumoto H. Serum leptin concentration positively correlates with body weight and total fat mass in postmenopausal Japanese women with osteoarthritis of the knee. Arthritis. 2011;2011:580632.

23. Altman RD. The classification of osteoarthritis. J Rheumatol Suppl 1995;43:42-3.

24. Xu S, Ma XX, Hu LW, Peng LP, Pan FM, Xu JH. Single nucleotide polymorphism of RANKL and OPG genes may play a role in bone and joint injury in rheumatoid arthritis. Clin Exp Rheumatol. 2014;32:697-704.

25. Kellgren JH, Lawrence JS. Radiological assessment of osteoarthrosis. Ann Rheum Dis. 1957;16:494-502.

26. Ducy P, Amling M, Takeda S, Priemel M, Schilling AF, Beil FT, et al. Leptin inhibits bone formation through a hypothalamic relay: a central control of bone mass. Cell. 2000;100:197-207.

27. Sato M, Takeda N, Sarui H, Takami R, Takami K, Hayashi M, et al. Association between serum leptin concentrations and bone mineral density, and biochemical markers of bone turnover in adult men. J Clin Endocrinol Metab. 2001;86:5273-6.

28. Kontogianni MD, Dafni UG, Routsias JG, Skopouli FN. Blood leptin and adiponectin as possible mediators of the relation between fat mass and BMD in perimenopausal women. J Bone Miner Res. 2004;19:546-51.

29. Martin A, de Vittoris R, David V, Moraes R, Bégeot M, Lafage-Proust MH, et al. Leptin modulates both resorption and formation while preventing disuse-induced bone loss in tail-suspended female rats. Endocrinology. 2005;146:3652-9.

30. Blain H, Vuillemin A, Guillemin F, Durant R, Hanesse B, de Talance N, et al. Serum leptin level is a predictor of bone mineral density in postmenopausal women. J Clin Endocrinol Meta. 2002;87:1030-5.

31. Weiss LA, Barrett-Connor E, von Mühlen D, Clark P. Leptin predicts BMD and bone resorption in older women but not older men: the rancho Bernardo study. J Bone Miner Res. 2006;21:758-64.

32. Värri M, Niskanen L, Tuomainen T, Honkanen R, Kröger H, Tuppurainen MT. Association of adipokines and estradiol with bone and carotid calcifications in postmenopausal women. Climacteric. 2016;19:204-11.

33. Barbour KE, Zmuda JM, Boudreau R, Strotmeyer ES, Horwitz MJ, Evans RW, et al. The effects of adiponectin and leptin on changes in bone mineral density. Osteoporos Int. 2012;23:1699-710.

34. Biver E, Salliot C, Combescure C, Gossec L, Hardouin P, Legroux-Gerot I, et al. Influence of adipokines and ghrelin on bone mineral density and fracture risk: a systematic review and meta-analysis. J Clin Endocrinol Metab. 2011;96:2703-13.

35. Oshima K, Nampei A, Matsuda M, Iwaki M, Fukuhara A, Hashimoto J, et al. Adiponectin increases bone mass by suppressing osteoclast and activating osteoblast. Biochem Biophys Res Commun. 2005;331:520-6.

36. Poonpet T, Honsawek S. Adipokines: biomarkers for osteoarthritis? World J Orthop. 2014;5:319-27.

37. Peng XD, Xie H, Zhao Q, Wu XP, Sun ZQ, Liao EY. Relationships between serum adiponectin, leptin, resistin, visfatin levels and bone mineral density, and bone biochemical markers in Chinese men. Clin Chim Acta. 2008;387:31-5.

38. Zhang H, Xie H, Zhao Q, Xie GQ, Wu XP, Liao EY, et al. Relationships between serum adiponectin, apelin, leptin, resistin, visfatin levels and bone mineral density, and bone biochemical markers in post-menopausal Chinese women. J Endocrinol Investig. 2010;33:707-11.

39. Oh KW, Lee WY, Rhee EJ, Baek KH, Yoon KH, Kang MI, et al. The relationship between serum resistin, leptin, adiponectin, ghrelin levels and bone mineral density in middle-aged men. Clin Endocrinol. 2005;63:131-8.

5

Uptake of the NICE osteoarthritis guidelines in primary care: a survey of older adults with joint pain

Emma Louise Healey[1]* (iD), Ebenezer K. Afolabi[1], Martyn Lewis[1,2], John J. Edwards[1], Kelvin P. Jordan[1,2], Andrew Finney[1,3], Clare Jinks[1], Elaine M. Hay[1] and Krysia S. Dziedzic[1]

Abstract

Background: Osteoarthritis (OA) is a leading cause of pain and disability. NICE OA guidelines (2008) recommend that patients with OA should be offered core treatments in primary care. Assessments of OA management have identified a need to improve primary care of people with OA, as recorded use of interventions concordant with the NICE guidelines is suboptimal in primary care. The aim of this study was to i) describe the patient-reported uptake of non-pharmacological and pharmacological treatments recommended in the NICE OA guidelines in older adults with a self-reported consultation for joint pain and ii) determine whether patient characteristics or OA diagnosis impact uptake.

Methods: A cross-sectional survey mailed to adults aged ≥45 years ($n = 28,443$) from eight general practices in the UK as part of the MOSAICS study. Respondents who reported the presence of joint pain, a consultation in the previous 12 months for joint pain, and gave consent to medical record review formed the sample for this study.

Results: Four thousand fifty-nine respondents were included in the analysis (mean age 65.6 years (SD 11.2), 2300 (56.7%) females). 502 (12.4%) received an OA diagnosis in the previous 12 months. More participants reported using pharmacological treatments (e.g. paracetamol (31.3%), opioids (40.4%)) than non-pharmacological treatments (e.g. exercise (3.8%)). Those with an OA diagnosis were more likely to use written information (OR 1.57; 95% CI 1.26,1.96), paracetamol (OR 1.30; 95% CI 1.05,1.62) and topical NSAIDs (OR 1.30; 95% CI 1.04,1.62) than those with a joint pain code. People aged ≥75 years were less likely to use written information (OR 0.56; 95% CI 0.40,0.79) and exercise (OR 0.37; 95% CI 0.25,0.55) and more likely to use paracetamol (OR 1.91; 95% CI 1.38,2.65) than those aged < 75 years.

Conclusion: The cross-sectional population survey was conducted to examine the uptake of the treatments that are recommended in the NICE OA guidelines in older adults with a self-reported consultation for joint pain and to determine whether patient characteristics or OA diagnosis impact uptake. Non-pharmacological treatment was suboptimal compared to pharmacological treatment. Implementation of NICE guidelines needs to examine why non-pharmacological treatments, such as exercise, remain under-used especially among older people.

Keywords: Osteoarthritis, Joint pain, General practice, NICE guidelines

* Correspondence: e.healey@keele.ac.uk
[1]Research Institute for Primary Care and Health Sciences, Keele University, Keele, Staffordshire ST5 5BG, UK
Full list of author information is available at the end of the article

Background

Osteoarthritis (OA) is a leading cause of pain and morbidity and, globally, is the fastest increasing cause of disability [1]. Evidence is accumulating about how primary care could reduce OA pain and disability: international guidelines address best evidence for components of this care but their impact on practice and behaviour is not clearly understood. In order to investigate this, we assessed uptake of one national (United Kingdom (UK)) OA management guideline by the general population.

The UK National Institute for Health and Care Excellence (NICE) produced OA management recommendations in 2008 [2], focused on the peripheral joint sites of the hip, knee, hand and foot. The NICE working definition of OA (here, "clinical OA") is based upon symptoms of activity-related joint pain rather than radiographic signs. The majority of self-reported joint pain in older adults has been determined to be due to clinical OA, with alternative clear diagnoses being relatively uncommon [3].

One-in-ten older people will consult primary care every year for clinical OA (diagnosed OA or recorded peripheral joint pain) [4]. NICE OA guidelines suggest that all core treatments (education, exercise, and weight loss) should be offered to everyone, irrespective of age, pain severity and co-morbidity [2]. Assessments of OA management have identified a need to improve primary care of people with OA, as recorded use of interventions concordant with the NICE guidelines is suboptimal [5]. The challenge for primary care is how best to manage OA for the majority of people [6, 7].

The aims of this study were, without prior hypothesis, i) to describe the patient-reported uptake of non-pharmacological and pharmacological treatments recommended in the NICE OA guidelines in a community-dwelling older adult population with a self-reported primary care consultation for joint pain, and, ii) to determine whether patient characteristics (age, sex, self-reported health, number of sites of disease, and overall morbidity burden) or a recorded formal diagnosis of OA were associated with uptake of these treatments.

Methods
Study design and population

This paper is one component of the 'Management of OSteoArthritis In ConsultationS' (MOSAICS) study [8, 9]. The data were derived from a cross-sectional population survey. A linked medical record review was conducted in order to estimate morbidity burden and identify the presence of any formal OA diagnosis. The findings are reported in line with the STROBE guidelines [10].

A 12 month period for diagnosis and consultation was selected to maximise accurate recall, to reflect those who had recently sought health care, and to include experience since the NICE guidelines had been published.

Data collection
The population survey

The population survey was mailed between May 2011 and April 2012 to all adults aged ≥45 years ($n = 28,443$) registered with eight general practices in the West Midlands and North West of England that varied in the size of the registered population, clinical staffing, urbanization and deprivation.

The survey used a two-stage mailing process. Prior to the mailing, General Practitioners (GPs) screened the list of potential participants and excluded people considered not eligible (e.g. those with psychiatric illness, recent bereavement). A letter of invitation to participate, study information, and the survey were sent to all eligible people. Individuals were invited to complete the survey and return it in a pre-paid envelope, indicating whether they consented to further contact and medical record review. A reminder letter and additional copy of the survey were sent to non-responders after 3 weeks. A telephone contact number provided recipients the opportunity to place questions and opt-out if they wished.

Survey responders provided socio-demographic and general health information and were asked to indicate whether they had experienced joint pain (hip, knee, hand and foot) in the previous 12 months. Those confirming the presence of joint pain were asked to report their consultation behaviours and treatment(s) used for their joint pain over the previous 12 months. Everyone who both reported a consultation for joint pain and consented to medical record review formed the study population for this analysis.

Survey responders were asked their gender, date-of-birth (for calculation of current age), height and weight, whether they lived alone, and work status (employed, unemployed, retired). General health was assessed using the SF-12 [11], a validated, generic measure with two summary scales: the physical component summary (PCS) and the mental component summary (MCS), standardised to scores from the general population of the United States (mean = 50, where lower scores indicate worse health).

Presence of joint pain over the previous 12 months was based on single questions for each of the peripheral joint sites of interest (hip, knee, hand and foot). For example, participants were asked, "Have you had any pain in the last year in or around the hip? (Yes/No)" (modified from Jinks et al., 2004) [12]. Those reporting pain in two or more of the four sites were classed as having multi-site joint pain.

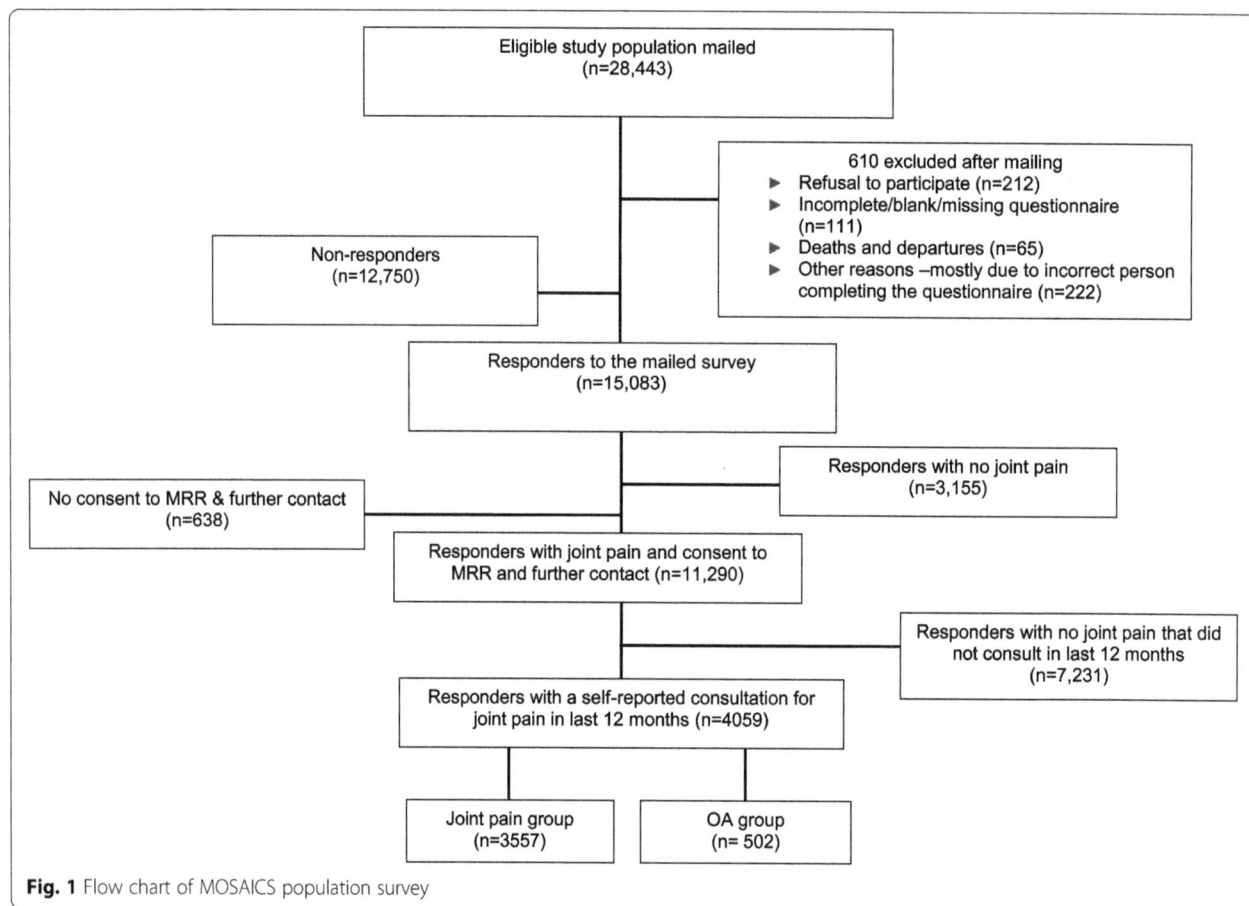

Fig. 1 Flow chart of MOSAICS population survey

Participants were asked if they had consulted their GP or practice nurse (PN) regarding joint pain over the previous 12 months. Self-reported information regarding the management of their joint pain over the previous 12 months was also collected. Participants were asked "In the past 12 months have you tried any of these for your joints?" Patients were asked to tick boxes to indicate which treatments had been used (modified from Jinks et al., 2004) [12]. Following this question was a list of options which linked to the NICE guidance e.g. joint operation, use of treatments such as core non-pharmacological treatments, and first- and second-line pharmacological treatments (see Table 2).

Medical record review

A retrospective medical record review in the study population was conducted to identify all Read codes recorded in consultations in the previous 12 months. Read codes are the most common way of recording morbidity in UK primary care. Anyone with a Read code from the N05 "Osteoarthritis and allied disorders" branch recorded in that period was classed as having a formal OA diagnosis.

To determine the morbidity burden, polypharmacy was employed as a simple proxy measure [13]. The count of unique drug types from the British National Formulary (BNF) prescribed in the previous 12 months was obtained from the medical record. Patients were dichotomised into two groups: < 10 and ≥ 10 drug types, based on previous work [14].

Statistical analysis

The study population was described in terms of socio-demographic factors, health status, recorded formal OA diagnosis in the last 12 months, morbidity burden, and number of self-reported joint pain sites (dichotomised into single or multiple). Uptake of recommended treatments was described in the study population, stratified by responder age-group.

Descriptive statistics were used, with mean and standard deviation (SD), frequency counts and percentages (as appropriate) presented. Age was grouped by decades and skewed data such as the SF12-PCS and SF12-MCS were categorised based on quartile scores to determine any association between health status and uptake of recommended treatments. A chi-squared test-for-trend was employed to estimate relationships between uptake of recommended treatments and age group.

Multivariable logistic regression analyses were carried out to estimate associations between participants' socio-demographic and health factors and the uptake of non-pharmacological and pharmacological treatments. The multivariate model was fully inclusive of all variables listed in Table 3. Results are shown as fully-adjusted odds ratios (AOR) with 95% confidence intervals (CI).

Data analysis was performed using IBM SPSS Statistics version 21 (Armonk, NY, USA) and STATA version 13 (StataCorp, 2013).

Results

Of the 28,443 people mailed the survey, 15,083 (53%) responded. Non-responders were more likely to be male (difference in response, 10.4%) and younger (mean difference 5.1 years). There were 11,290 participants with relevant self-reported joint pain who consented to medical record review (75%). 4059 (36%) reported consulting primary care for their joint pain in the previous 12 months and these formed the study population for this paper (Fig. 1). 502 (12.4%) were found to have a formal OA diagnosis in their medical record in the previous 12 months. Table 1 shows the characteristics of participants included in the study population.

Table 2 describes the uptake of all of the NICE-recommended treatments in the previous 12 months. Overall the uptake of the core non-pharmacological treatments was considerably lower than the first-line pharmacological treatments. For example, only 9.4 and 3.8% of patients used weight loss or aerobic fitness training respectively, whereas 31.3 and 26.0% of patients used paracetamol or topical non-steroidal anti-inflammatory drugs (NSAIDs) respectively.

The multivariable analysis demonstrated that various patient characteristics were associated with uptake of recommended treatments (see Table 3): women, compared to men, were more likely to report use of written information (AOR 1.28, 95% CI 1.09,1.50) and weight loss (AOR 1.54, 95% CI 1.16,2.04). Older individuals (≥75 compared to age 45–54) were less likely to report use of written information (AOR 0.56, 95% CI 0.40,0.79) and exercise (AOR 0.37, 95% CI 0.25,0.55), but more likely to report use of paracetamol (AOR 1.91, 95% CI 1.38,2.65). Multi-site joint pain was associated with greater provision of information only. Those with a greater morbidity burden (≥10 BNF count of unique drug types compared to < 10) were more likely to use exercise (AOR 1.44, 95% CI 1.16,1.77) and weight management (AOR 1.87, 95% CI 1.37,2.57) and both first-line pharmacological treatments. Worse scores on

Table 1 Characteristics of the eligible population

Characteristic	Participants (n = 4059)
Gender	
Female	2300 (56.7)
Male	1759 (43.3)
Age (years)	
45–54	770 (19.0)
55–64	1136 (28.0)
65–74	1225 (30.2)
75 and above	928 (22.8)
[a]Employment status	
Employed	1105 (27.9)
Unemployed	596 (15.1)
Retired	2253 (57.0)
[a]BMI (kg/m^2)	
Not overweight (< 25.0)	1161 (29.6)
Overweight (25.0–29.9)	1583 (40.3)
Obese (≥30.0)	1184 (30.1)
No. of pain sites	
Single site	777 (19.1)
Multi-site	3282 (80.9)
Morbidity burden (BNF drug count)	
< 10 count	2222 (54.7)
≥ 10 count	1837 (45.3)
SF12 - Physical health, mean (SD)	43.6 (12.4)
SF12 - Mental health, mean (SD)	49.5 (10.5)
OA diagnosis	
Yes	502 (12.4)
No	3557 (87.6)

[a]Distribution based on valid response (missing data: 105, 2.6% (employment status); 131, 3.2% (BMI); 107, 2.6% (SF-12))

the SF-12 PCS (below lower quartile score compared to above upper quartile score) were associated with greater use of information (AOR 2.13, 95% CI 1.63,2.77), exercise (AOR 1.64, 95% CI 1.20,2.24), and both first-line pharmacological treatments. A similar comparison for the SF-12 MCS suggested greater use of information, weight loss and both pharmacological treatments in people with worse scores. Those with a recorded diagnosis of OA were more likely to report use of information and both first-line pharmacological treatments.

Discussion
Summary

This study examined one example of a national guideline of best primary care for OA and found evidence that those with OA report a lack of guideline-based advice and treatment; a finding that was particularly predominant in the oldest ages. This is similar to treatment

Table 2 Uptake of the NICE recommended treatments in the past 12 months, overall and stratified by age groups

	Total (n = 4059)		45-54y n (%)	55-64y n (%)	65-74y n (%)	≥75y n (%)
	n	% (95% CI)				
Core treatments						
***Written information[a]	934	23.0 (21.7,24.3)	190 (24.7)	298 (26.2)	267 (21.8)	179 (19.3)
**Muscle strengthening exercises	532	13.1 (12.1,14.1)	113 (14.7)	172 (15.1)	150 (12.2)	97 (10.5)
*Aerobic fitness exercise	154	3.8 (3.2,4.4)	36 (4.7)	44 (3.9)	55 (4.5)	19 (2.0)
Dieting to lose weight[b]	261	9.4 (8.3,10.5)	37 (7.1)	90 (10.9)	99 (11.4)	35 (6.4)
1st and 2nd line pharmacological treatment						
***Paracetamol	1270	31.3 (29.9,32.7)	149 (19.4)	283 (24.9)	395 (32.2)	443 (47.7)
***Anti-inflammatory creams/gels e.g. topical NSAIDs	1055	26.0 (24.7,27.4)	150 (19.5)	243 (21.4)	341 (27.8)	321 (34.6)
*Capsaicin cream	66	1.6 (1.2,2.0)	4 (0.5)	22 (1.9)	21 (1.7)	19 (2.0)
***Anti-inflammatory tablets e.g. oral NSAIDs	1276	31.4 (30.0,32.8)	306 (39.7)	406 (35.7)	366 (29.9)	198 (21.3)
***Stronger painkillers e.g. opioids, compound analgesics	1641	40.4 (38.9,41.9)	263 (34.2)	416 (36.6)	535 (43.7)	427 (46.0)
Intra-articular corticosteroid injection	463	11.4 (10.4,12.4)	81 (10.5)	146 (12.9)	131 (10.7)	105 (11.3)
Adjunctive treatment						
Warmth, heat or cold application	334	8.2 (7.4,9.0)	57 (7.4)	105 (9.2)	95 (7.8)	77 (8.3)
***Walking aids	676	16.7 (15.6,17.8)	64 (8.3)	122 (10.7)	179 (14.6)	311 (33.5)
***Assistive devices	301	7.4 (6.6,8.2)	24 (3.1)	44 (3.9)	75 (6.1)	158 (17.0)
Transcutaneous electric nerve stimulation (TENS)	127	3.1 (2.6,3.6)	22 (2.9)	41 (3.6)	37 (3.0)	27 (2.9)
Shock-absorbing shoes or insoles	247	6.1 (5.4,6.8)	41 (5.3)	63 (5.5)	81 (6.6)	62 (6.7)
Appliances and support and braces	265	6.5 (5.7,7.3)	52 (6.8)	80 (7.0)	59 (4.8)	74 (8.0)
Service use						
Joint arthroplasty/operation	365	9.0 (8.1,9.9)	73 (9.5)	105 (9.2)	102 (8.3)	85 (9.2)
***Manual therapy	998	24.6 (23.3,25.9)	219 (28.4)	311 (27.4)	282 (23.0)	186 (20.0)

[a]Written information is a composite variable derived from the addition of responses of participants who used information about treatments, information about self-management and information about OA when they consulted with joint pain
[b]Restricted to obese/overweight participants (n = 2767)
Treatment association with age is indicated by: *p < 0.05, **p < 0.01, ***p < 0.001 (by chi square test for trend)

patterns for knee pain demonstrated prior to 2008 [15]. Semi-structured interviews with older adults with knee pain in a 2008 study had identified an early reliance on pharmacological treatments and underuse of non-pharmacological interventions in early treatment choices [15]. Exercise of any type for OA has also previously been found to be under-used in primary care [16].

Strengths and limitations

A strength of this survey is the large sample size achieved ensuring greater precision in estimates and sufficient power to test statistical associations. Use of self-reported information has some advantages to medical record use as non-pharmacological interventions and over-the-counter drug use are poorly-recorded in medical records. The heterogeneity of practice characteristics across the sample increases the generalisability of the findings to the UK population as a whole. Due to the nature of the data collection, one potential limitation of this study is recall bias. A recall period of up to 12 months may have affected participants' ability to accurately self-report information about

their consultation behaviours and treatments used. As the study focused on treatments over the previous 12 months, it was also impossible to determine whether other treatments had been tried prior to moving onto further treatments (e.g. a trial of non-pharmacological treatments prior to first-line pharmacological options). It is not known whether people reporting use of treatments were responding to clinical recommendations or acting independently; for those not using treatments, they may not have been advised to do so or chosen not to. Although we performed multiple comparisons, the main conclusions rest on plausible and consistent associations across ages and comparable aspects of care. The NICE 2008 guidelines have been updated in 2014 [17]. Although the patient survey data were collected before the 2014 update, there is no reason to suspect that clinical practice would be particularly different since the guideline update, especially since the emphasis on non-pharmacological strategies is retained in the 2014 update. The issues raised by the findings of this survey remain very relevant.

Table 3 Uptake of the recommended NICE core non-pharmacological and first line pharmacological treatments (N = 4059)

Characteristic	Written information[a]		Muscle strengthening/aerobic fitness exercise		Dieting to lose weight[b]		Paracetamol		Topical NSAIDs	
	n (%)	AOR (95% CI)	n (%)	AOR (95% CI)	n (%)	AOR (95% CI)	n (%)	AOR (95% CI)	n (%)	AOR (95% CI)
Total	934		618		261		1270		1055	
Gender										
Male	353 (20.1)	1	244 (13.9)	1	92 (7.1)	1	511 (29.1)	1	424 (24.1)	1
Female	581 (25.3)	1.28^(xx) (1.09, 1.50)	374 (16.3)	1.12 (0.93, 1.35)	169 (11.5)	1.54^(xx) (1.16, 2.04)	759 (33.0)	1.09 (0.94, 1.27)	631 (27.4)	1.13 (0.97, 1.32)
Age group (years)										
45–54	190 (24.7)	1	133 (17.3)	1	37 (7.1)	1	149 (19.4)	1	150 (19.5)	1
55–64	298 (26.2)	1.02 (0.80, 1.29)	192 (16.9)	0.78 (0.60, 1.03)	90 (10.9)	1.52 (0.97, 2.36)	283 (25.0)	1.12 (0.87, 1.45)	243 (21.4)	0.96 (0.74, 1.24)
65–74	267 (21.8)	0.76 (0.56, 1.03)	183 (14.9)	0.55^(xx) (0.38, 0.78)	99 (11.4)	1.64 (0.94, 2.86)	395 (32.2)	1.29 (0.94, 1.76)	341 (27.8)	1.20 (0.88, 1.64)
≥75	179 (19.3)	0.56^(xx) (0.40, 0.79)	110 (11.9)	0.37^(xxx) (0.25, 0.55)	35 (6.4)	0.74 (0.39, 1.40)	443 (47.7)	1.91^(xxx) (1.38, 2.65)	321 (34.6)	1.32 (0.94, 1.84)
Employment status										
Employed	277 (25.1)	1	171 (15.5)	1	56 (7.1)	1	203 (18.4)	1	197 (17.8)	1
Unemployed	143 (24.0)	0.74^(x) (0.58, 0.98)	102 (17.1)	1.03 (0.77, 1.38)	49 (12.8)	1.06 (0.67, 1.66)	195 (32.7)	1.16 (0.90, 1.51)	157 (26.3)	1.17 (0.90, 1.52)
Retired	494 (21.9)	0.91 (0.71, 1.18)	327 (14.5)	1.17 (0.87, 1.58)	149 (9.7)	0.92 (0.58, 1.45)	841 (37.3)	1.15 (0.89, 1.50)	667 (29.6)	1.12 (0.86, 1.46)
No. of pain sites										
Single site	116 (14.9)	1	106 (13.6)	1	31 (6.4)	1	180 (23.2)	1	151 (19.4)	1
Multi-site	818 (24.9)	1.59^(xxx) (1.26, 2.00)	512 (15.6)	0.98 (0.77, 1.26)	230 (10.1)	1.08 (0.70, 1.68)	1090 (33.2)	1.10 (0.88, 1.35)	904 (27.5)	1.15 (0.93, 1.43)
Morbidity burden (BNF drug count)										
<10 counts	501 (22.5)	1	294 (13.2)	1	87 (5.9)	1	451 (20.3)	1	419 (18.9)	1
≥10 counts	433 (23.6)	0.91 (0.75, 1.08)	324 (17.6)	1.44^(xx) (1.16, 1.77)	174 (13.5)	1.87^(xxx) (1.37, 2.57)	819 (44.6)	1.88^(xxx) (1.60, 2.23)	636 (34.6)	1.61^(xxx) (1.35, 1.91)
BMI (Kg/m²)										
Not overweight (< 25.0)	253 (21.8)	1	170 (14.6)	1	n/a	n/a	343 (29.5)	1	287 (24.7)	1
Overweight (25.0–29.9)	355 (22.4)	1.01 (0.83, 1.23)	246 (15.5)	1.02 (0.82, 1.27)	84 (5.3)	1	482 (30.4)	1.05 (0.87, 1.27)	420 (26.5)	1.12 (0.93, 1.35)
Obese (≥30.0)	295 (24.9)	0.96 (0.78, 1.18)	180 (15.2)	0.80 (0.63, 1.02)	177 (15.0)	2.48^(xxx) (1.85, 3.32)	388 (32.8)	0.95 (0.78, 1.16)	311 (26.3)	0.91 (0.74, 1.12)
SF12 – Physical health (Quartile)										
Worst to 27.58	273 (27.7)	2.13^(xxx) (1.63, 2.77)	168 (17.0)	1.64^(xx) (1.20, 2.24)	102 (14.2)	1.44 (0.89, 2.32)	467 (47.4)	2.64^(xxx) (2.04, 3.41)	344 (34.9)	1.67^(xxx) (1.28, 2.16)
27.59–38.36	249 (25.4)	1.76^(xxx) (1.38, 2.25)	167 (17.0)	1.67^(xxx) (1.26, 2.23)	75 (11.0)	1.29 (0.81, 2.05)	361 (36.8)	2.24^(xxx) (1.75, 2.87)	290 (29.6)	1.60^(xxx) (1.25, 2.04)
38.37–48.26	231 (23.1)	1.53^(xxx) (1.21, 1.93)	155 (15.5)	1.47^(xx) (1.12, 1.93)	42 (6.2)	0.86 (0.53, 1.40)	261 (26.1)	1.70^(xxx) (1.33, 2.16)	225 (22.5)	1.26 (0.99, 1.61)
48.27–71.88	166 (16.9)	1	115 (11.7)	1	34 (5.5)	1	139 (14.1)	1	156 (15.8)	1
SF12 – Mental health (Quartile)										
Worst to 39.93	275 (28.5)	1.42^(xx) (1.12, 1.78)	176 (18.2)	1.11 (0.85, 1.44)	100 (14.0)	1.90^(xx) (1.26, 2.84)	404 (41.9)	1.59^(xxx) (1.28, 1.97)	314 (32.5)	1.51^(xxx) (1.21, 1.89)
39.94–49.55	231 (23.5)	1.18 (0.95, 1.48)	140 (14.3)	0.97 (0.75, 1.26)	68 (10.6)	1.64^(x) (1.08, 2.48)	337 (34.3)	1.34^(xx) (1.08, 1.65)	290 (29.5)	1.48^(xxx) (1.18, 1.84)
49.56–57.11	207 (21.4)	1.14 (0.91, 1.43)	144 (14.9)	1.04 (0.80, 1.35)	43 (6.9)	1.10 (0.70, 1.74)	233 (24.1)	1.04 (0.84, 1.30)	203 (21.0)	1.09 (0.87, 1.37)
57.12 to 74.46	206 (19.8)	1	145 (14.0)	1	42 (5.8)	1	254 (24.5)	1	208 (20.0)	1

Table 3 Uptake of the recommended NICE core non-pharmacological and first line pharmacological treatments ($N = 4059$) (*Continued*)

Characteristic	[a]Written information		Muscle strengthening/ aerobic fitness exercise		[b]Dieting to lose weight		Paracetamol		Topical NSAIDs	
	n (%)	AOR (95% CI)	n (%)	AOR (95% CI)	n (%)	AOR (95% CI)	n (%)	AOR (95% CI)	n (%)	AOR (95% CI)
OA diagnosis										
Yes	146 (29.1)	1.57[xxx] (1.26, 1.96)	88 (17.5)	1.31[x] (1.00, 1.70)	31 (8.9)	0.79 (0.52, 1.21)	203 (40.4)	1.30[x] (1.05, 1.62)	166 (33.1)	1.30[x] (1.04, 1.62)
No	788 (22.2)	1	530 (14.9)	1	230 (9.5)	1	1067 (30.0)	1	889 (25.0)	1

n is the number of participants who used core treatments out of 4059 eligible respondents. Number in the subcategories do not always sum to the total number of who used treatment due to missing data. % figures represent valid percent (i.e. excluding missing data)

AOR adjusted odds ratio

[a]Written information is a composite variable derived from the addition of responses of participants who used information about treatments, information about self-management and information about OA when they consulted with joint pain; [b]Restricted to obese/overweight participants. $n = 3742$ in final multivariable analysis

[x]$p < 0.05$, [xx]$p < 0.01$, [xxx]$p < 0.001$

Comparison with existing literature

This survey considered everyone with a self-reported consultation for joint pain in the previous 12 months. Only 12.4% of the study population had a recorded OA diagnosis in their medical record during this period, though study participants may have received an OA diagnosis prior to this. People with recorded peripheral joint pain have previously been identified to have a similar preponderance of radiographic OA compared to those with an OA diagnosis [18] and so it is reasonable to consider that the OA guidelines would apply to the whole study population.

In the adjusted models, which accounted inter alia for sex, age, morbidity burden, and clinical severity (through the SF-12 PCS and multi-site pain variable, as multi-site pain is associated with symptom severity [19]), the main variable associated with lower likelihood of use of the core non-pharmacological treatments was older age. The association between older age and reduced use of information may reflect a duration effect, if older people had used it previously, though it could also be due to other factors.

It is possible that the lower use of exercise was due to patient or clinician beliefs about the appropriateness of exercise in the elderly. It has previously been identified that only 16% of men and 12% of women aged ≥65 in the general population achieve recommended physical activity levels [20], therefore while this finding is not surprising, it is in contrast to the NICE universal recommendation for exercise in people with OA despite age.

Increasing age was also associated with greater use of paracetamol. Strauss et al. [21] demonstrated that patients with a preference towards the pharmacological options were generally older, though in this study it is not known if greater paracetamol use is influenced by patient- or clinician-level management. Clinical severity, measured by the SF-12 PCS and the multisite pain variable, appears to be associated with greater use of information. Worse physical function was also associated with greater use of exercise and first-line pharmacotherapy. The latter finding is unsurprising but it is encouraging that people with worse physical function reported greater use of exercise.

Implications for research and/or practice

This study indicates the potential importance of an OA diagnosis. People with such a diagnosis recently recorded were more likely to report having used treatments recommended in the NICE OA guidelines, i.e. certain core non-pharmacological treatments (exercise and provision of written information) and the first-line pharmacological treatments. This corresponds with previous work by our group which showed that those with an OA diagnosis were more likely to have clinician-recorded quality indicators of care than those with a joint pain symptom code [22]. It raises the possibility that, when GPs themselves are clearer about the diagnosis, there may be better uptake of the treatments that are recommended in the NICE OA guidelines by the patient, which reflects other findings about the nature of OA consultations in primary care [23].

Clinically, the known benefits of exercise [24] and weight loss [25] for hip and knee OA need to be better integrated into routine clinical practice to help reduce the apparent suboptimal uptake in the population with joint pain at large, and in the elderly in particular. Patients and clinicians need to be aware of the benefits of non-pharmacological interventions, to access these early in the course of OA and avoid reliance on pharmacological management.

A particular challenge will be to determine how to maximise patient participation in and adherence to exercise in the long-term. Evidence of barriers and facilitators of exercise adherence related to OA is not strong, although systematic reviews have highlighted the importance of educational and behavioural strategies as well as regular individualised exercise, supervision and follow-up [26, 27]. Future interventions incorporating these components should be tested to find the best way of increasing and maintaining exercise levels in this population in the long-term.

Conclusions

This is the first survey conducted to identify self-reported use of non-pharmacological and pharmacological treatments recommended in the NICE OA guidelines within primary care. Non-pharmacological treatment uptake was found to be suboptimal and lower than pharmacological treatment, especially in older people. Effective strategies to promote guideline adherence in all ages need to be identified, with a particular emphasis on non-pharmacological management in older age groups.

Abbreviations

AOR: Adjusted Odds Ratio; BNF: British National Formulary; CI: Confidence Interval; GP: General Practitioner; MCS: Mental Component Summary; MOSAICS: Management of OSteoArthritis In ConsultationS study; NICE: National Institute for Health & Care Excellence; NSAIDs: Non-steroidal anti-inflammatory drugs; OA: Osteoarthritis; PCS: Physical Component Summary; PN: Practice Nurse; SD: Standard Deviation; UK: United Kingdom

Acknowledgements

The authors would like to thank the OA Research Users' Group and the network, nursing, health informatics and administrative staff at Keele University's Arthritis Research UK Primary Care Centre, and Keele CTU for all their support and assistance with this study. Particular thanks go to Professors Peter Croft, Pauline Ong and Chris Main. NIHR West Midlands CRN Primary Care, study coordinators and research nurses. The authors would like to give special thanks to all of the staff and patients at the participating general practices and the GP facilitators, who provided support to the general practices involved in the study.

Funding

This paper presents independent research funded by the National Institute for Health Research (NIHR) Programme Grant [Grant number RP-PG-0407-10386]. The views expressed in this paper are those of the author(s) and not necessarily those of the NHS, the NIHR or the Department of Health and Social Care. This research was also funded by the Arthritis Research UK Centre in Primary Care Grant (Grant Number 18139). KD, ELH and CJ are part-funded by the National Institute for Health Research (NIHR) Collaborations for Leadership in Applied Health Research and Care West Midlands. KD is part-funded by a Knowledge Mobilisation Research Fellowship (KMRF-2014-03-002) from the NIHR. AF was supported by an NIHR Doctoral, Clinical Academic Training Fellowship. JJE was supported by the NIHR through an In-Practice Fellowship. EMH is a NIHR Senior Investigator.

Authors' contributions

ELH, EA, ML, JJE, KPJ, AF, CJ, EMH and KS made substantial contributions to conception and design of the study along with analysis and interpretation of data. ELH, EA, ML, JJE, KPJ, AF, CJ, EMH and KS have been involved in the drafting of the manuscript and have given final approval of the version to be published.

Consent for publication

Not Applicable.

Competing interests

Dr. Clare Jinks is a member of the editorial board for BMC Musculoskeletal Disorders. The remaining authors declare that they have no other conflicts of interest.

Author details

[1]Research Institute for Primary Care and Health Sciences, Keele University, Keele, Staffordshire ST5 5BG, UK. [2]Keele Clinical Trials Unit, David Weatherall Building, Keele University, Staffordshire, UK. [3]School of Nursing and Midwifery, Keele University, Staffordshire, UK.

References

1. Vos T, Flaxman AD, Naghavi M, et al. Years lived with disability (YLDs) for 1160 sequelae of 289 diseases and injuries 1990-2010: a systematic analysis for the global burden of disease study 2010. Lancet. 2012;380(9859):2163–96.
2. National Institute for Health & Clinical Excellence. NICE clinical guideline [CG59] osteoarthritis: the care and management of osteoarthritis in adults. London: National Institute for Health & Clinical Excellence; 2008.
3. Thomas E, Peat G, Croft P. Defining and mapping the person with osteoarthritis for population studies and public health. Rheumatology (Oxford, England). 2014;53(2):338–45.
4. Jordan KP, Joud A, Bergknut C, et al. International comparisons of the consultation prevalence of musculoskeletal conditions using population-based healthcare data from England and Sweden. Ann Rheum Dis. 2014; 73(1):212–8.
5. Hagen KB, Smedslund G, Osteras N, et al. Quality of community-based osteoarthritis care: a systematic review and meta-analysis. Arthritis Care Res (Hoboken). 2016;68(10):1443–52.
6. Mamlin LA, Melfi CA, Parchman ML, et al. Management of osteoarthritis of the knee by primary care physicians. Arch Fam Med. 1998;7(6):563–7.
7. Rosemann T, Wensing M, Joest K, et al. Problems and needs for improving primary care of osteoarthritis patients: the views of patients, general practitioners and practice nurses. BMC Musculoskelet Disord. 2006;7:48.
8. Dziedzic KS, Healey EL, Porcheret M, et al. Implementing the NICE osteoarthritis guidelines: a mixed methods study and cluster randomised trial of a model osteoarthritis consultation in primary care--the management of OsteoArthritis in consultations (MOSAICS) study protocol. Implement Sci. 2014;9(1):95.
9. Dziedzic KS, Healey EL, Porcheret M, et al. Implementing Core NICE guidelines for osteoarthritis in primary care with a model consultation: MOSAICS a cluster randomised controlled trial. Osteoarthr Cartil. 2018;26(1): 43 53. https://doi.org/10.1016/j.joca.2017.09.010
10. von Elm E, Altman DG, Egger M, et al. The strengthening the reporting of observational studies in epidemiology (STROBE) statement: guidelines for reporting observational studies. J Clin Epidemiol. 2008;61(4):344–9.
11. Ware J Jr, Kosinski M, Keller SD. A 12-item short-form health survey: construction of scales and preliminary tests of reliability and validity. Med Care. 1996;34(3):220–33.
12. Jinks C, Jordan K, Ong BN, et al. A brief screening tool for knee pain in primary care (KNEST). 2. Results from a survey in the general population aged 50 and over. Rheumatology (Oxford, England). 2004;43(1):55–61.
13. Brilleman SL, Salisbury C. Comparing measures of multimorbidity to predict outcomes in primary care: a cross sectional study. Fam Pract. 2013;30(2):172–8.
14. Hovstadius B, Hovstadius K, Astrand B, et al. Increasing polypharmacy - an individual-based study of the Swedish population 2005-2008. BMC Clin Pharmacol. 2010;10:16.
15. Porcheret M, Jordan K, Jinks C, et al. Primary care treatment of knee pain--a survey in older adults. Rheumatology (Oxford, England). 2007;46(11):1694–700.
16. Cottrell E, Roddy E, Foster NE. The attitudes, beliefs and behaviours of GPs regarding exercise for chronic knee pain: a systematic review. BMC Fam Pract. 2010;11:4.
17. National Institute for Health & Clinical Excellence. NICE clinical guideline [CG177] osteoarthritis: the care and management of osteoarthritis in adults. London: National Institute for Health & Clinical Excellence; 2014.
18. Jordan KP, Tan V, Edwards JJ, et al. Influences on the decision to use an osteoarthritis diagnosis in primary care: a cohort study with linked survey and electronic health record data. Osteoarthritis Cartilage. 2016;24(5):786–93.
19. Keenan AM, Tennant A, Fear J, et al. Impact of multiple joint problems on daily living tasks in people in the community over age fifty-five. Arthritis Rheum. 2006;55(5):757–64.
20. Craig R, Mindell J, Hirani V. Health survey for England 2008: physical activity and fitness. 2009.
21. Strauss VY, Carter P, Ong BN, et al. Public priorities for joint pain research: results from a general population survey. Rheumatology. 2012;51:20752082. https://doi.org/10.1093/rheumatology/kes179.
22. Edwards JJ, Jordan KP, Peat G, et al. Quality of care for OA: the effect of a point-of-care consultation recording template. Rheumatology (Oxford, England). 2015;54(5):844–53.
23. Paskins Z, Sanders T, Hassell AB. Comparison of patient experiences of the osteoarthritis consultation with GP attitudes and beliefs to OA: a narrative review. BMC Fam Pract. 2014;15:46.
24. Uthman OA, van der Windt DA, Jordan JL, et al. Exercise for lower limb osteoarthritis: systematic review incorporating trial sequential analysis and network meta-analysis. BMJ. 2013;347:f5555.
25. Christensen R, Bartels EM, Astrup A, et al. Effect of weight reduction in obese patients diagnosed with knee osteoarthritis: a systematic review and meta-analysis. Ann Rheum Dis. 2007;66(4):433–9.
26. Jordan JL, Holden MA, Mason EE, et al. Interventions to improve adherence to exercise for chronic musculoskeletal pain in adults. Cochrane Database Syst Rev. 2010;1:CD005956.
27. Larmer PJ, Reay ND, Aubert ER, et al. Systematic review of guidelines for the physical management of osteoarthritis. Arch Phys Med Rehabil. 2014;95(2):375–89.

6

Linguistic validation, validity and reliability of the British English versions of the Disabilities of the Arm, Shoulder and Hand (DASH) questionnaire and QuickDASH in people with rheumatoid arthritis

Alison Hammond[1]* iD, Yeliz Prior[1] and Sarah Tyson[2]

Abstract

Background: Although the Disabilities of the Arm, Shoulder and Hand (DASH) questionnaire is widely used in the UK, no British English version is available. The aim of this study was to linguistically validate the DASH into British English and then test the reliability and validity of the British English DASH, (including the Work and Sport/Music DASH) and QuickDASH, in people with rheumatoid arthritis (RA).

Methods: The DASH was forward translated, reviewed by an expert panel and cognitive debriefing interviews undertaken with 31 people with RA. Content validity was evaluated using the ICF Core Set for RA. Participants with RA ($n = 340$) then completed the DASH, Health Assessment Questionnaire (HAQ), Short Form Health Survey v2 (SF36v2) and Measure of Activity Performance of the Hand (MAPHAND). We examined internal consistency and concurrent validity for the DASH, Work and Sport/Music DASH modules and QuickDASH. Participants repeated the DASH to assess test-retest reliability.

Results: Minor wording changes were made as required. The DASH addresses a quarter of Body Function and half of Activities and Participation codes in the ICF RA Core Set. Internal consistency for DASH scales were consistent with individual use (Cronbach's alpha = 0.94–0.98). Concurrent validity was strong with the HAQ ($r_s = 0.69$–0.91), SF36v2 Physical Function ($r_s = -0.71 - -0.85$), Bodily Pain ($r_s = -0.71 - -0.74$) scales and MAPHAND ($r_s = 0.71$–0.93). Test-retest reliability was good ($r_s = 0.74$–0.95).

Conclusions: British English versions of the DASH, QuickDASH and Work and Sport/Music modules are now available to evaluate upper limb disabilities in the UK. The DASH, QuickDASH, Work and Sport/Music modules are reliable and valid to use in clinical practice and research with British people with RA.

Keywords: Patient reported outcomes, Upper limb assessment, Rehabilitation, Rheumatoid arthritis

* Correspondence: a.hammond@salford.ac.uk; hammond116@btinternet.com
[1]Centre for Health Sciences Research (OT), L701 Allerton, University of Salford, Frederick Road, Salford M6 6PU, UK
Full list of author information is available at the end of the article

Background

Rheumatoid arthritis (RA) impacts on hand and upper limb function. Within two years of diagnosis, 93% of people with RA report hand pain, 82% hand stiffness, 73% hand muscle weakness, 70% have at least one hand impairment and 50% experience shoulder joint tenderness and have reduced shoulder function [1–3]. Rehabilitation therefore includes maintaining and improving hand and upper limb function [4]. Using reliable, valid outcome measures is important to ensure problems are accurately identified and treatment benefits demonstrated.

The Disabilities of the Arm, Shoulder and Hand (DASH) questionnaire is a widely used patient reported outcome measure (PROM) of upper limb function used in musculoskeletal conditions [5]. Its purpose is to detect upper limb disorders of differing severity, assess changes over time and evaluate outcomes of interventions [6]. It is one of the best upper limb measures clinimetrically [7, 8]. The QUICKDASH, a shorter, more quickly administered version derived from the DASH, was developed using Rasch analysis [9–11]. Both also include optional modules for those whose jobs require a lot of upper limb performance (WORKDASH) and for sports people and musicians (sports and music: SPAMDASH).

The DASH was originally published in Canadian/ North American English. Outcome measures should be linguistically validated (i.e. translated and culturally adapted) into the language of the target country and psychometrically tested with target population(s) before being used in that country [12, 13]. There are English versions of the DASH for Australia, Hong Kong and South Africa [14] but a British English version has not yet been linguistically validated and psychometrically tested in the United Kingdom (UK). Currently, the Canadian/North American English version is being used in rheumatology clinical practice and research. Whilst much of the North American English DASH is understandable to British English speakers, clinicians and patients regularly comment that some activities included are: unclear, e.g. "yard work"; not in common usage e.g. "transportation"; infrequently performed in the UK, e.g. "wash walls." Additionally, some phrases and sentences could be shortened to reflect Plain English usage. Consequently, a British English version is required that is then psychometrically tested in populations it is commonly used with.

The DASH consists of 30 items evaluating upper limb-related activities, participation and symptoms [11]. There has been some debate as to whether the DASH is unidimensional. Factor analysis of the original Canadian/North American [11] and also Dutch [15], Japanese [16] and Chinese [17] versions of the DASH identified a single factor and thus all items can be summed to form a total score. However, studies using factor and /or Rasch analysis with the Canadian/North American DASH in the UK identified two factors [18] while the French [19], Italian [20] and Canadian /North American [21] versions revealed three factors. Psychometric testing of measures should include a combination of classical testing and item response theory (e.g. Rasch analysis) to establish psychometric properties, including unidimensionality [22].

The overall aims of this study were to: linguistically validate the DASH into British English; investigate content validity of the DASH in RA; and evaluate the psychometrics of the British English DASH and QuickDASH amongst people with RA in the UK. The psychometrics assessed were: concurrent and discriminant validity, internal consistency, test retest reliability, sensitivity to change, compliance (amount of missing data) and floor and ceiling effects of the British English DASH and Quick-DASH amongst British people with RA.

Alongside this, we also investigated construct validity of the British English DASH and QuickDASH using Rasch analysis. This is reported separately [Prodinger B, Hammond A, Tennant A, Prior Y, Tyson S. Deconstructing the Disabilities of the Arm, Shoulder and Hand (DASH) and QuickDASH in Rheumatoid Arthritis, submitted].

Methods

Ethical approval was obtained from the National Research Ethics Service Committee North West - Greater Manchester North (12/NW/0841) and the University of Salford's School of Health Sciences Ethics Panel. All participants provided written, informed consent.

Participants

Participants were recruited: by research nurses screening for eligibility in 17 Rheumatology out-patient clinics (either in clinic or identified from departmental databases); and from amongst participants in a previous outcome measure study we conducted, who had consented to be contacted for future studies. All were recruited from the same Rheumatology out-patient clinics originally and with whom eligibility was re-checked prior to consent. Participants were eligible if they: had a confirmed diagnosis of RA; were able to read, write and understand English; and had not (or were not about to) altered their disease-modifying medication regimen in the last three months (which could affect test-retest reliability).

Linguistic and cross-cultural validation

The adaptation procedures devised by the Institute of Work and Health for DASH translation were followed [23]. This consists of six steps:

(1) *forward translation*: two translators (AH: a rheumatology rehabilitation researcher familiar with the DASH) and a non-health professional unfamiliar

with the DASH (JG: an experienced teacher) independently reviewed the DASH to identify any words that needed to be changed into British English (e.g. transportation is termed transport) and use of Plain English (i.e. simplifying words and phrases).

(2) *translation synthesis*: an independent recorder assisted the two translators agreeing any recommended changes

(3) *backward translation*: was not required as the translation was into another form of English.

(4) *expert committee review*: The committee included: the two translators (AH, JG); synthesis recorder (YP); an experienced Rheumatology occupational therapist familiar with using the DASH (AJ); an English language expert (GMcL); a Canadian English-speaking researcher (KH); and an experienced outcome measures researcher (ST). The committee discussed the synthesised translation, made additional recommendations and agreed and approved the wording of the draft British English DASH. This process ensures semantic, idiomatic, experiential and conceptual equivalence.

(5) *field testing of the adapted DASH with people with RA*: Cognitive debriefing interviews are commonly used during PROM development to investigate the appropriateness of items and to gain insight into participants' understanding of the content of measures [12, 24]. Participants with RA were recruited from four Rheumatology out-patient clinics. They completed the draft British English DASH (including the two optional modules if applicable) in their own time and were interviewed within two weeks about the relevance and comprehensibility of items. The results were discussed with the expert committee and, if necessary, further changes in wording made and the final British English DASH agreed. Finally, the Flesch Reading Ease score was calculated using Microsoft Word to check its readability is similar to the original DASH. Content validity: we systematically linked the DASH items (and sub-items, where applicable) to the International Classification of Functioning, Disability and Health (ICF) Core Set for RA [25, 26]. DASH items have previously been linked to the ICF [27].

(6) *psychometric testing of the British English DASH with people with RA in the UK.*

After each of steps 4, 5 and 6 reports were sent to the Institute of Work and Health for translation approval before proceeding to the next step [23].

Psychometric testing procedures

Participants were mailed a questionnaire booklet which collected data to describe the recruited population: demographic and disease data: age, gender, marital, educational and employment status, disease duration and RA disease-modifying medication as well as the measures described below. Two to three weeks later, participants were mailed the British English DASH to complete at home a second time (to evaluate test-retest reliability). Two reminders were sent for each mailing, as necessary.

Measurement instruments
The British English DASH

The DASH consists of 30 items, measured using five-point Likert scales (1–5): 21 regarding daily activity; five regarding symptoms; three about participation (the impact of the condition on daily life); and one about confidence in abilities [28]. The QUICKDASH was derived from the DASH and consists of 11 items (six of daily activity ability; two about symptoms (pain and tingling); and three about participation) [11]. The two optional modules (SPAM- and WORK-DASH) were also included.

The medical outcomes survey 36 item short-from health survey version 2 (SF36v2)

From which sub-scales of Physical Function, Bodily Pain and Vitality (fatigue) scales were selected [29, 30]. QualityMetric Health Outcomes™ Scoring Software 4.5 was used to manage missing SF36v2 data and calculate norm-based scores converted to 0–100 scale for each sub-scale [31]. Lower scores denote worse health states.

The health assessment questionnaire (HAQ)

Indicates ability to perform 20 daily activities rated on a 0–3 scale (0 = not at all difficult; 3 = unable to do) [32], scored using the HAQ20 method, in which the total score is obtained by summing all 20 items (0–20 = mild; 21–40 = moderate; 41–60 = severe disability) [33, 34]. This method was used as the HAQ20 does not weight items worse if an assistive device is used, as occurs when normally scoring the HAQ. Higher scores denote greater activity limitations.

The hand HAQ

Seven items of upper limb function derived from the HAQ (i.e. Dressing; Cutting meat/food; Lifting a full cup or glass; Opening a new milk carton; Opening car doors; Opening jars which have been previously opened; Turning taps on and off [35]. The score is the sum of the seven items, with higher scores denoting greater activity limitations.

The British English measure of activity performance of the hand (MAP-HAND)

Eighteen items of activity ability requiring hand use, each measured on a 0–3 scale (0 = not at all difficult; 3 = unable to do) [36, 37]. The total score is obtained by summing the 18 items, with higher scores denoting greater activity limitations.

Symptom 10-point numeric rating scales (NRS)
Evaluating: hand pain on activity; and self-reported disease activity level, general pain at rest, general pain on movement, stiffness, movement limitations, from the Evaluation of Daily Activity Questionnaire [38].

RA quality of life scale (RAQOL)
Thirty items about quality of life (QoL) answered yes (=1) or no (=0), with yes items summed to give a total score. Higher scores indicate worse QoL [39].

Perceived change in health status
At Test 2 only, this was measured using a 5-point NRS by asking "*Overall, how much is your arthritis troubling you now compared to when you last completed this questionnaire?*" (1 = much less; 2 = somewhat less; 3 = about the same; 4 = somewhat more; 5 = much more).

We hypothesised that there would be strong correlations between the four DASH scales and these measures.

Sample size
As Rasch analysis was also being used to assess construct validity of the British English DASH, a sample size of at least 250 was recruited [Prodinger B, Hammond A, Tennant A, Prior Y, Tyson S. Deconstructing the Disabilities of the Arm, Shoulder and Hand (DASH) and QuickDASH in Rheumatoid Arthritis, submitted]. This number was determined from the need to ensure a uniform distribution of patients across the construct of upper limb function, so that the precision of the estimate of both persons and items, across the construct, remains similar [40]. At least 79 sets of repeated responses were required to demonstrate that a test-retest correlation of 0.7 differs from a background correlation (constant) of 0.45, with 90% power at the 1% significance level. A test-retest correlation of 0.7 is deemed a minimum acceptable level [41].

Statistical analyses
Rasch analyses of both the DASH and QUICKDASH indicated that, using a testlet approach taking account of local dependency, both can be considered as unidimensional and total raw scores, standardised to 0–100, can therefore be used [Prodinger B, Hammond A, Tennant A, Prior Y, Tyson S. Deconstructing the Disabilities of the Arm, Shoulder and Hand (DASH) and QuickDASH in Rheumatoid Arthritis, submitted]. DASH and Quick-DASH standardised scores can be converted to a Rasch metric interval scale when required for parametric analyses [Prodinger B, Hammond A, Tennant A, Prior Y, Tyson S. Deconstructing the Disabilities of the Arm,

Shoulder and Hand (DASH) and QuickDASH in Rheumatoid Arthritis, submitted].

For both the DASH and QUICKDASH, standardised (0–100) scores are calculated by:

$$\text{DASH DISABILITY/SYMPTOM SCORE} = \frac{[(\text{sum of n responses})-1]}{n} \times 25$$

(where n is the number of completed responses). A higher score represents worse ability/symptoms. The DASH score cannot be calculated if there are more than three missing items, nor the QUICKDASH if more than one missing item.

The WORK- and SPAM-DASH were scored by: adding the assigned values for each response, dividing by 4 (number of items); subtracting 1; and multiplying by 25 to convert to a 0–100 scale. Optional module scores cannot be calculated if there are missing items.

The Statistical Package for the Social Sciences v20 was used for analyses [42], apart from linear weighted kappas, calculated using MedCalc [43]. As all measures consist of ordinal data, non-parametric statistical tests were used to assess the psychometrics.

Concurrent validity
Of the four DASH scores was assessed using Spearman's correlations with measures of related constructs (i.e. SF36v2 sub-scales, HAQ20, Hand HAQ, MAP-HAND, RAQOL, and symptom NRSs). Correlations of 0.8–1.00 were deemed very strong; 0.6–0.79 strong; 0.4–0.59 moderate; 0.20–0.39 weak; and 0–0.19 are very weak [44].

Discriminant validity
Was assessed using Kruskal-Wallis tests to evaluate differences in scores between participants with different degrees of disease activity, using the disease activity NRS (low disease activity = 0–3; moderate = 4–6; high = 7–10).

Internal consistency
Was assessed using Cronbach's alpha. Results of ≥0.8 were deemed good to excellent [44]. A value of ≥0.85 is consistent with individual use and > 0.7 with group-level use.

Test-retest reliability
Was assessed, in those stating their condition was "the same" at Test 2, using Spearman's correlations and intra-class correlation coefficients (ICC (2,1): two-way random consistency, average measures model). An ICC ≥ 0.75 was considered excellent [45]. Reliability of individual DASH items was calculated using linear weighted kappa. Levels of agreement are interpreted as < 0.20 = poor; 0.21–0.40 = fair; 0.41–0.60 = moderate; 0.61–0.80 = good; 0.81–1.00 = very good [46].

Sensitivity to change

Was assessed by calculating Standard Error of Measurement (SEM) and the Minimal Detectable Change$_{95}$ (MDC$_{95}$) scores, i.e. a statistical estimate of the smallest detectable change corresponding to change in ability [47, 48].

The formulae used were: $SEM = s \sqrt{(1 - r)}$, where s = the mean and standard deviation (SD) of Test 1 and Test 2 (retest), r = the reliability coefficient for the test, i.e. Pearson's correlation co-efficient between Test and Test 2 values. Thereafter the MDC$_{95}$ was calculated using the formula: $MDC_{95} = SEM \times \sqrt{2} \times 1.96$ [48].

Compliance (missing data)

The number of missing data items were reviewed to identify the percentage of the four DASH scales which could not be scored, and the commonest missing items.

Floor and ceiling effects

Were considered present if > 15% of participants achieved either the lowest or highest scores in the four DASH scales [49, 50].

Results

Steps 1 to 5: Linguistic validation and cross-cultural adaptation

The expert panel agreed several changes to simplify language: "perform" was changed to "do"; "estimate" to "guess"; "household chores" to "household jobs"; "wash floors" to "clean floors"; "put on a pullover sweater" to "put on a jumper"; "transportation" to "transport"; "using your usual technique for your work" to "doing your work in your usual way"; "using your usual technique for playing your instrument or sport" to "playing your instrument or sport in your usual way"; "yard work" to "outdoor property work" (as this was identified as meaning outdoor property maintenance in Canada); "wash walls" to "wash windows" (as the former is a rare activity and washing windows requires a similar action); and for "carry a heavy object (over 10lbs)" we added "or 5 kg" to provide a rough metric equivalent.

Cognitive debriefing interviews were conducted with 26 women and five men (see Table 1). Minor changes to clarify were suggested for seven items. Five participants were unsure whether the instruction "ability to do the following activities..." referred to ability with or without aids and adaptations, as they might answer differently using these. The panel agreed not to change instructions as these are consistent across all language versions of the DASH. For the activity items, only two raised interpretation concerns. Five interpreted "Make a bed" (item 9) as completely changing the bed linen. In British English, "make a bed" describes the daily tidying or straightening bedding and was interpreted as such by other participants. Discussion with Canadians indicated that

Table 1 DASH study participant characteristics (n = 340)

Participant Characteristics	Cognitive debriefing Participants (n = 31)	Psychometric testing: Participants (n = 340)
Age:(Mean (SD)	63.42 (12.04)	61.96 (12.09)
Gender (M:F)	5:26	89:251
Condition duration (years) (Mean (SD):	15.71 (12.61)	14.44 (11.73)
Marital status: n (%)		
Married/living with partner	23 (74%)	241 (71%)
Living status: n (%)		
Family/significant other	24 (77%)	245 (72%)
Children living at home	4 (13%)	36 (11%)
Employment status		
Paid employment	3 (10%)	108 (32%)
Retired	22 (71%)	204 (60%)
Other	6 (19%)	28 (8%)
Education level (ISCED)		
Secondary education only	19 (61%)	182 (54%)
Current medication		
Not on DMARDs	2 (6%)	34 (10%)
Monotherapy	10 (32%)	91 (27%)
Combination therapy	10 (32%)	190 (56%)
Biologic drugs	9 (29%)	25 (7%)

this means the same in Canadian/North American English. Nine queried whether "manage transport needs" (item 20) referred specifically to driving, getting a lift or using public transport, as each required different levels of upper limb activity, or to multiple transport methods. Other participants interpreted this related to their own travel circumstances. For symptom severity, eight participants indicated it was difficult differentiating between "arm, shoulder or hand pain severity" (item 24), and pain severity "when you do any specific activity" (item 25) as their pain usually lasts some time without changing with different activities. However, the other participants could identify activities inducing/ exacerbating pain and thus rate these items separately. Five were unable to identify whether the "weakness in their arms, shoulder or hand" (item 27) was any different in the last week than usual, as their upper limb was constantly weak. Thirteen were unsure if they could solely attribute sleeping problems to arm, shoulder or hand pain (item 29) as they either had multiple painful joints or widespread pain, although they did answer the question. The panel discussed these items and decided not to make further changes. The Flesch Reading Ease score for the British English DASH was 62.8, i.e. similar to the Canadian DASH (61.5), indicating a reading age of 13 to 15-year olds is required [51].

Content validity

Using the Brief ICF Core Set for RA, the DASH addresses: 5/24 Body Functions codes, 0/13 Body Structures codes; 15/26 Activities and Participation codes; and 0/5 Environmental Factors codes. Eight items were linked to either fine hand use (d440) or hand and arm use (d445) and allocated to carrying, moving and handling, other (d449). Five DASH items were not linked to the Brief ICF Core Set: gardening (item 8); interference with social activities (item 22); tingling (item 26); weakness (item 27); and feeling less capable (item 30), as the Core Set does not include Personal Factors. (See Additional file 1: Table S1).

Step 6: Psychometric testing
Participants

Overall, 595 people were screened for eligibility, 423 consented and 340 returned the Test 1 questionnaire booklet and 273 the Test 2 booklet (see Fig. 1). Participant characteristics are shown in Table 1 and health status, activity limitations and quality of life measures descriptive data are shown in Table 2. The mean time between tests was 34.6 (SD 13.07) days.

Concurrent validity

The DASH correlated strongly with all disease activity, symptom, function and quality of life measures ($r_s = 0.61-0.99$); as did the QuickDASH ($r_s = 0.61-0.91$). WORKDASH correlations were mainly strong ($r_s = 0.53-0.80$); and SPAMDASH correlations moderate to strong ($r_s = 0.52-0.78$) (see Table 3).

Discriminant validity

There were significant differences between the three levels of perceived disease activity for the DASH, Quick-DASH, WORKDASH and SPAMDASH, with

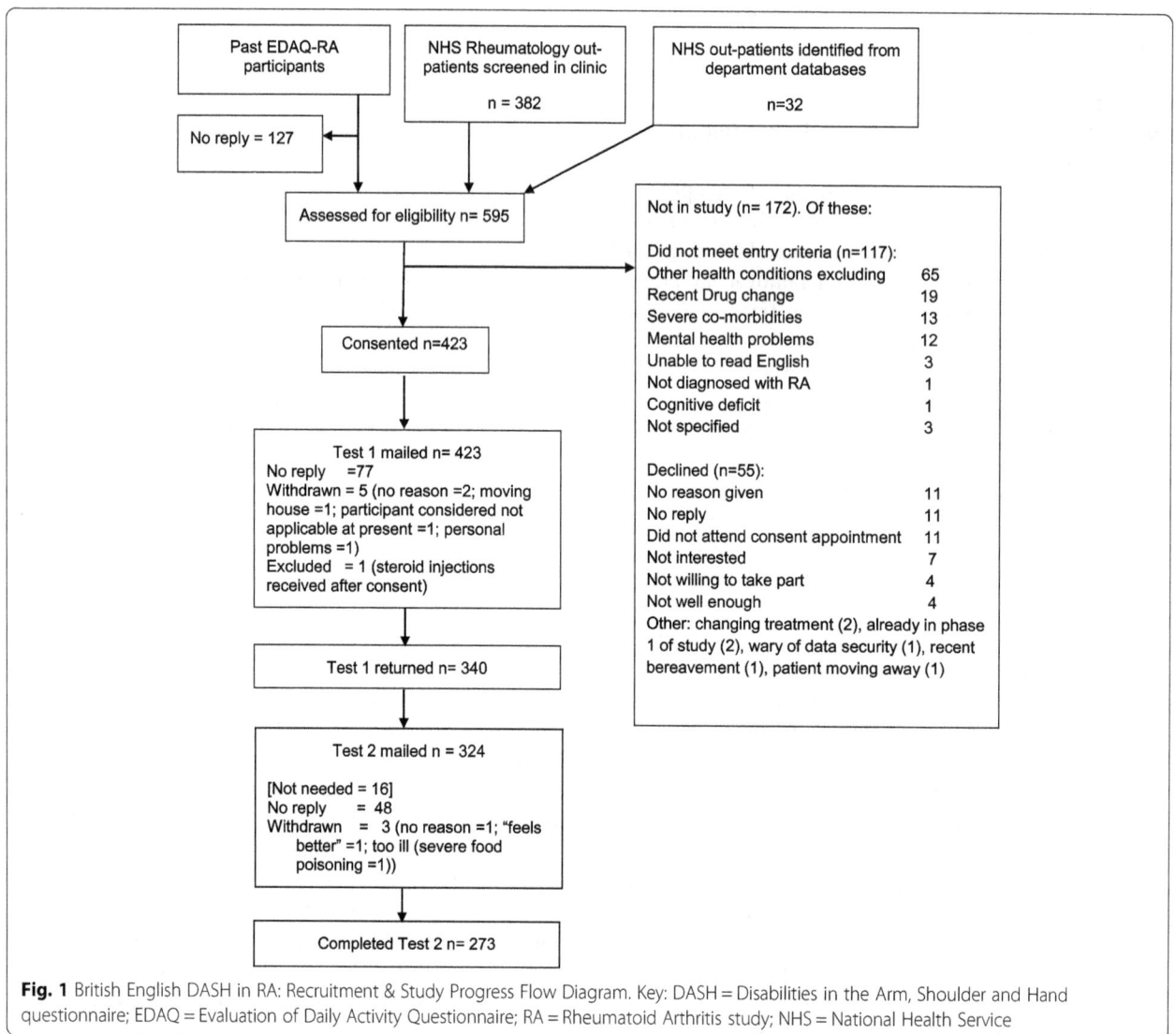

Fig. 1 British English DASH in RA: Recruitment & Study Progress Flow Diagram. Key: DASH = Disabilities in the Arm, Shoulder and Hand questionnaire; EDAQ = Evaluation of Daily Activity Questionnaire; RA = Rheumatoid Arthritis study; NHS = National Health Service

Table 2 Descriptive data for health status measures ($n = 340$)

Health status measures (median (IQR))	Test 1 ($n = 340$)	Test 2 ($n = 273$)
DASH (range 0–100)	35.34 (18.33–56.35)	36.67 (16.95–55.00)
QuickDASH (range 0–100)	34.09 (15.91–50.0)	36.36 (18.18–56.81)
WORKDASH (0–100)	25 (6.25–43.75) ($n = 158$)	25 (0–39.06) ($n = 118$)
SPAMDASH (range 0–100)	25 (12.50–59.38) ($n = 57$)	31.25 (18.75–75.0) ($n = 39$)
Test 1 only:		
Disease activity level NRS (range 0–10)	4 (2–6)	
Pain when moving NRS (range 0–10)	5 (2–7)	
SF36v2 Bodily Pain (range 0–100)	42.24 (34.18–47.48)	
Hand pain on activity NRS (range 0–10)	4 (2–7)	
Fatigue NRS (0–10)	6 (4–8)	
SF36v2 Vitality (range 0–100)	43.69 (34.77–49.63)	
HAQ20 (0–60)	13 (4–23)	
Hand HAQ (range 0–21)	5 (1.75–10)	
MAPHAND (range 0–54)	17 (8.25–27)	
SF36v2 Physical Function (range 0–100)	36.49 (26.93–46.06)	
RAQOL (range 0–30)	10.50 (4–19)	

participants with higher perceived disease activity scoring worse on the DASH scales (see Table 4).

Internal consistency
Cronbach's alpha values for the four DASH scales were excellent ranging from 0.94 (WORKDASH) to 0.98 (DASH) (see Table 5).

Test-retest reliability
Data for those participants reporting they were "the same" at Test 2 as at Test 1 were analysed. For all four DASH measures, correlations between Test 1 and Test 2 scores were strong ($r_s = 0.74–0.95$). For the DASH and QuickDASH, ICC(2,1) were excellent (see Table 5). As there are no Rasch transformation tables available for the WORK-and SPAMDASH, ICC(2,1) could not be calculated. For individual items in the DASH and

QuickDASH, reliability was moderate ($n = 9$) or good ($n = 21$); for the WORKDASH moderate ($n = 3$) and good ($n = 1$); and SPAMDASH for all four items were good. (See Additional file 1: Table S2).

Sensitivity to change
Using Rasch transformed scores, for the DASH, SEM = 1. 78 and MDC$_{95}$ = 4.94; and Quick DASH SEM = 1.65 and MDC$_{95}$ = 4.57. As there are no Rasch transformation tables available for the WORK-AN|D SPAMDASH, SEM and MDC$_{95}$ could not be calculated.

Missing data
All 30 DASH items were answered by 226/340 (67%). One item was unanswered by 76 participants (23%); two by 20 (7%); three items by 4 (1%); and five items by 4 (1%). Three participants (1%) returned the DASH uncompleted.

Table 3 Concurrent validity of the DASH, WORKDASH and SPAMDASH with health status, activity limitation and quality of life measures

	Disease activity NRS	Pain on movement NRS	Fatigue NRS	Hand pain on activity NRS	HAQ20	Hand HAQ	MAPHAND	RAQOL	SF36v2 Physical Function	SF36v2 Bodily Pain	SF36v2 Vitality
DASH ($n = 340$)	0.61**	0.70**	0.64**	0.75**	0.91**	0.88**	0.93**	0.80**	-0.85**	-0.74**	-0.63**
QuickDASH ($n = 340$)	0.61**	0.70**	0.65**	0.76**	0.87**	0.84**	0.91**	0.79**	-0.82**	-0.73**	-0.62**
WORKDASH ($n = 158$)	0.54**	0.62**	0.62**	0.69**	0.80**	0.74**	0.74**	0.74**	-0.71**	-0.71**	-0.53**
SPAMDASH ($n = 57$)	0.52**	0.55**	0.48**	0.57**	0.69**	0.60**	0.71**	0.78**	-0.74**	-0.71**	-0.61**

Key: Spearman's correlations; ** $p < 0.001$; *NRS* numeric rating scale

Table 4 Discriminant validity: DASH ($n = 327$), QuickDASH ($n = 334$), WORKDASH ($n = 157$) and SPAMDASH ($n = 57$) median (IQR) scores and differences between perceived disease activity groups

	Low disease activity (0–3)	Moderate disease activity (4–6)	High disease activity (7–10)	Chi-square	df	p
DASH	19.58 (9.58–36.32)	42.81 (27.29–58.33)	57.50 (43.33–72.50)	399.40	332	0.007
QuickDASH	15.91 (6.82–36.36)	40.91 (25.00–52.27)	56.82 (39.77–65.91)	214.00	102	0.000
WORKDASH	12.50 (0–29.69)	28.13 (18.75–50.0)	50.0 (31.25–68.75)	71.37	28	0.000
SPAMDASH	25 (0–37.5)	56.25 (31.25–87.50)	100 (75.00–100)	50.02	28	0.006

Scores could not be generated because of missing data for the following: DASH, 11 participants (3%); QuickDASH, 3 participants (< 1%); WORKDASH, 4 participants (2%); and SPAMDASH, two participants (3%). There were no significant differences in the characteristics, disease activity, symptom, function or quality of life scores of those for whom any DASH scores could be completed or not. However, those participants with missing data were more likely to be older (65.27 (SD 10.49) years vs 60.28 (SD 12.50) years, $t = 3.66$; $p < 0.001$); and to be single, divorced/separated or widowed/widowered (chi-square 9.25; df = 3; $p = 0.03$). Items unanswered by more than 5% of participants were: sexual activities ($n = 56$ (16%)); and recreational activities requiring little effort ($n = 18$ (5%)). Those not answering the sexual activities item were significantly: older (67.25 (SD10.25) years vs 60.91 (SD 12.15) years; $t = 3.65$; $p < 0.001$); and more likely to be living alone (chi-square 15.65, df = 1; $p < 0.001$) than those who did answer. This therefore reflected which participants were most likely to have missing data, as sexual activities was the commonest unanswered question.

Floor and ceiling effects

There were no floor or ceiling effects for the DASH (2% scored 0; 0.3% scored 100) or the QuickDASH (5.6% scored 0, 0% scored 100). However, for the WORK- and SPAM-DASH there were floor effects: 21 and 17.5% respectively. There were no ceiling effects for the WORK-DASH (2%) but there were for the SPAMDASH (15.8%).

Discussion

Linguistically validated British English versions of the DASH and QuickDASH are now available for use in the UK. These British-English translations demonstrated good psychometric properties in a sample of people with RA and can be used in both clinical practice and research.

We ensured linguistic and cross-cultural validity of the DASH by using the IWH DASH translation process, while gaining the developers' approval throughout. During cognitive debriefing, some participants were unsure if "ability to do the following activities…" referred to ability with or without aids and adaptations, as ability can differ when using these. Clarifying this, to ensure respondents answer in the same way, could be beneficial. However, the 50 language versions currently available do not specify this, so these changes were not made.

In terms of content validity, the DASH scales address some of the Body Functions and over half of the Activities and Participation items in the Brief ICF Core Set for RA and those not covered by the DASH are mostly those not relevant to the arm, shoulder and hand. Some core issues are potentially relevant and not reflected in the DASH. These include: body image (1801), as many people can be disturbed by their hand appearance in RA [52]; muscle endurance (b740) and maintaining a body position (d415), as DASH ICF linking did not specifically identify prolonged and/or static actions [27]; and using communication devices and techniques (d360), as the use of smart/mobile phones and computers/tablets is now ubiquitous, compared to when the DASH was developed in 1995. However, participants did not raise such issues in the cognitive debriefing interviews suggesting the DASH adequately reflects their main problems. As device use is a common source of upper limb pain in those with high-frequency use, it may be time to update the DASH and include this as a new item, thus reflecting modern-day life. Potentially, it could replace an existing item which is now less common, e.g. change a lightbulb overhead, as the advent of LED bulbs means this activity is now less frequently performed.

Table 5 Internal consistency and test-retest reliability of the DASH, QuickDASH, WORKDASH and SPAMDASH (for those reporting "the same" at Test 2)

	Cronbach's alpha	n for test-retest	Test 1 score (median, IQR)	Test 2 score (median, IQR)	Spearman's Correlation (r_s)	ICC(2,1) (95% CI)
DASH	0.98	170	30.83 (15.83–55.00)	30.00 (12.50–53.33)	0.95**	0.97 (0.96,0.98)
QuickDASH	0.94	180	29.55 (13.63–47.73)	30.00 (13.63–53.41)	0.93**	0.95 (0.94,0.96)
WORKDASH	0.94	53	25.00 (6.25–37.50)	25.00 (0–37.50)	0.74**	–
SPAMDASH	0.97	19	25.00 (12.50–48.44)	25.00 (18.75–75.00)	0.92**	–

Key: Spearman's correlations; ** $p < 0.001$

Concurrent validity of the DASH scales was strong for the DASH, QuickDASH and WORKDASH and moderate to strong for the SPAMDASH, which may have been affected by the small sample size. Psychometric testing in RA has been conducted in three other language versions of the DASH in RA (Swedish, Turkish and Dutch) [6, 53, 54]. Results of the test-retest reliability indicate the DASH and Quick DASH can be used for both group and individual measurement in RA. Additionally, sensitivity to change (MDC_{95}) indicated DASH and QuickDASH changes of about 5 (on a 0–100 scale) are similar to those reported by Kennedy et al. [11]. However, the MDC_{95} for the WORK- and SPAM-DASH could not be calculated as we do not have Rasch transformation tables available for these two modules. Rasch analysis also identified that the DASH and QuickDASH can be considered unidimensional and thus summed or standardised scores can be used [Prodinger B, Hammond A, Tennant A, Prior Y, Tyson S. Deconstructing the Disabilities of the Arm, Shoulder and Hand (DASH) and QuickDASH in Rheumatoid Arthritis, submitted]. A strength of this study is that we had a large sample of people with RA recruited from a wide variety of rheumatology out-patient clinics, meaning the results are representative for people with RA.

The limitations of this study are that we only tested the DASH and QuickDASH in people with RA. Further testing is recommended in other upper limb conditions to investigate psychometric properties. Responsiveness (i.e. longitudinal validity) still needs to be tested and minimal clinically important differences (MCID) also need to be established. Construct validity of the WORK-DASH and SPAMDASH using Rasch analysis is also warranted.

Conclusions

Overall, psychometric testing of the British English versions of the DASH, QuickDASH, WORKDASH and SPAM-DASH demonstrated good validity and reliability in a British English speaking sample of people with RA in the UK. These four British English DASH scales meet most of the recommendations of the Consensus-based Standards for the selection of health Measurement Instruments (COS-MIN) checklist [22, 55]. Accordingly, the British English DASH, QuickDASH, WORK-and SPAMDASH can be used in clinical practice and research in the UK and are available from the Institute of Work and Health DASH website [56, 57].

Abbreviations
DASH: Disabilities of the Arm, Shoulder and Hand Questionnaire; HAQ: Health Assessment Questionnaire; ICC: Intra-class correlation coefficient; ICF: International Classification of Functioning, Disability and Health; MAPHAND: Measure of activity performance of the hand questionnaire; MDC: Minimum detectable change; NRS: Numeric rating scale; PROM: Patient reported outcome measure; RA: Rheumatoid arthritis; RAQOL: Rheumatoid arthritis quality of life scale; SF36v2: Medical outcomes survey 36 item short form health survey version 2; SPAMDASH: Sport and music module of the disabilities of the arm, shoulder and hand questionnaire; WORKDASH: Work module of the disabilities of the arm, shoulder and hand questionnaire

Acknowledgements
The authors wish to thank: all the study participants for their time in completing questionnaires; the expert panel members for their time in supporting the translation process: John Grogan (translator), Kris Hollands (Canadian-English speaking health researcher, University of Salford); Angela Jackson (Rheumatology occupational therapist, Stepping Hill Hospital, Stockport); Graham McLeish (English language expert, Services for Export and Language, University of Salford); Professor Alan Tennant (University of Leeds and Swiss Paraplegic Institute) for advice during the planning of the project; Robert Peet and Kate Woodward-Nutt, Centre for Health Sciences, University of Salford, for assistance with data collection and data entry; and all the Principal Investigators, rheumatology consultants, rheumatology and research nurses and occupational therapists assisting with participant recruitment and study support at the participating sites: Prof Terry O'Neill, Ann McGovern, Jennifer Green, Angharad Walker (Salford Royal Hospital); Prof Ian Bruce, Lindsey Barnes, Elizabeth Beswick, Sarah Evans (Manchester Royal Infirmary); Dr. Leena Dass, Dr. Sophia Naz, Lorraine Lock (North Manchester General Hospital); Dr. Chris Deighton, Alison Booth, Jo Morris (Royal Derby Hospital); Prof David Walsh, Debbie Wilson, Jayne Smith (Kings Mill Hospital, Sherwood Forest Hospitals NHS Foundation Trust); Dr. Chetan Mukhtyer, Loretta Dean, Susan Rowell (Norfolk and Norwich Hospitals); Dr. Bela Szenbenyi, Carol Gray (Diana Princess of Wales, Grimsby); Dr. Mike Green, Anne Gill, Lisa Carr (York Hospital); Dr. Kirsten Mackay, Julie Easterbrook, Liz Burnett (Torbay Hospital); Dr. Mike Green, Alison Miernik, Rachel Bailey-Hague (Harrogate District Hospital); Dr. Atheer Al-Ansari, Jayne Edwards, Julia Nicholas (Robert Jones & Agnes Hunt Hospital, Oswestry); Dr. Wendy Holden, Janet Cushnaghan, Angie Dempster, Hayley Paterson (Basingstoke and North Hampshire Hospital); Mr. David Johnson, Lindsey Barber, Jan Smith (Stepping Hill Hospital); Dr. Karen Douglas, Lucy Kadiki, Chitra Ramful, Daljit Kaur (Russell Hall Hospital, Dudley); Dr. Anca Ghiurlic, Christine Graver (Royal Hampshire Hospital, Winchester); Dr. Frank McKenna, Jane McConiffe (Trafford Hospitals); Dr. Sophia Naz and Lorraine Lock (Fairfield Hospital).

Funding
This project was funded by Arthritis Research UK [Grant No: 20031]. NHS service support costs were secured from the Greater Manchester Comprehensive Local Research Network (the Lead CLRN).

Authors' contributions
AH was the chief investigator, overseeing all stages of the research and writing up. AH and ST designed the study. AH and YP initiated the study and YP was the study co-ordinator and conducted cognitive debriefing interviews in Stage 1. AH conducted the statistical analyses. AH, YP and ST were all members of the Study Management Group reviewing progress and discussing findings. All authors contributed to and approved the final manuscript.

Competing interests
The authors declare that they have no competing interests.

Author details
[1]Centre for Health Sciences Research (OT), L701 Allerton, University of Salford, Frederick Road, Salford M6 6PU, UK. [2]Division of Nursing, Midwifery & Social Work, University of Manchester, Manchester, UK.

References
1. Horsten NCA, Ursum J, Roorda LD, van Schaardenburg D, Dekker J, Hoeksma AF. Prevalence of hand symptoms, impairments and activity limitations in rheumatoid arthritis in relation to disease duration. J Rehabil Med. 2010;42:916–21.

2. Olofsson Y, Book C, Jacobsson LT. Shoulder joint involvement in patients with newly diagnosed rheumatoid arthritis. Prevalence and associations. Scand J Rheumatol. 2003;32:25–32.

3. Bilberg A, Bremmell T, Baolgh I, Mannerkorpi K. Significantly impaired shoulder function in the first years of rheumatoid arthritis: a controlled study. Arth Res Ther. 17:261.

4. National Collaborating Centre for Chronic Conditions. Rheumatoid arthritis: national clinical guidelines for management and treatment in adults. London: Royal College of Physicians; 2009.

5. Beaton DE, Davis AM, Hudak P, McConnell S. The DASH (disabilities of the arm, shoulder and hand) outcome measure: what do we know about it now? Brit J Hand Ther. 2001;6(4):109–18.

6. Bilberg A, Bremmell T, Mannerkorpi K. Disability of the arm, shoulder and hand questionnaire in Swedish patients with rheumatoid arthritis: a validity study. J Rehabil Med. 2012;44:7–11.

7. Bot SD, Terwee CB, van der Windt DA, Bouter LM, Dekker J, de Vet HC. Clinimetric evaluation of shoulder disability questionnaires: a systematic review of the literature. Ann Rheum Dis. 2004;63:335–41.

8. Angst F, Schwyzer H-K, Aesclimann A, Simmen BR, Goldhahn J. Measures of adult shoulder function: disabilities of the arm, shoulder, and hand questionnaire (DASH) and its short version (QuickDASH), shoulder pain and disability index (SPADI), American shoulder and elbow surgeons (ASES) society standardized shoulder assessment form, constant (Murley) score (CS), simple shoulder test (SST), Oxford shoulder score (OSS), shoulder disability questionnaire (SDQ), and western Ontario shoulder instability index (WOSI). Arthritis Care Res. 2011;63(S11):S174–88.

9. Beaton DE, Wright JG, Katz JN. Development of the QuickDASH: comparison of three item-reduction approaches. J Bone Joint Surg Am. 2005;87:1038–46.

10. Gummesson C, Ward MM, Atroshi I. The shortened disabilities of the arm, shoulder and hand questionnaire (quick DASH): validity and reliability based on responses within the full-length DASH. BMC Musculoskelet Disord. 2006; 7(44):1–7.

11. Kennedy CA, Beaton DE, Solway S, McConell S, Bombardier C. The DASH and QuickDASH outcome measure user's manual. 3rd ed: Toronto, Institute for Work & Health; 2011.

12. Acquadro C, Joyce CRB, Patrick DL, Ware JE, Wu AW. Linguistic validation manual for patient-reported outcomes (PRO) instruments. Lyon: Mapi Research Trust; 2004. https://store.mapigroup.com/.

13. Beaton DE, Bombardier C, Guillemin F, Marcos Bozi F. Guidelines for the process of cross-cultural adaptation of self-report measures. Spine. 2004;25: 3186–91.

14. Institute for Work and Health. DASH: Available Translations. http://www. dash.iwh.on.ca/available-translations. Downloaded on 23.7.17.

15. Veehof MM, Sleegers EJA, van Veldhoven NHJM, Schuurman AH, van Meeteren NLU. Psychometric qualities of the Dutch language version of the disabilities of the arm, shoulder and hand questionnaire (DASH-DLV). J Hand Ther. 2002;15:347–54.

16. Imaeda T, Toh S, Nakao Y, Nishida J, Hirata H, Ijichi M, Kohri C, Nagano A. Validation of the Japanese Society of Surgery for the hand version of the disability of the arm, shoulder and hand questionnaire. J Orthop Sci. 2005; 10:353–9.

17. Lee EWC, Chung MMH, Li APS, Lo SK. Construct validity of the Chinese version of the disabilities of the arm, shoulder and hand questionnaire (DASH HK-PWH). J Hand Surg (Br). 2005;30B(1):29–34.

18. Rodrigues J, Zhang W, Scammell B, Russell P, Chakrabarti I, Fullilove S, Davidson D, Davis T. Validity of the disabilities of the arm, shoulder and hand patient reported outcome measure (DASH) and the QuickDASH when used on Dupuytren's disease. J Hand Surg (Eur). 2016;41E:589 99.

19. Fayad F, Lefevre-Colau M-M, Mace Y, Fermanian J, Mayoux-Benhamou A, Roren A, Rannou F, Roby-Brami A, Gautheron V, Revel M, Poiradeau S. Validation of the French version of the disability of the arm, shoulder and hand questionnaire (F-DASH). Joint Bone Spine. 2008;75:195–200.

20. Franchignoni F, Giordano A, Sartorio F, Vercelli S, Pascariello B, Ferriero G. Suggestions for refinement of the disabilities of the arm, shoulder and hand outcome measure: (DASH): a factor analysis and rasch validation study. Arch Phys Med Rehabil. 2010;91:1370–7.

21. Lehman LA, Woodbury M, Velozo CA. Examination of the factor structure of the disabilities of the arm, shoulder and hand questionnaire. Am J Occ Ther. 2011;65:169–78.

22. Mokkink LB, Terwee CB, Patrick DL, Alonso J, Stratford PW, Knol DL, et al. The COSMIN checklist for assessing the methodological quality of studies on measurement properties of health status measurement instruments: an international Delphi study. Qual Life Res. 2010;19:539–49.

23. Beaton DE, Bombardier C, Guillemin F, Ferraz MB. Recommendations for the Cross-Cultural Adaptation of the DASH & QuickDASH Outcome Measures. Toronto: Institute of Work and Health; 2007. http://www.dash.iwh.on.ca/translation-guidelines. Downloaded 23.7.17.

24. Willis GB, Miller K. Cross cultural cognitive interviewing: seeking comparability and enhancing understanding. Field Methods. 2011;23(4):331–41.

25. Stucki G, Cieza A, Geyh S, Battistella L, Lloyd J, Simmons D, Kostansjek N, Schouten J. ICF Core set for rheumatoid arthritis. J Rehabil Med Suppl. 2004; 44:87–93.

26. International Classification of Functioning, Disability and Health (ICF) Core Sets for Musculoskeletal Conditions (RA) (2013). Geneva: ICF Research Branch. https://www.icf-research-branch.org/download/send/7-musculoskeletalconditions/126-comprehensiveandbrieficfcoresetsrheumatoidarthritis. Accessed 31.7.17.

27. Drummond AS, Sampaio RF, Mancini MC, Kirkwood RN, Stamm TA. Linking the disabilities of arm, shoulder and hand to the international classification of functioning, disability and health. J Hand Ther. 2007;20:336–44.

28. Hudek PL, Amadio PC, Bombardier C. The upper extremity collaborative group. Development of an upper extremity outcome measure: the DASH (disabilities of the arm, shoulder and hand). Am J Ind Med. 1995; 29(5):602–8.

29. Ware JE, Sherbourne CD. The MOS 36-item short-form health survey (SF-36). I. Conceptual framework and item selection. Med Care. 1992;30:473–83.

30. Ware JE. SF-36 health survey update. Spine. 2000;25:3130–9.

31. QualityMetric Health Outcomes™ Scoring Software 4.5. Lincoln, RI: QualityMetric, Incorporated. 24 Albion Road, Bldg 400. Lincoln, R.I. 02865, U.S.A.

32. Kirwan JR, Reeback JS. Stanford health assessment questionnaire modified to assess disability in British patients with rheumatoid arthritis. Br J Rheumatol. 1986;25:26–9.

33. Tennant A, Hillman M, Fear J, Pickering A, Chamberlain MA. Are we making the most of the Stanford health assessment questionnaire? Br J Rheumatol. 1996;35:574–8.

34. Wolfe F. Which HAQ is best? A comparison of the HAQ, MHAQ and RA-HAQ, a difficult 8 item HAQ (DHAQ), and a rescored 20 item HAQ (HAQ20): analyses in 2491 rheumatoid arthritis patients following leflunomide initiation. J Rheumatol. 2001;28:982–9.

35. Johnsson PM, Eberhardt K. Hand deformities are important signs of disease severity in patients with early rheumatoid arthritis. Rheumatology. 2009;48:1398–401.

36. Prior Y, Hammond A, Tyson S, Tennant A. Development and testing of the British English measure of activity performance of the HAND (MAP_HAND) questionnaire in rheumatoid arthritis. Ann Rheum Dis. 2015; 74(Suppl 2):1324.

37. Prior Y, Tennant A, Hammond A, Tyson S. Psychometric testing of measure of activity performance in the hand (map-hand) questionnaire in rheumatoid arthritis: Rasch analysis. Clin Rehabil. 2015;29(10):1014.

38. Hammond A, Tennant A, Tyson A, Nordenskiold U, Hawkins R, Prior Y. The reliability and validity of the English version of the evaluation of daily activity questionnaire for people with rheumatoid arthritis. Rheumatology. 2015;54(9):1605–15.

39. De Jong Z, van der Heijde D, McKenna SP, Whalley D. The reliability and construct validity of the RAQoL: a rheumatoid arthritis-specific quality of life instrument. Br J Rheumatol. 1997;36:878–83.

40. Teresi JA, Kleinman M, Ocepek-Welikson K. Modern psychometric methods for detection of differential item functioning: application to cognitive assessment measures. Stat Med. 2000;19(11–12):1651–83.

41. Nunnally JC. Psychometric theory. New York: McGraw-Hill; 1978.

42. IBM Corp. IBM SPSS statistics for windows, version 20.0. IBM Corp. Released: Armonk; 2011.

43. MedCalc for Windows. Version 16.2, vol. 1. Belgium: MedCalc Software, Ostend; 2016.

44. Evans JD. Straightforward statistics for the behavioural sciences. In: Pacific grove (CA):brooks/Cole publishing; 1996.

45. Cichetti DV. Guidelines, criteria and rules of thumb for evaluating normed and standardised assessment instrument in psychology. Psychol Assessment. 1994;6:284–90.

46. Altman DG. Practical statistics for medical research. London: Chapman Hall; 1991.

47. Stratford PW. Getting more from the literature: estimating the standard error of measurement from reliability studies. Physiother Can. 2004;56:27–30.

48. Donoghue D. PROP group and stokes E. How much change is true change? The minimum detectable change of the berg balance scale in elderly people. J Rehabil Med. 2009;41:343–6.

49. Fitzpatrick R, Davey C, Buxton MJ, Jones DR. Evaluating patient-based outcome measures for use in clinical trials. Health Technol Assess. 1998; 2(14). NHS R&D HTA Programme. https://lra.le.ac.uk/bitstream/2381/1389/1/mon214.pdf. Accessed 28 July 17.

50. Terwee CB, Bot SDM, de Boer MR, et al. Quality criteria were prosed for measurement properties of health status questionnaires. J Clin Epidemiol. 2007;60:34–42.

51. Kincaid JP, Fishburne RP Jr, Rogers RL, Chissom BS. Derivation of new readability formulas (Automated Readability Index, Fog Count and Flesch Reading Ease Formula) for Navy enlisted personnel. Research Branch Report, 8–75. Millington: Naval Technical Training, U. S. Naval Air Station, Memphis, TN; 1975.

52. Vamos M, White GL, Caughey DE. Body image in rheumatoid arthritis: the relevance of hand appearance to desire for surgery. Br J med Psychol. 1990; 63:267–77.

53. Aktekin LA, Eser F, Baskan BM, Sivas F, Malhan S, Oksuz E, Bodur H. Disability of arm shoulder and hand questionnaire in rheumatoid arthritis patients: relationship with disease activity, HAQ, SF-36. Rheum Internat. 2011;31(6):823–6.

54. Raven EEJ, Haverkamp D, Sierevelt IN, van Montfoort DO, Poll RG, Blankevoort L, Tak PP. Construct validity and reliability of the disability of arm, shoulder, hand questionnaire for upper extremity complaints in rheumatoid arthritis. J Rheumatol. 2008;35:2334–8.

55. Mokkink LB, Terwee CB, Patrick DL, Alonso J, Stratford PW, Knol DL, Bouter LM, Devet HCW. COSMIN Checklist manual v1 2012. http://www.cosmin.nl/cosmin_checklist.html. Accessed 31 July 17.

56. Hammond A, Prior Y, Tyson S. Disabilities of the Arm, Shoulder and Hand – British English. http://www.dash.iwh.on.ca/sites/dash/public/translations/DASH_English_UK.pdf Accessed 30 July 17.

57. Hammond A, Prior Y, Tyson S. The QuickDASH – British English. http://www.dash.iwh.on.ca/sites/dash/public/translations/QuickDASH_English_UK.pdf. Accessed 30 July 17.

7

Comparison of mesenchymal stem cells obtained by suspended culture of synovium from patients with rheumatoid arthritis and osteoarthritis

Yuji Kohno[1], Mitsuru Mizuno[1], Nobutake Ozeki[1], Hisako Katano[1], Koji Otabe[1], Hideyuki Koga[2], Mikio Matsumoto[3], Haruka Kaneko[3], Yuji Takazawa[3] and Ichiro Sekiya[1*]

Abstract

Background: Mobilization of mesenchymal stem cells (MSCs) from the synovium was revealed using a "suspended synovium culture model" of osteoarthritis (OA). The pathology of rheumatoid arthritis (RA) differs from that of OA. We investigated whether mobilization of MSCs from the synovium also occurred in RA, and we compared the properties of synovial MSCs collected from suspended synovium culture models of RA and OA.

Methods: Human synovium was harvested during total knee arthroplasty from the knee joints of patients with RA ($n = 8$) and OA ($n = 6$). The synovium was suspended in a bottle containing culture medium and a culture dish at the bottom. Cells were harvested from the dish and analyzed.

Results: No significant difference was observed between RA and OA in the harvested cell numbers per g of synovium. However, the variation in the number of cells harvested from each donor was greater for RA than for OA. The harvested cells were multipotent and no difference was observed in the cartilage pellet weight between RA and OA. The surface epitopes of the cells in RA and OA were similar to those of MSCs.

Conclusion: Mobilization of MSCs from the synovium was demonstrated using a suspended synovium culture model for RA. The harvested cell numbers, chondrogenic potentials, and surface epitope profiles were comparable between the RA and OA models.

Keywords: Synovial mesenchymal stem cell (synovial MSC), MSC mobilization, Suspended synovium culture model, Rheumatoid arthritis, Osteoarthritis, Harvested cell number, Chondrogenic potential

Background

Mesenchymal stem cells (MSCs) are seldom detected in samples of synovial fluid from the knees of healthy volunteers [1–3]. However, the number of MSCs in the synovial fluid increases with the radiologic grade of osteoarthritis (OA) [2]. The cell morphology and gene profiles of MSCs from the synovial fluid of patients with OA have a stronger resemblance to those from the synovium than from the bone marrow, suggesting an intriguing possibility that MSCs found in synovial fluid originate from the synovium and that OA can trigger the release of MSCs from the synovium into the synovial fluid [1]. We have recently demonstrated a "suspended synovium culture model" in which MSCs from the synovium of patients with OA were mobilized into a non-contacted culture dish through culture medium [4].

MSCs are also found in the synovial fluid of patients with rheumatoid arthritis (RA), an autoimmune condition characterized by inflammation, usually in bilateral joints, and systemic features such as fatigue or fever [5–7]. However, an unanswered question is whether the synovium of patients with RA directly releases MSCs into the synovial fluid, as occurs in patients with OA, because the pathological conditions of RA and OA are different. A further

* Correspondence: sekiya.arm@tmd.ac.jp
[1]Center for Stem Cells and Regenerative Medicine, Tokyo Medical and Dental University, 1-5-45 Yushima, Bunkyo-ku, Tokyo 113-8510, Japan
Full list of author information is available at the end of the article

possibility is that the use of anti-inflammatory drugs in patients with RA may affect the synovium as a source of MSCs in the synovial fluid.

The primary aim of this study was to evaluate the possible release of MSCs from the synovium in a suspended synovium culture model of RA. Since some properties of synovial MSCs may vary depending on disease etiology, a secondary aim was to compare the properties of synovial MSCs obtained from the suspended synovium culture models of RA and OA.

Methods

Synovium harvest and 'suspended synovium culture'

This study was approved by local institutional review boards (the Medical Research Ethics Committee of Tokyo Medical and Dental University and the Hospital Ethics Committee of Juntendo University Hospital), and informed consent was obtained from all study subjects. Human synovium was harvested during total knee arthroplasty from knee joints of patients with RA (8 donors) and OA (6 donors). The patients ranged in age from 49 to 79 years for RA donors and from 55 to 78 years for OA donors. Patient demographics are listed in Table 1.

The synovium was cut into six approximately 1 g pieces with a surgical knife and washed thoroughly with phosphate-buffered saline (PBS; Invitrogen, Carlsbad, CA) to remove blood traces. Each synovium piece was sutured with 4–0 nylon thread and suspended in a 100 mL bottle (Sarstedt, Numbrecht, Germany) containing a 35-mm-diameter culture dish (Thermo Fisher Scientific, Yokohama, Japan) placed at the bottom. The

culture dish contained 40 mL of a-modified Eagle medium (a-MEM; Invitrogen) with 10% fetal bovine serum (Invitrogen), and 1% penicillin/streptomycin (Invitrogen) (Fig. 1).

After culturing for 7 days at 37 °C, three dishes were stained with 0.5% crystal violet (Wako, Osaka, Japan) in 10% formalin for 5 min, washed twice with distilled water, and the cell colonies were observed by light microscopy. The synovium before and 7 days after suspended culture was examined histologically.

The other three dishes from each donor were left in the bottles with the suspended synovium for 14 days, and passage 0 cells were collected for cell counting. The cells were then replated, cultured for a further14 days, and analyzed for differentiation and surface epitopes.

Histological analysis

The synovium before and 7 days after suspended culture was fixed in 10% formalin, embedded in paraffin wax, sectioned at 5 μm, and stained with hematoxylin and eosin. Each sample was assigned to one of three grades according to the thickness of the synovial intima: grade 1 = synovial intima less than four cells thick; grade 2 = synovial intima four to six cells thick; and grade 3 = synovial intima seven or more cells thick [8, 9].

Differentiation assay

For chondrogenesis, 2.5×10^5 cells were transferred to a 15 ml tube (BD Falcon) and cultured in chondrogenic induction medium containing 10 ng/ml transforming growth factor-β3 (Miltenyi Biotec Japan, Tokyo, Japan)

Table 1 Patient demographics

Group	Patient number	Age	Sex	CRP (mg/dl)	ESR (mm)	Medicine		
						PSL (mg /day)	DMARDs other than biologics	Biologics
RA	#1	49	F	0.1	17	2	MTX	ETN
	#2	79	F	5.7	98			
	#3	65	F	0.02	39	5	TCR, IGU	TCZ
	#4	55	F	2.3	47	2	MTX, SASP	TCZ
	#5	79	F	0.1	12	2.5	BUC, SASP	
	#6	38	F	0.0		2	MTX	TCZ
	#7	50	F	2.5	52		MTX, AZA	
	#8	73	F	0.3	2	2		ETN
OA	#9	62	M	0.1	5			
	#10	72	F	0.1	5			
	#11	78	F	0.0	19			
	#12	72	M	0.0	8			
	#13	55	F	0.2	20			
	#14	73	F	0.1	15			

The mean of age was 61 years old in RA group, and 69 years old in OA group: no significant difference between them ($p = 0.56$ by Mann-Whitney's U test). *PSL* Prednisolone, *MTX* Methotrexate, *TCR* Tacrolimus, *IGU* Iguratimod, *SASP* Salazosulfapyridine, *BUC* Bucillamine, *AZA* Azathioprine, *ETN* Etanercept, *TCZ* Tocilizumab

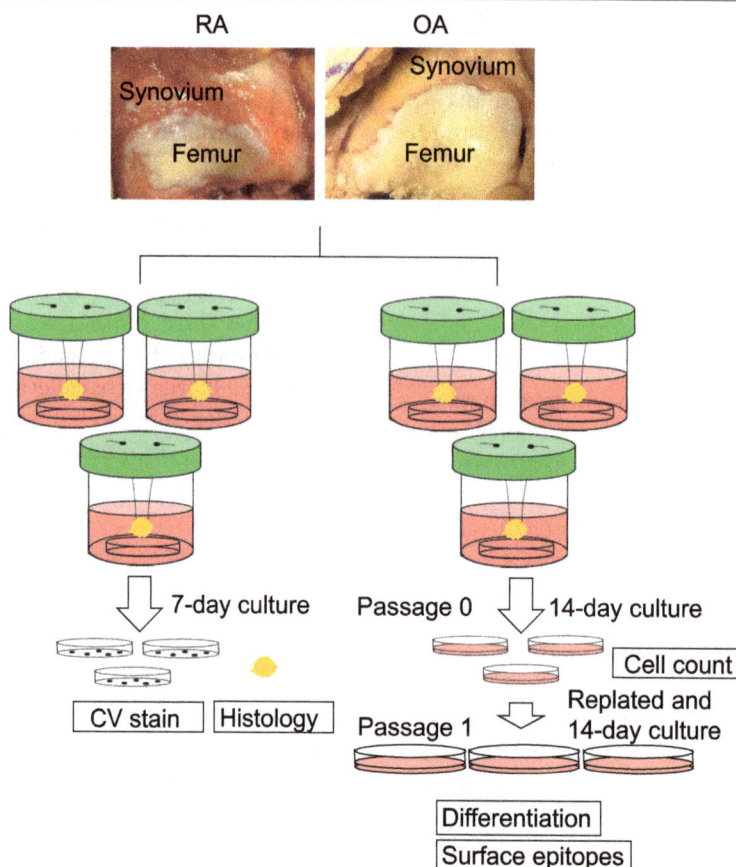

Fig. 1 Suspended synovium culture protocol. Human synovium was harvested during total knee arthroplasty from knee joints of patients with rheumatoid arthritis (RA; n = 8) and osteoarthritis (OA; n = 6). Approximately 1 g of synovium from each donor was suspended in each of six bottles that contained culture medium and a culture dish placed at the bottom of the bottle. After seven days of suspended synovium culture, three dishes were stained with 0.5% crystal violet and the suspended synovium was also examined histologically. After fourteen days of suspended synovium culture, the harvested cell numbers were evaluated from the remaining three dishes for each donor. The cells were passaged again and used for differentiation assays and analysis of surface epitope expression

and 500 ng/ml bone morphogenetic protein 2 (BMP-2, Infuse; Medtronic, Minneapolis, MN); this medium was changed every 3–4 days. After 21 days, the cell pellets were embedded, sectioned and stained with safranin O and fast green (Wako, Tokyo, Japan).

Calcification was studied by plating 100 cells in a 60 cm^2 dish and culturing for 14 days in α-MEM with 10% fetal bovine serum. Adherent cells were subsequently cultured in an osteogenic induction medium containing 50 μg/ml ascorbic acid 2-phosphate (Wako), 10 nM dexamethasone (Wako), and 10 mM β-glycerophosphate (Sigma-Aldrich); this medium was changed every 3–4 days. After 14 days, calcification was assessed by alizarin red (Merck Millipore, Billerica, MA) staining.

Adipogenesis was evaluated by plating 100 cells in a 60 cm^2 dish and culturing for 14 days to allow colony formation. Adherent cells were cultured in an adipogenic induction medium supplemented with 100 nM dexamethasone, 0.5 mM isobutylmethylxanthine (Sigma-Aldrich), and 50 mM indomethacin (Wako) for an

additional 14 days; this medium was changed every 3–4 days. Adipocyte colonies were stained with oil red O (Muto Pure Chemicals, Tokyo, Japan).

Flow cytometry analysis

Passage 2 cells were suspended in Hank's Balanced Salt Solution (HBSS) at a density of 5×10^5 cells/mL and stained for 30 min on ice with the following antibodies: CD11b-PE, CD11c-PE-Cy7, CD14-APC, CD31-FITC, CD44-APCH7, CD45-FITC, CD73-BV421, CD90-PE, CD105-PerCP-Cy5.5, CD206-FITC, and HLADR-APC (BD, Franklin Lakes, NJ). Cell surface antigens were analyzed using a triple-laser FACS Verse™ system (BD).

Statistical analysis

The results were analyzed using Mann-Whitney's U test with GraphPad Prism 6 (GraphPad Software, La Jolla, CA, USA). P values < 0.05 were considered significant.

Results

After seven days of suspended synovium culture, cell colonies were observed in the dishes in both the RA and OA samples (Fig. 2a). No significant difference was noted for the passage 0 cell numbers between the RA and OA cultures: the passage 0 harvested cell numbers after 14 days of suspended synovium culture was $2.6 \times 10^5 \pm 2.0 \times 10^5$ cells/g synovium for the RA and $2.4 \times 10^5 \pm 0.7 \times 10^5$ cells/g synovium for the OA samples (Fig. 2b). However, the passage 0 cell numbers varied greatly among the RA samples depending on the donor, whereas these numbers were similar in the OA samples. An F-test analysis revealed a significant difference in this variation ($P = 0.04$) (Fig. 2b). The harvested cell numbers for passage 1 were $3.2 \times 10^6 \pm 2.0 \times 10^6$ cells/g synovium for the RA and $3.7 \times 10^6 \pm 2.1 \times 10^6$ cells/g synovium for the OA samples (Fig. 2c); this difference was not statistically significant ($P > 0.05$).

Histological analysis of the synovium before and after 7 days of suspended culture was conducted after assigning each synovium to one of three grades according to the number of cells in the synovial intima (Fig. 3a). The synovial intima grade decreased after suspended culture in four RA donors, remained constant in three RA donors, and increased in one RA donor, whereas it decreased in two OA donors and remained constant in four OA donors (Fig. 3b).

Differentiation assays confirmed that passage 1 cells formed cartilage pellets that positively stained with safranin O (Fig. 4a) when cultured in chondrogenic medium. The cartilage pellet weight was 4.6 ± 1.1 mg for RA cultures and 4.4 ± 0.9 mg for OA cultures, and this difference was not statistically significant ($P > 0.05$) (Fig. 4b). Passage 1 cells calcified (Fig. 4c) and differentiated into adipocytes (Fig. 4d) when cultured in differentiation media.

The surface epitopes expressed by passage 1 cells included the MSC markers CD44, CD73, and CD90 at high level ($> 90\%$) and CD105 at a moderate or high level ($> 60\%$) (Fig. 5). Passage 1 cells also expressed the hematopoietic markers CD11b, CD11c, CD14, CD31 & 45, CD206 and HLA-DR at low levels ($< 10\%$). The expression profiles appeared similar between the RA and OA cells.

Discussion

MSCs are characterized by their colony-forming ability and their multipotency for differentiating in vitro into chondrocytes, adipocytes, and osteoblasts [10]. In this study, suspended synovium culture resulted in the appearance of colony forming cells in the dish at the base of the culture bottle. These cells showed characteristics of MSCs, including the potential for multilineage differentiation and expression of surface epitopes common to

MSCs. The colony forming cells obtained from the suspended synovium culture therefore appeared to be MSCs.

These MSCs, when derived from the synovium from RA donors, mobilized through culture medium to a culture dish. Marinova-Mutafchieva et al. detected MSCs in the synovial fluid of patients with RA [7]. Yan et al. demonstrated that intraarticular injection of MSCs improved cartilage condition in a murine collagen-induced arthritis model [11]. Taken together, these findings indicate that MSCs are mobilized from the synovium into the synovial fluid and that they participate in tissue repair by ensuring replacement of the mature cells that are lost during the course of disease in RA patients.

The MSCs obtained from the suspended synovium cultures from RA and OA donors had similar mean harvested cell numbers at passage 0 and passage 1, chondrogenic potential, and surface epitope profiles. We previously reported similar results for a comparison of the properties of synovial MSCs obtained using digested synovial cells from RA and OA donors in a standard cell culture [12]. This similarity between the current findings from suspended synovium culture and our previous results from standard cell culture is interesting because migrated cells from synovium and digested cells in synovium are seemed to have similar properties.

The number of cells harvested following suspended synovium culture at passage 0 varied greatly among the RA samples from different donors. We noted a similar response in our previous study that used standard cell culture and determined that the variations were due to differences in nucleated cell numbers per synovium weight between samples obtained from RA and OA donors [12]. The present finding was also due to a wider variation in the nucleated cell numbers per synovium weight among the RA samples when compared to the OA samples.

The changes in the synovial intima grade (Fig. 3) and the harvested cell number (Fig. 2) were not correlated. We had expected that the synovial intima grade would decrease following suspended culture because the synovial intima cells moved through the medium from the suspended synovium into the dish. Two reasons may explain why the synovial intima grade did not decrease in all donors. One reason may be that the same area of the synovium could not be evaluated histologically before and after the suspension. A second reason may be that both synovial intima cells and subsynovial cells may have moved through the medium into the dish.

We previously demonstrated a relationship between the synovitis score and the total yield of synovial MSCs in a rat carrageenan-induced arthritis model [13]. In the current human study, C-reactive protein (CRP) levels were over 2 mg/dl, and erythrocyte sedimentation rate

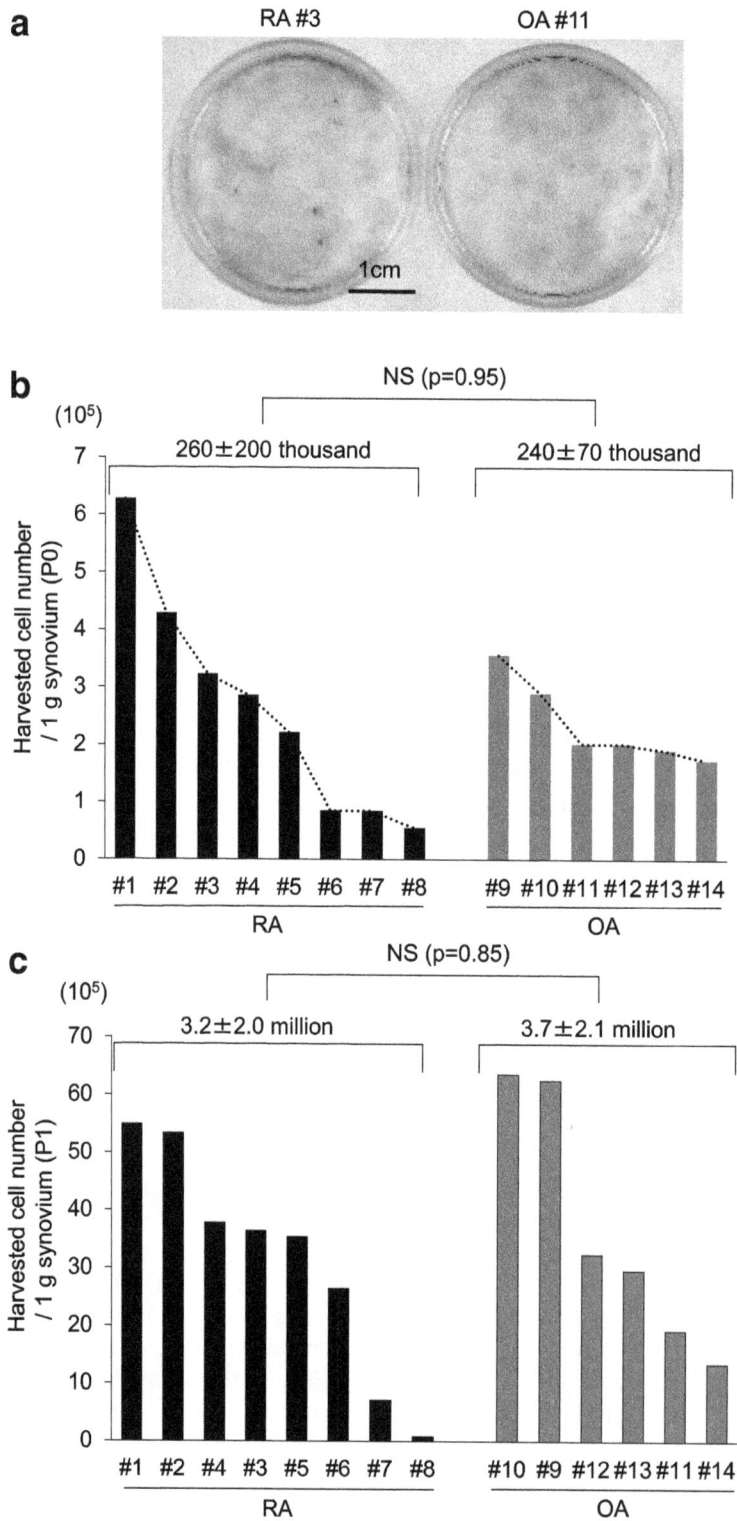

Fig. 2 Cell colonies and harvested cell numbers after suspended culture of synovium from patients with rheumatoid arthritis (RA; $n = 8$) and osteoarthritis (OA; $n = 6$). **a** Representative cell colonies stained with crystal violet after 7 days of suspended synovium culture. **b** Passage 0 cell numbers/g synovium after 14 days of suspended synovium culture. **c** Passage 1 cell numbers/g synovium after 14 days of culture of passage 0 cells. Average values with standard deviation are shown (RA, $n = 8$; OA, $n = 6$). NS: not significant

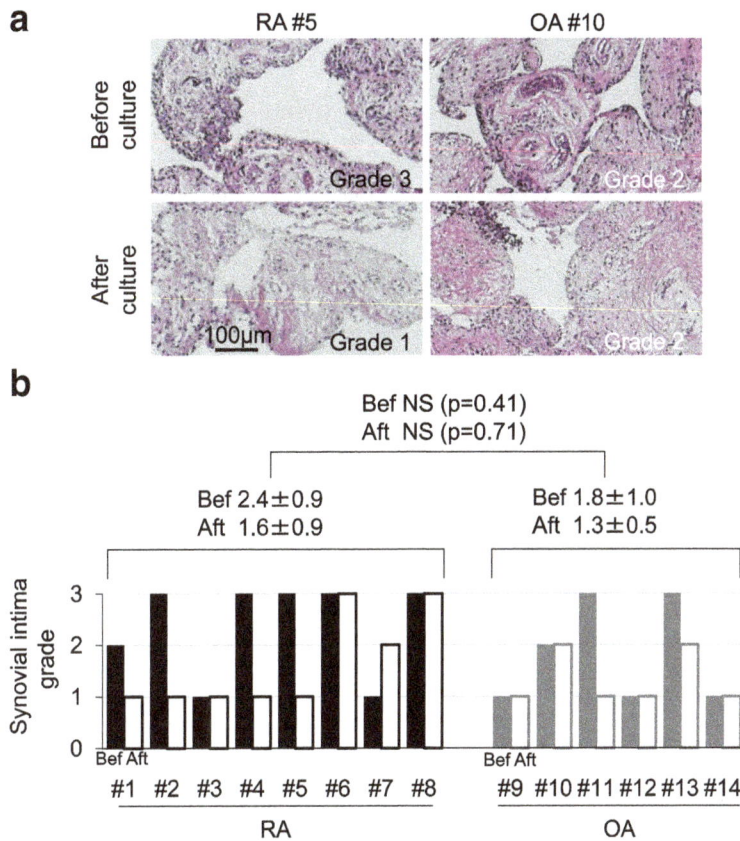

Fig. 3 Histological analysis of synovium from patients with rheumatoid arthritis (RA; $n = 8$) and osteoarthritis (OA; $n = 6$) before and after 7 days of suspended culture. **a** Representative sections stained with hematoxylin and eosin. Each synovium was assigned to one of three grades according to the thickness of the synovial intima: grade 1 = synovial intima less than four cells thick; grade 2 = synovial intima four to six cells thick; and grade 3 = synovial intima seven or more cells thick. **b** Synovial intima grade before and after 7 days of suspended synovium culture. Bef: before, Aft: after, NS: not significant

(ESR) levels were over 40 mm in RA donors #2, #4, and #7, whereas these levels were within the normal limits in all patients with OA (Table 1). In only RA #7 were the harvested cell numbers of both P0 and P1 lower (Fig. 2b, c) and the synovial intima grade determined to be lower by histological analysis (Fig. 3). Therefore, serological inflammation levels did not affect the harvested cell number after suspended synovium culture, and these levels did not seem to affect the synovial intima grade determined by histological analysis. Drugs used to treat RA might affect these outcomes.

In the current study, synovium was suspended in the culture medium containing FBS. This raised the question whether MSCs would also mobilize from the synovium if synovial fluid from the patients was used instead of culture medium. We previously found a greater expansion of synovial MSCs derived from OA donors when the MSCs were cultured in a two-dimensional system containing autologous synovial fluid than in a culture medium containing FBS [14]. This suggests that synovial MSCs would also

mobilize into synovial fluid in the suspended synovium culture model.

In this study, mobilization of MSCs from the synovium was demonstrated by the "suspended synovium culture model." We observed a direct migration of the cells from the synovium to a dish placed on the bottom of the culture bottle using time-lapse video (data not shown). The movie showed that many cells were released from the synovium just after the culture started, the cells migrated to the dish, and some of the cells formed cell colonies.

Inherent synovial fibroblasts play an important role, especially in RA. In the suspended culture model, two possibilities arose: the mobilized cells could be exclusively MSCs or they could be a mixture of MSCs and fibroblasts. The time-lapse movie indicated that the suspended synovium releases both fibroblasts and synovial MSCs, and that after 14 days of culture, most of the cells are MSCs because MSCs are remarkably different from fibroblasts in terms of their high proliferative potential and colony forming ability.

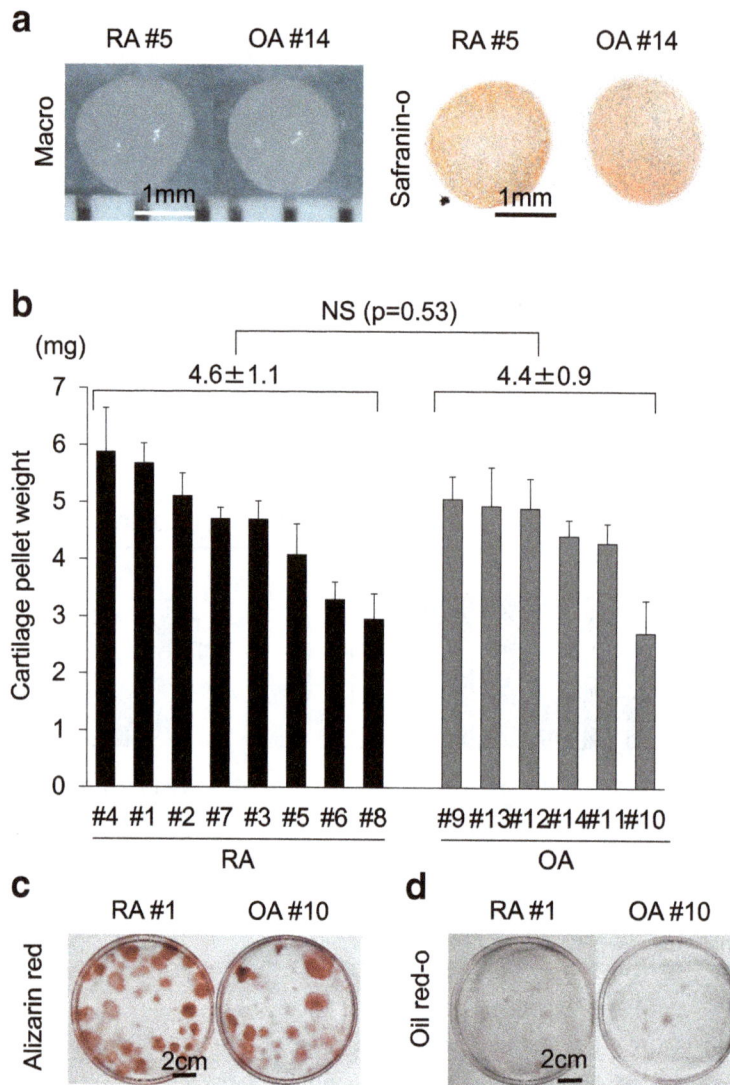

Fig. 4 Differentiation assays of the cells passaged after suspended culture of synovium from patients with rheumatoid arthritis (RA; $n = 8$) and osteoarthritis (OA; $n = 6$). **a** Chondrogenesis. Representative macro pictures and histological sections stained with safranin O are shown. **b** Cartilage pellet weight. Average values with standard deviation are shown. NS: not significant. **c** Calcification. Representative cell colonies stained with alizarin red are shown. **d** Adipogenesis. Representative cell colonies stained with oil red O are shown

We did not show unstimulated cells as controls for the differentiation assays. We have previously reported that MSCs do not differentiate into chondrocytes unless cultured in a chondrogenic medium [15, 16]. The MSCs also do not differentiate into adipocytes without an adipogenic medium [17]. Many papers have reported that MSCs are not calcified without a calcification medium [18]. Therefore, we did not prepare unstimulated cells as controls for the differentiation assays.

In this paper, we used the term "calcification" rather than "osteogenesis." We had previously investigated gene expression profiles of MSCs during chondrogenesis, adipogenesis, and "osteogenesis." The expression of chondrogenesis-related genes, such as Sox9, Aggrecan, and COL2A1, increased during chondrogenesis [19], as did the expression of adipogenesis-related genes, such as PPARγ, LPL, and FABP4, during adipogenesis [17]. However, we were unable to confirm a significant increase in the expression of osteogenesis-specific genes, such as Osterix, Runx2, and Osteocalcin, during "osteogenesis," despite the positive staining of the MSCs with alizarin red (data not shown). For that reason, we have used the term "calcification" instead of "osteogenesis" [1, 3, 12].

We propose three limitations for the model and this study. One limitation was the small sample number, which precluded the performance of detailed analyses. The second limitation was the varied treatment histories of the patients with RA, which precluded a full analysis

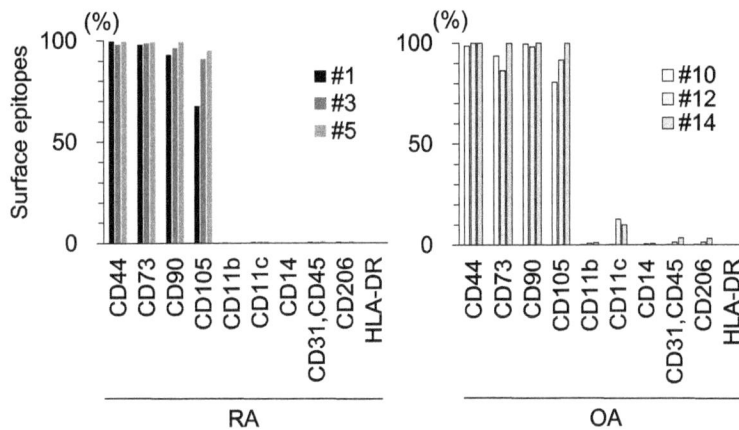

Fig. 5 Cell surface markers expressed by synovial cells passaged after suspended culture of synovium from patients with rheumatoid arthritis (RA; $n = 8$) and osteoarthritis (OA; $n = 6$)

of the effects of drugs. The third limitation was the low yield of passage 0 synovial MSCs, which prevented analysis of differentiation and surface epitope expression. One additional passage of passage 1 synovial MSCs may reduce the differences observed in the properties of synovial MSCs obtained from RA and OA donors.

Conclusion

We revealed a mobilization of MSCs from suspended synovium from a RA donor through culture medium into a culture dish. The harvested cell numbers at passage 0 showed a greater variation for RA samples than for OA samples. The mean harvested cell numbers at passage 0 and 1, chondrogenic potential, and MSC surface epitope expression were similar for synovium from RA and OA donors.

Abbreviations
BMP-2: Bone morphogenetic protein 2; CRP: C-reactive protein; ESR: Erythrocyte sedimentation rate; MSCs: Mesenchymal stem cells; OA: Osteoarthritis; RA: Rheumatoid arthritis; α-MEM: Alpha minimum essential medium

Acknowledgements
We thank all the members of the Center for Stem Cells and Regenerative Medicine, Tokyo Medical and Dental University, and especially Mr. Keiichiro Komori and Ms. Shizuka Fujii for flow cytometry analysis and cell culture, Dr. Kenta Katagiri for experiment instruction, and Ms. Mika Watanabe and Ms. Kimiko Takanashi for the management of our laboratory. We also thank Dr. Takeshi Muneta, Ms. Moe Takenoshita, and Ms. Ellen Roider for proofreading the manuscript. This study was supported by JSPS KAKENHI Grant Number 15 K10463 and 17 K16676.

Funding
HKat was funded from JSPS KAKENHI Grant Number 15 K10463, and KO was funded from JSPS KAKENHI Grant Number 17 K16676.

Authors' contributions
YK designed the study, performed all experiments, and wrote the manuscript. MMi, NO, and HKat provided ideas and revised the manuscript. KO and HKo obtained informed consent, collected human tissues, and revised the manuscript. MMa, HKan, and YT obtained informed consent, collected human tissues, and proofread the manuscript. IS provided ideas, organized the data, and completed the manuscript. All authors read and approved the submitted draft of the paper.

Consent for publication
Not applicable.

Competing interests
The authors declare that they have no competing interests.

Author details
[1]Center for Stem Cells and Regenerative Medicine, Tokyo Medical and Dental University, 1-5-45 Yushima, Bunkyo-ku, Tokyo 113-8510, Japan. [2]Department of Joint Surgery and Sports Medicine, Tokyo Medical and Dental University, 1-5-45 Yushima, Bunkyo-ku, Tokyo 113-8510, Japan. [3]Department of Orthopaedics, Juntendo University School of Medicine, 3-1-3 Hongo, Bunkyo-ku, Tokyo 113-8431, Japan.

References
1. Morito T, Muneta T, Hara K, Ju YJ, Mochizuki T, Makino H, et al. Synovial fluid-derived mesenchymal stem cells increase after intra-articular ligament injury in humans. Rheumatology (Oxford). 2008;47(8):1137–43. https://doi.org/10.1093/rheumatology/ken114.
2. Sekiya I, Ojima M, Suzuki S, Yamaga M, Horie M, Koga H, et al. Human mesenchymal stem cells in synovial fluid increase in the knee with degenerated cartilage and osteoarthritis. J Orthop Res. 2012;30(6):943–9. https://doi.org/10.1002/jor.22029.
3. Matsukura Y, Muneta T, Tsuji K, Koga H, Sekiya I. Mesenchymal stem cells in synovial fluid increase after meniscus injury. Clin Orthop Relat Res. 2014; 472(5):1357–64. https://doi.org/10.1007/s11999-013-3418-4.
4. Katagiri K, Matsukura Y, Muneta T, Ozeki N, Mizuno M, Katano H, et al. Fibrous synovium releases higher numbers of mesenchymal stem cells than adipose synovium in a suspended synovium culture model. Arthroscopy. 2017;33(4):800–10. https://doi.org/10.1016/j.arthro.2016.09.033.
5. McInnes IB, Schett G. The pathogenesis of rheumatoid arthritis. N Engl J Med. 2011;365(23):2205–19. https://doi.org/10.1056/NEJMra1004965.
6. Jones EA, English A, Henshaw K, Kinsey SE, Markham AF, Emery P, et al. Enumeration and phenotypic characterization of synovial fluid multipotential mesenchymal progenitor cells in inflammatory and degenerative arthritis. Arthritis Rheum. 2004;50(3):817–27. https://doi.org/10.1002/art.20203.
7. Marinova-Mutafchieva L, Taylor P, Funa K, Maini RN, Zvaifler NJ. Mesenchymal cells expressing bone morphogenetic protein receptors are present in the rheumatoid arthritis joint. Arthritis Rheum. 2000;43(9):2046–55. https://doi.org/10.1002/1529-0131(200009)43:9<2046::AID-ANR16>3.0.CO;2-8.

8.   Richardson D, Pearson RG, Kurian N, Latif ML, Garle MJ, Barrett DA, et al. Characterisation of the cannabinoid receptor system in synovial tissue and fluid in patients with osteoarthritis and rheumatoid arthritis. Arthritis Res Ther. 2008;10(2):R43. https://doi.org/10.1186/ar2401.

9.   Haywood L, McWilliams DF, Pearson CI, Gill SE, Ganesan A, Wilson D, et al. Inflammation and angiogenesis in osteoarthritis. Arthritis Rheum. 2003;48(8): 2173–7. https://doi.org/10.1002/art.11094.

10. Dominici M, Le Blanc K, Mueller I, Slaper-Cortenbach I, Marini F, Krause D, et al. Minimal criteria for defining multipotent mesenchymal stromal cells. The International Society for Cellular Therapy position statement. Cytotherapy. 2006;8(4):315–7. https://doi.org/10.1080/14653240600855905.

11. Yan M, Liu X, Dang Q, Huang H, Yang F, Li Y. Intra-articular injection of human synovial membrane-derived mesenchymal stem cells in murine collagen-induced arthritis: assessment of immunomodulatory capacity in vivo. Stem Cells Int. 2017;2017:9198328. https://doi.org/10.1155/2017/9198328.

12. Kohno Y, Mizuno M, Ozeki N, Katano H, Komori K, Fujii S, et al. Yields and chondrogenic potential of primary synovial mesenchymal stem cells are comparable between rheumatoid arthritis and osteoarthritis patients. Stem Cell Res Ther. 2017;8(1):115. https://doi.org/10.1186/s13287-017-0572-8.

13. Matsukura Y, Muneta T, Tsuji K, Miyatake K, Yamada J, Abula K, et al. Mouse synovial mesenchymal stem cells increase in yield with knee inflammation. J Orthop Res. 2015;33(2):246–53. https://doi.org/10.1002/jor.22753.

14. Zhang S, Muneta T, Morito T, Mochizuki T, Sekiya I. Autologous synovial fluid enhances migration of mesenchymal stem cells from synovium of osteoarthritis patients in tissue culture system. J Orthop Res. 2008;26(10): 1413–8. https://doi.org/10.1002/jor.20659.

15. Sekiya I, Colter DC, Prockop DJ. BMP-6 enhances chondrogenesis in a subpopulation of human marrow stromal cells. Biochem Biophys Res Commun. 2001;284(2):411–8. https://doi.org/10.1006/bbrc.2001.4898.

16. Shirasawa S, Sekiya I, Sakaguchi Y, Yagishita K, Ichinose S, Muneta T. In vitro chondrogenesis of human synovium-derived mesenchymal stem cells: optimal condition and comparison with bone marrow-derived cells. J Cell Biochem. 2006;97(1):84–97. https://doi.org/10.1002/jcb.20546.

17. Sekiya I, Larson BL, Vuoristo JT, Cui JG, Prockop DJ. Adipogenic differentiation of human adult stem cells from bone marrow stroma (MSCs). J Bone Miner Res. 2004;19(2):256–64. https://doi.org/10.1359/JBMR.0301220.

18. Morimoto D, Kuroda S, Kizawa T, Nomura K, Higuchi C, Yoshikawa H, et al. Equivalent osteoblastic differentiation function of human mesenchymal stem cells from rheumatoid arthritis in comparison with osteoarthritis. Rheumatology (Oxford). 2009;48(6):643–9. https://doi.org/10.1093/rheumatology/kep044.

19. Sekiya I, Vuoristo JT, Larson BL, Prockop DJ. In vitro cartilage formation by human adult stem cells from bone marrow stroma defines the sequence of cellular and molecular events during chondrogenesis. Proc Natl Acad Sci U S A. 2002;99(7):4397–402. https://doi.org/10.1073/pnas.052716199.

8

Human osteochondritis dissecans fragment-derived chondrocyte characteristics ex vivo, after monolayer expansion-induced de-differentiation, and after re-differentiation in alginate bead culture

Matthias Aurich[1,2,3], Gunther O. Hofmann[2], Florian Gras[2] and Bernd Rolauffs[4,5]*

Abstract

Background: Autologous chondrocyte implantation (ACI) is a therapy for articular cartilage and osteochondral lesions that relies on notch- or trochlea-derived primary chondrocytes. An alternative cell source for ACI could be osteochondritis dissecans (OCD) fragment-derived chondrocytes. Assessing the potential of these cells, we investigated their characteristics ex vivo and after monolayer expansion, as monolayer expansion is an integral step of ACI. However, as monolayer expansion can induce de-differentiation, we asked whether monolayer-induced de-differentiation can be reverted through successive alginate bead culture.

Methods: Chondrocytes were isolated from the OCD fragments of 15 patient knees with ICRS grades 3–4 lesions for ex vivo analyses, primary alginate bead culture, monolayer expansion, and alginate bead culture following monolayer expansion for attempting re-differentiation. We determined yield, viability, and the mRNA expression of aggrecan and type I, II, and X collagen.

Results: OCD fragment-derived chondrocyte isolation yielded high numbers of viable cells with a low type I:II collagen expression ratio (< 1) and a relatively high aggrecan and type II and X collagen mRNA expression, indicating chondrogenic and hypertrophic characteristics. As expected, monolayer expansion induced de-differentiation. Alginate bead culture of monolayer-expanded cells significantly improved the expression profile of all genes investigated, being most successful in decreasing the hypertrophy marker type X collagen to 1.5% of its ex vivo value. However, the chondrogenic phenotype was not fully restored, as the collagen type I:II expression ratio decreased significantly but remained > 1.

Conclusion: OCD fragment derived human chondrocytes may hold not yet utilized clinical potential for cartilage repair.

Keywords: Chondrocyte, Articular cartilage, De-differentiation, Re-differentiation, Monolayer expansion, Alginate bead culture

* Correspondence: berndrolauffs@googlemail.com
[4]G.E.R.N. Tissue Replacement, Regeneration & Neogenesis, Department of Orthopedics and Trauma Surgery, Medical Center - Albert-Ludwigs-University of Freiburg, Faculty of Medicine, Albert-Ludwigs-University of Freiburg, Hugstetter Straße 55, 79106 Freiburg, Germany
[5]Massachusetts Institute of Technology, Center for Biomedical Engineering, 500 Technology Sq, Cambridge, MA 02139, USA
Full list of author information is available at the end of the article

Background

Articular cartilage (AC) provides a low-friction interface for joint movement and distributes the forces that occur within the musculoskeletal system to the underlying subchondral bone. AC lesions are a common clinical problem because they do not heal spontaneously and often progress to higher grade AC lesions and, over time, to osteoarthritis (OA) [1]. Consequently, higher grade AC lesions are the target of many clinical therapies and basic science studies that aim to restore the AC layer with tissue engineered implants or induced hyaline-like AC. The use of autologous chondrocytes from non-weight bearing regions of AC that are seeded into a scaffold for implantation is one such method, termed autologous chondrocyte implantation (ACI). ACI is a clinically successful therapy for AC [2] and osteochondral lesions [3, 4]. However, as large-scale, degenerative AC and osteo-chondral lesions are a major focus of our field [5], the improvement of currently used ACI techniques and materials and the assessment of novel cell sources will gain more importance.

A crucial step in generating implants for ACI is the expansion of primary chondrocytes in monolayer culture to increase the number of available chondrocytes that are seeded into an implantable scaffold. Chondrocyte de-differentiation in extended monolayer expansion [6] limits the time of monolayer expansion, and, thus, the amount of chondrocytes that can be generated for ACI. In this context, alternative cell sources that could be used instead or in combination with autologous chondrocytes from classically used biopsy sites such as the intercondylar notch are highly interesting. Other studies focused on lesion chondrocytes [7], OA-chondrocytes [8–10], and on progenitor cells [11], as these can be differentiated in vitro into desired lineages [12–14]. Potentially, an attractive source for autologous chondrocytes for knee ACI could be the osteochondral fragment that dislocates from an osteochondritis dissecans (OCD) lesion, as an older study reported that a large OCD defect of the weight-bearing knee joint surface was treated by transplantation of an autogeneic osteochondral fragment [15]. In this context, we have previously demonstrated that human chondrocytes isolated from OCD fragments are viable [16] and, compared to notch chondrocytes from the same human joints, have an comparable mRNA expression of AC tissue engineering-relevant types I and II collagen [17]. Also, the ratio of type I to II collagen, which presents the balance between a chondrogenic vs. a de-differentiated phenotype, was comparable between OCD fragment and notch chondrocytes, indicating a chondrogenic phenotype in both OCD fragment and notch chondrocytes [17]. However, monolayer expansion, which represents an important step for producing the cell numbers needed for generating ACI implants, changed the mRNA expression profiles of clinically used notch chondrocytes but also of OCD fragment chondrocytes towards a de-differentiated phenotype [17].

In the present study, we asked the question whether human OCD fragment-derived chondrocytes, after they were intentionally de-differentiated through monolayer-expansion, can be re-differentiated using the alginate bead system [18] as a three-dimensional (3D) ACI model. Thus, we investigated ex vivo chondrocyte yield, viability, morphology, and the aggrecan and types I, II, and X collagen mRNA expression profiles of human OCD fragment-derived chondrocytes. We compared these ex vivo characteristics with those after monolayer expansion, after primary alginate bead culture, and after alginate bead culture following monolayer expansion. Collectively, such information is relevant for using human OCD fragment-derived chondrocytes for clinical ACI but, unfortunately, this information has been unavailable until now.

Methods
Articular cartilage

AC grade 4 according to the International Cartilage Repair Society (ICRS) classification system [19] from the dissected OCD fragments of the knee joints of 15 OCD patients was used (Fig. 1). The associated demographic data of these patients are shown in Table 1. Routine MRI was used to confirm OCD diagnosis and general recommendations on inclusion and exclusion criteria were respected [2, 20]. During the initial knee arthroscopy for generating AC biopsies for ACI, OCD-fragments were harvested (Fig. 1) and transferred in standard medium to our research laboratory for further analyses. As routine surgical therapy, the OCD-affected bone was restored if necessary and matrix-associated ACI was used as previously described [21] using Novocart® 3D (TETEC, Reutlingen, Germany).

Cell isolation and culture

Chondrocytes were isolated from the biopsy material designated to this study by sequential protease digestion for 1 h in 0.2% pronase, followed by overnight digestion in 0.025% collagenase-P in DMEM / F-12 medium (GIBCO BRL; Life Technologies, Grand Island, New York), supplemented with 5% autologous serum and 50 µg gentamicin / ml. The released cells were counted manually and cell viability was assayed by Trypan blue exclusion. The chondrocytes were washed three times in phosphate-buffered saline (PBS). An aliquot of 10,000 cells was dissolved in RNA extraction buffer (TRIzol Reagent; Life Technologies, Gaithersburg, Maryland) for molecular analysis (analysis 1 ex vivo). Other isolated chondrocytes were cultured in alginate beads (see below) for 3 weeks, followed by successive analysis (analysis 2

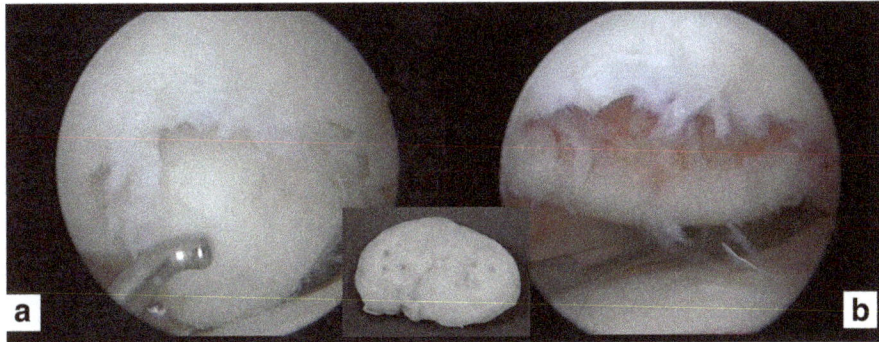

Fig. 1 Arthroscopic images of an osteochondritis dissecans (OCD) lesion ICRS grade 4 of the medial femoral condyle in a 24 year old male patient. **a** Gives the initial finding at arthroscopy. **b** Illustrates the lesion after debridement and the insert shows a representative image of an dislocated and arthroscopically removed OCD fragment

alginate). The remaining isolated chondrocytes that were not used for alginate culture were seeded in low-density monolayer culture for 3 weeks, comparable to the chondrocyte expansion routinely performed for ACI. This corresponded to approximately 2–3 passages. The chondrocytes in alginate and monolayer were cultured at 37 °C and 5% CO2 in standard DMEM / F12 feeding medium supplemented with 5% autologous serum and 50 µg gentamicin. The medium was changed every other day. At the time of confluence the monolayer chondrocytes were liberated by trypsin digestion and washed three times in PBS. An aliquot of 10,000 chondrocytes was dissolved in RNA extraction buffer (TRIzol Reagent) for molecular analysis (analysis 3 monolayer). The remaining monolayer-expanded chondrocytes were cultured in alginate beads (see below) for another 3 weeks followed by subsequent analyses (analysis 4 monolayer & alginate).

Preparation and culture of alginate beads
The isolated chondrocytes were encapsulated in alginate beads at a density of 4×10^6 cells / ml of alginate gel, as described by [22] modified by [18]. Briefly, the cells were suspended in sterile 0.15 M NaCl containing low-viscosity alginate gel (1.2%), then slowly pressed through a 22 gauge needle in a dropwise fashion into a 102 mM $CaCl_2$ solution. After instantaneous gelation the beads were allowed to polymerize further for a period of 10 min in the $CaCl_2$ solution. After 1 wash in 10 volumes of 0.15 M NaCl and 3 washes in 10 volumes of Ham's F12 / DMEM medium,

the beads were finally placed in standard culture medium (Ham's F-12 / DMEM medium (50 / 50) with 10% FBS, 50 mg / ml gentamicin and 25 mg / ml ascorbic acid). Each bead contained an average chondrocyte number of $44 \pm 2 \times 10^3$ cells / bead. Nine beads were cultured per well of a 24-well plate. The cells were incubated at all stages in a humidified atmosphere of 5% CO_2 at 37 °C and maintained by medium change 3 times per week with 1.5 ml medium/well. After 3 weeks, the beads were dissolved with 1 ml of 55 mM sodium citrate, 0.15 M NaCl, pH 6.05, at 25 °C for 20 min and the chondrocytes were recovered by centrifugation [18].

Quantitative real-time polymerase chain reaction (qRT-PCR)
Chondrocytes were dissolved in RNA extraction buffer (1 ml TRIzol Reagent), and Chloroform (200 µl) was added. After shaking and incubation for 3 min at room temperature, the samples were centrifuged for 15 min at 12000 g (4 °C) for phase separation. Total RNA was then precipitated from the aqueous phase with isopropyl alcohol (0.5 ml, 10 min, room temperature), and centrifuged for 10 min at 12000 g and 4 °C. Subsequently, the RNA was washed twice with 700 µl of 75% ethanol, dried at 42 °C, and re-dissolved in nuclease-free water, followed by digestion of genomic DNA using RNase free DNase (Qiagen, Hilden, Germany). Total RNA yield was assessed by spectrophotometry at 260 nm. The cDNA was synthesized from 1 µg of total RNA using the Omniscript RT Kit (Qiagen, Hilden, Germany) according to the manufacturer's protocol. Quantitative real-time PCR was performed in an iCycler iQ (Bio-Rad Laboratories, Hercules, California) in 20 µl reaction volume containing 9.4 µl cDNA, 0.3 µl forward primer, 0.3 µl reverse primer and 10 µl iQ SYBR Green supermix (Bio-Rad Laboratories). All investigated target genes and the sequences of their corresponding primers are listed in Table 2. The primers were validated by gel analysis, are listed in the NCBI reference sequence database and have

Table 1 Details of the specimens used in this study

Number of knees	15
Mean age (years) (range)	28 (16–49)
Male: female	10: 5
Site of OCD	11 medial, 4 lateral
Mean defect size (cm^2) (range)	4.6 (3–8)

Table 2 Primers used for the polymerase chain reaction (PCR); F: forward primer sequence, R: reverse primer sequence

Gene Name	PubMed Accession Number	Sequence
GAPDH	BT006893	F: CAT CAC TGC CAC CCA GAA GA
		R: CCT GCT TCA CCA CCT TCT TG
Type X collagen	X98568	F: CCT CTT GTT AGT GCC AAC CAG
		R: GAG CCA CTA GGA ATC CTG AG
Type I collagen (COL1A2)	XM_029245	F: CTC TGC GAC ACA AGG AGT CT
		R: ATC TTC ACC AGC CTT GCC AG
Type II collagen (COL2A1)	X16711	F: CAA CAC TGC CAA CGT CCA GAT
		R: CTG CTT CGT CCA GAT AGG CAA T
Aggrecan	NM_013227	F: ACT TCC GCT GGT CAG ATG GA
		R: TCT CGT GCC AGA TCA TCA CC

been used in our previous studies [16, 17, 23]. The sequence specificity was confirmed by BLAST searches. The reactions were run with appropriate controls (no template) to assess cross-contamination. The cycling parameters were: 95 °C for 3 min; 40 cycles: 94 °C for 20 s, annealing at 60 °C for 20 s, extension at 72 °C for 20 s; and 95 °C for 1 min. The PCR was evaluated by melting curve analysis. Data were calculated by the cycle threshold method (expressed as $2^{-\Delta Ct}$), normalized to glyceraldehyde phosphate dehydrogenase (GAPDH) mRNA expression, and are presented as ratios. Amplification efficiencies and GAPDH stable expression as reference gene were confirmed for our previous studies [16, 17, 23], in which the same protocol was used.

Histology

A representative AC sample was fixed in 4% paraformaldehyde and embedded in paraffin. Paraffin sections of 5 μm thickness were prepared. Conventional staining included a routine dual stain with hematoxylin / eosin for cellular distribution and safranin-O / fast green for proteoglycan content. Alkaline phosphatase detection was performed using a commercially available kit according to the manufacturer's protocol (Pierce). Immunohistochemistry was performed with a mouse monoclonal antibody against human type I collagen (Oncogene Research Products, Boston, Massachusetts) and a rabbit polyclonal antibody against human type II collagen (Abcam, Cambridge, UK) and type X collagen (kindly provided by Klaus von der Mark, University of Erlangen, Germany), as described earlier in our and other studies [16, 24].

Statistical analyses

Analyses were performed using SigmaPlot 11.0 and SigmaStat 3.0 (SPSS Inc., Chicago, USA). Analysis of variance (ANOVA) and normality testing were performed for all groups. Differences between the groups before or after cell culture were assessed with the Kruskal–Wallis one-way ANOVA on ranks. If the ANOVA tests for comparing chondrocytes before vs. after cell culture were statistically significant, an all-pairwise multiple comparison procedure (Student-Newman-Keuls Test) was performed to isolate the group or groups that differed from the others. Correlations were tested for significance by the Spearman's rank order correlation test. A $p < 0.05$ was considered statistically significant.

Results

Histology and immunohistochemistry

The histological characteristics of a representative OCD AC fragment derived from the medial femoral condyle are shown in Fig. 2. Two overviews at 5× magnification depict the irregular superficial zone stained with hematoxylin and eosin and with safranin-O and fast green (Fig. 2a,b), illustrating a homogenous chondrocyte distribution throughout the extracellular matrix. The safranin-O and fast green stain (Fig. 2b) revealed that the central part of the fragment contained proteoglycans, whereas the superficial zone was depleted. Interestingly, there was an increased pericellular staining in the deep zone, indicating in increased proteoglycan deposition I in that zone (insert in B). Note the presence of a fibrous-appearing layer covering the superficial zone (Fig. 2a insert), whose immunostaining for type I and II collagen is depicted in Fig. 2c,d, revealing that type I collagen was present within the superficial zone and the fibrous layer and that collagen type II was present throughout the tissue. The phase contrast pictures (inserts in C and D) depict the entire section. Interestingly, alkaline phosphatase was detected throughout the tissue (Fig. 2e) in the pericellular area (insert in E), which was also true for type X collagen (Fig. 2f). Collectively, these images demonstrated that the examined OCD fragment contained the types I, II, and X collagen.

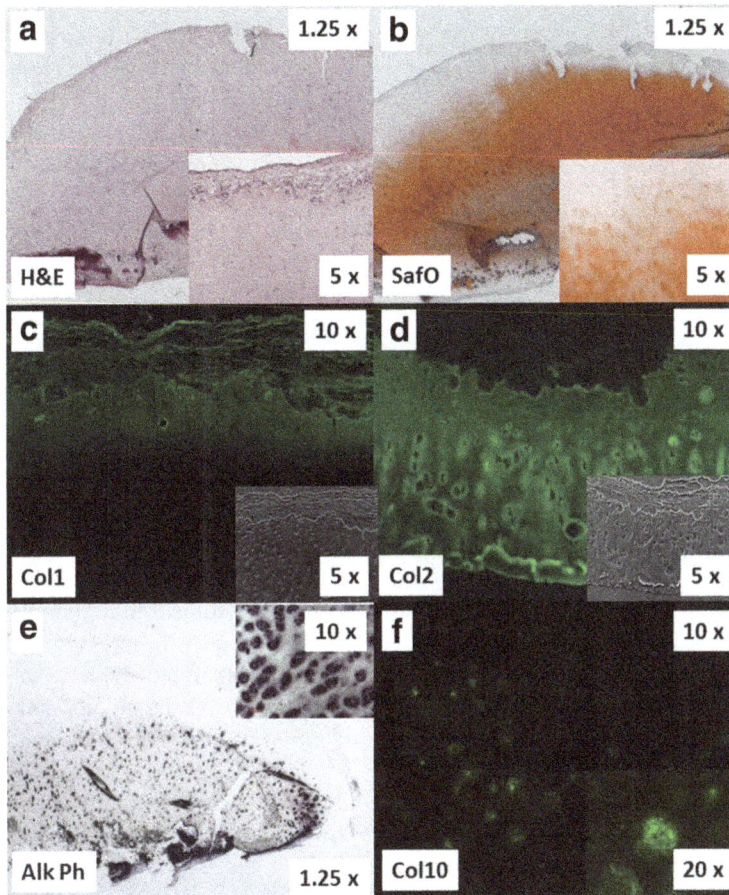

Fig. 2 Histology of a representative OCD fragment from the debrided ICRS grade 4 lesion of the medial condyle of a 22 year old patient. **a** Depicts a hematoxylin / eosin stain and (**b**) a safranin-O / fast green stain. **c, d** Shows immunostaining for types I (**c**) and II collagen (**d**) together with phase contrast images as inserts. **e** Shows alkaline phosphatase staining. **f** Shows immunostaining for type X collagen. Original magnifications of 1.25 x (**a, b**), 10 x (**c-f**) and insert magnifications of 5 x (**a-d**), 10 x (**e, f**)

Chondrocyte yield, viability, and morphology

Approximately $0.73 \pm 0.33 \times 10^6$ chondrocytes per gram wet weight were extracted. The mean cell viability was in all groups above 88% and no significant differences between the groups were noted. After isolation the suspended chondrocytes depicted a round phenotype but once seeded onto a tissue culture plate in low density the morphology had changed as expected to a more irregular and fibroblastic-appearing phenotype. After 3 weeks of monolayer expansion, the chondrocytes had regained this phenotype. During subsequent cultivation in alginate beads for another 3 weeks, the chondrocytes had changed to a round morphology. The number of isolated cells per OCD fragment and the viability of the individual cell cultures that were derived from these fragments is given in Table 3.

Molecular analyses

Molecular analyses revealed patient-specific mRNA expression variation on the order of magnitudes. Aggrecan mRNA expression (Fig. 3A) was comparable immediately after cell isolation (analysis 1) and after primary culture in alginate beads (analysis 2), which increased the expression 1.08-fold but without any significant difference between the two groups. After expansion in monolayer culture (analysis 3), aggrecan mRNA expression was decreased to 0.007-fold, compared to cell isolation and to alginate bead culture, and the difference was significant ($p < 0.001$), compared to both groups. After alginate bead culture following monolayer expansion (analysis 4), aggrecan mRNA expression was significantly increased 10.2-fold ($p < 0.001$), compared to monolayer expansion only (analysis 3). However, the expression levels were significantly lower than after isolation (0.07-fold, $p < 0.001$) or 3D culture I (0.07-fold, $p < 0.001$). Additional information on mRNA expression and cell viavility can be found in the supplementary file (Additional file 1).

Type I collagen mRNA expression (Fig. 3B) was increased after monolayer culture expansion (analysis 3), compared to ex vivo (analysis 1, 24.1-fold) and to alginate bead culture (analysis 2, 24.8-fold), and the difference was significant

Table 3 Number of isolated cells per OCD fragment and viability of the individual cell cultures that were derived from these fragments

OCD Fragment	Cell number (× 100.000/g wet weight)	Viability after Cell Culture (% of total)			
		Analysis 1	Analysis 2	Analysis 3	Analysis 4
1	0.72	91	89	93	92
2	0.36	86	88	87	89
3	0.8	75	79	81	85
4	0.56	96	95	94	91
5	1.24	90	96	90	93
6	0.42	89	85	93	89
7	1.01	93	93	85	89
8	0.77	82	91	87	85
9	0.9	87	85	89	96
10	0.61	93	87	94	95
11	1.23	95	94	92	93
12	0.31	96	97	95	91
13	0.37	87	92	89	84
14	0.41	91	93	92	90
15	1.22	92	93	90	92

($p < 0.001$), compared to both groups. After alginate bead culture following monolayer expansion (analysis 4), type I collagen mRNA expression was significantly decreased to 0.5-fold ($p < 0.001$), compared to monolayer expansion only (analysis 3). However, the expression levels were significantly higher than ex vivo (analysis 1, 12.5-fold, $p < 0.001$) or after alginate bead culture (analysis 2, 12.9-fold, $p < 0.001$).

Type II collagen mRNA expression (Fig. 3C) was not significantly different after primary culture in alginate beads (analysis 2) vs. ex vivo (analysis 1). After expansion in monolayer culture (analysis 3), type II collagen mRNA expression was decreased to 0.003-fold, compared to ex vivo (analysis 1) and 0.004-fold compared to alginate bead culture (analysis 2). The difference was significant ($p < 0.001$), compared to both groups. After alginate bead culture following monolayer expansion (analysis 4), type II collagen mRNA expression was significantly increased to 4.5-fold ($p < 0.001$), compared to monolayer expansion (analysis 3). However, the expression levels were significantly lower than ex vivo (analysis 1, 0.012-fold, $p < 0.001$) or alginate bead culture (analysis 2, 0.019-fold, $p < 0.001$).

Type X collagen mRNA expression (Fig. 3D) was not significantly changed after alginate bead culture (analysis 2), compared to ex vivo (analysis 1). After monolayer expansion (analysis 3), the type collagen X mRNA expression was significantly decreased to 0.03-fold, compared to ex vivo (analysis 1, $p < 0.001$). It further decreased after

alginate bead culture following monolayer expansion (analysis 4, $p < 0.001$) by 0.6-fold, compared to monolayer expansion (analysis 3), or decreased 0.01-fold, compared to ex vivo (analysis 1).

The ratio of type I to II collagen mRNA expression (Fig. 3E), which we calculated for each OCD fragment from the types I and II collagen mRNA expression values, was comparable ex vivo (analysis 1, 0.026 ± 0.035) and after alginate bead culture (analysis 2, 0.054 ± 0.09, 3D culture I), as the trend towards a 0.49-fold decrease after alginate bead culture did not reach significance. For both groups the ratio values were < 1, indicating a higher type II than I collagen mRNA expression and, thus, a healthy chondrocyte function. After monolayer expansion (analysis 3), the ratio was increased to 69.61 ± 47.7 and the increase was significant, compared to both groups ($p < 0.001$). After alginate bead culture following monolayer expansion (analysis 4), the ratio value was 7.23 ± 4.2, which indicated a significant recovery of the ratio, compared to monolayer expansion (analysis 3, $p < 001$, Fig. 3).

We also analyzed the data to uncover potential differences between medial and lateral defect locations. However, the mRNA expression data obtained from analyses 1 to 4 for chondrocytes from the medial vs. lateral defect locations were not significantly different (except type I collagen expression in the group analysis 2).

Correlation analyses

Ex vivo aggrecan mRNA expression levels (analysis 1) correlated significantly and positively with those after culture in alginate beads (analysis 2, $p < 0.001$, correlation coefficient cc: 0.988). Moreover, the ex vivo mRNA expression of collagen type I (analysis 1) correlated significantly and positively with the expression levels in primary alginate bead culture (analyses 2, $p = 0.005$, cc: 0.682). The same was true for the collagen types II ($p < 0.001$, cc: 0.989) and X ($p < 0.001$, cc: 0.986) expression levels, indicating that a high ex vivo expression of aggrecan, collagen types I, II, and X were associated with a high expression in primary alginate culture.

Interestingly, the mRNA expression levels after monolayer expansion (analysis 3) of all genes of interest correlated significantly and positively with the expression levels after alginate bead culture following monolayer expansion (analysis 4; aggrecan: $p < 0.001$, cc: 0.913; collagen type I: $p < 0.001$, cc: 0.973; collagen type II: $p < 0.001$, cc: 0.987; collagen type x: $p < 0.001$, cc: 0.981). This indicated that OCD fragment-derived chondrocytes with a relatively high mRNA expression of these genes in monolayer culture had also high expression levels in subsequent alginate bead culture following monolayer expansion. Together, these data indicated that patient-specific mRNA

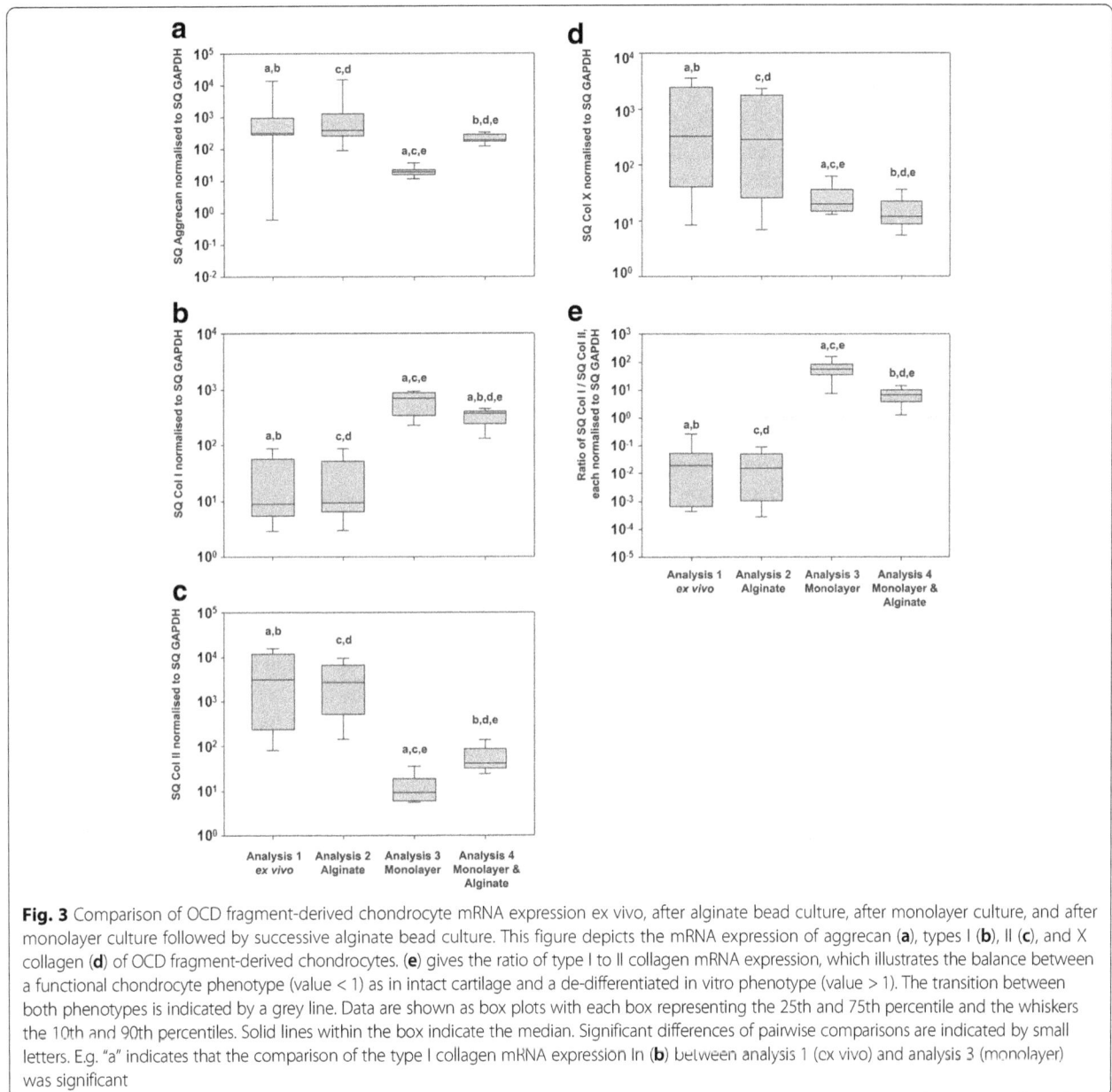

Fig. 3 Comparison of OCD fragment-derived chondrocyte mRNA expression ex vivo, after alginate bead culture, after monolayer culture, and after monolayer culture followed by successive alginate bead culture. This figure depicts the mRNA expression of aggrecan (**a**), types I (**b**), II (**c**), and X collagen (**d**) of OCD fragment-derived chondrocytes. (**e**) gives the ratio of type I to II collagen mRNA expression, which illustrates the balance between a functional chondrocyte phenotype (value < 1) as in intact cartilage and a de-differentiated in vitro phenotype (value > 1). The transition between both phenotypes is indicated by a grey line. Data are shown as box plots with each box representing the 25th and 75th percentile and the whiskers the 10th and 90th percentiles. Solid lines within the box indicate the median. Significant differences of pairwise comparisons are indicated by small letters. E.g. "a" indicates that the comparison of the type I collagen mRNA expression in (**b**) between analysis 1 (ex vivo) and analysis 3 (monolayer) was significant

expression level variations were maintained across the culture systems used.

Discussion

The present study asked whether intentionally in monolayer de-differentiated human OCD fragment-derived chondrocytes can be re-differentiated by using the alginate bead system [18] as an in vitro 3D ACI model. First, we demonstrated that chondrocytes can be isolated from the dissected OCD fragments of human patients with a sufficient yield and viability that was consistent with the literature [16]. Furthermore, ex vivo OCD fragment-derived chondrocytes displayed a functional chondrocyte phenotype, which was determined by calculating the ratio

of type I to II collagen mRNA expression. The ratio was comparable to those of chondrocytes from the notch and from AC lesions of human knee joints [7], suggesting a comparable chondrogenic phenotype of cells from these three AC locations. As expected, monolayer expansion led to chondrocyte de-differentiation [6], based on an irregular and fibroblastic-appearing phenotype and a decreased aggrecan and type II collagen mRNA expression and simultaneous increases in the type I collagen mRNA expression and the type I to II collagen expression ratio, compared to ex vivo. Subsequent alginate bead culture of the monolayer-expanded, de-differentiated OCD fragment-derived chondrocytes led to changes in cell morphology and mRNA expression that were consistent with re-differentiating the de-differentiated OCD fragment-derived chondrocytes. However, although we noted increased aggrecan and type II collagen mRNA expression levels and decreases in the type I collagen mRNA expression and the type I to II collagen expression ratio, the resulting mRNA expression values were significantly different from those measured ex vivo. Thus, induced re-differentiation was only partially successful in recovering the mRNA expression profiles. Interestingly, the type X collagen mRNA expression of OCD fragment-derived chondrocytes was lowest after re-differentiation of monolayer-induced de-differentiation in alginate beads, compared to primary alginate bead culture, monolayer expansion, and even compared to ex vivo. That monolayer expansion led to a significant reduction in the type X collagen mRNA expression or, as an alternative explanation, to the selection of a less hypertrophic cell pool was consistent with our previous study [17]. Collectively, this study demonstrated that ex vivo OCD fragment-derived chondrocytes were characterized by a chondrogenic but also hypertrophic phenotype, based on the low type I to II collagen expression ratio, and at the same time the high type X collagen mRNA expression. After monolayer expansion, the re-differentiation through alginate bead culture was most effective in modulating the mRNA expression of type X collagen and, to a lesser extent, of aggrecan but was not effective in lowering the collagen type I to II expression ratio to values below 1. Thus, induced re-differentiation led to a marked reduction of the hypertrophic phenotype to approximately 1.5% of its ex vivo value but did not fully restore the chondrogenic phenotype, measured as type I to II collagen expression ratio. Collectively, OCD fragment-derived cells are interesting chondrogenic but also hypertrophic chondrocytes, whose re-differentiation with the here described method was effective in modulating hypertrophic but not chondrogenic characteristics. Subsequent procedures for improving the chondrogenic properties of OCD-fragment-derived cells would greatly enhance their clinical potential.

For inducing chondrocyte re-differentiation, previous studies have used alginate bead and pellet culture [25], alginate bead culture combined with serum or growth factor cocktails [26], hypoxic pellet culture [27], porous scaffold surfaces for the co-culture with mesenchymal stromal cells [28], agarose [29] and photocrosslinkable hydrogels [30], as well as the chimeric Activin A / BMP2 ligand AB235 [31]. These studies investigated the re-differentiation of human OA-chondrocytes obtained during joint replacement procedures [25–27, 30, 31] and of porcine and bovine chondrocytes [28, 29]. As human chondrocytes derived from dislocated OCD fragments have not been investigated, the present study added an important part to the literature on chondrocyte re-differentiation. Re-differentiation in 3D can be enhanced by adding human serum or transforming growth factor

beta1 and insulin-transferrin-selenium-linoleic acid-bovine serum albumin [26] or human mesenchymal stromal cells [28], by using hypoxic conditions [27], by varying adhesion site density but not stiffness [29], and by choosing re-differentiation-supporting biomaterials such as hyaluronic acid hydrogels [30]. In the present study, the re-differentiation-associated changes in mRNA expression were comparable to [25], in which changes in mRNA expression were induced via 3D alginate bead cultures after chondrocyte de-differentiation. In line with our study, [25] reported a significantly decreased type X collagen mRNA expression and increased types I and II collagen and aggrecan expression. In this respect, the effects of alginate bead culture for re-differentiating OCD fragment-derived chondrocytes appeared comparable to human OA-chondrocytes obtained during joint replacement procedures.

A recent study investigated the frequency of OCD fragment chondrocyte cultures and reported that it was possible to culture chondrocytes from traumatic osteochondral fragments within a year of injury but not from fragments due to OCD [32]. This interesting study suggested that the time elapsed between loose body formation and fragment excision was the main factor affecting the cell culture setup. Our data does not allow drawing a direct comparison, as we did not record the time between loose body formation and cell isolation. However, we noted two methodological differences between the studies. Whereas [32] used enzymatic digestion with collagenase-A overnight, the present study used a sequential digestion for 1 h in pronase, followed by overnight digestion in collagenase-P. Another independent study [33] used the same sequential digestion used here and reported a comparably high viability in each studied OCD fragment but did not attempt cell culture. Additionally, the culture conditions between [32] and our study differed, as [32] used 10% of fetal bovine serum and the present study used 5% autologous serum. Together, these methodological differences may explain in part the difference in the number of successfully established OCD fragment-derived chondrocyte cultures. Thus, a head-to-head comparison of these different methods together with information on time since disease onset as suggested by [32] may help to determine the optimal conditions and the expected frequency of successfully established OCD fragment-derived chondrocytes.

It is worthwhile to mention that recent research on healthy (porcine) AC identified GAPDH as one of the most stably expressed genes [34], whereas it is considered a less stable reference gene in full osteoarthritis (human) patients older than 60 years [35]. As the choice of the appropriate reference gene depends on the individual experimental set-up [36], we had confirmed the suitability of the chosen reference gene for our previous studies. However, the method could be improved upon because MIQE guidelines encourage using more than one reference gene [37]. Generally, the methodology of the present study was chosen to allow better comparisons to our previous studies [16, 17, 23, 38]. A previous study comparing the here chosen method of SYBR Green based detection to TaqMan based detection found TaqMan to be more sensitive and to generate lower calculated expression levels than the SYBR Green assay, suggesting that any discussion of gene expression levels needs to be linked to the qPCR method used in the analysis [39]. However, this was not of great concern in the present study because our main conclusions were based on the *expression ratio* of type I to II collagen as well as *relative* changes in aggrecan and types II and X collagen mRNA expression. Also in a methods context, it is worth mentioning that de-differentiation of monolayer cultured chondrocytes is a progressive process that depends on passage and culture time [26, 40]. Thus, one can chose either time or passage number for culture standardization. Here, we chose a standardized culture time of 3 weeks, according to [26], which corresponded to approximately 2–3 passages. We did not analyze the re-differentiation status as a function of chondrocyte passage number, although this would be interesting data.

Although we calculated the number of isolated cells per OCD fragment wet weight, we did not record the total number of cells that were contained within the fragment at the time of isolation because we allocated the cell suspension into 4 cell culture groups. Thus, we cannot directly assess whether all OCD fragments would have qualified for ACI, based on cell numbers. However, the sparse literature on this topic documents that a range of cell densities is being used for ACI [41]. Additionally, in the personal experience of the authors OCD fragments can be processed for later ACI as a future therapy option, regardless of the initial cell number.

As the cell quality affects the clinical outcome of ACI [42], it is helpful to mention that OCD fragment-derived chondrocyte exhibited a patient-specific variation of the mRNA expression that was on the order of magnitudes. Specifically, the chondrocytes from certain donors had a more chondrogenic mRNA expression profile than the cells from other donors. These variations were not associated with any patient demographics. However, we noted through our correlation analyses that the patient-specific variations in the mRNA expression levels were maintained across the culture systems used. This indicated that patient-specific expression characteristics measured ex vivo were maintained in vitro throughout de-differentiation and induced re-differentiation. Whether such patient-specific expression characteristics can potentially be preserved after implantation is not known. In the context of cell quality, it appears also important to choose an appropriate cell source for ACI. Studies that examine joint locations are valuable, as chondrocytes from diverse locations differ in many

characteristics. For example, their metabolic characteristics vary across joints [10, 43]. Moreover, the cellular distribution within the native tissue varies between individual joints [44] and even joint surfaces within the same joint [44, 45] and between different stages of OA [46]. In clinical routine, ACI utilizes biopsies of macroscopically intact cartilage from non-weight bearing areas of the (knee) joint [47] such as the intercondylar notch and the trochlea. To determine the "best cell source" for regenerative cartilage therapies, one study investigated chondrocytes isolated from AC lesions vs. from healthy AC [48]. Interestingly, chondrocytes from the AC lesion performed better than from healthy AC and it was concluded that AC lesions could be viable donor sites for ACI. In this regard, chondrocytes from alternative cell sources such as AC lesions [48] may hold clinical potential for AC repair but need further investigation, as – in the case of AC lesions – conflicting evidence has been reported [49]. However, in the case of knee OCD fragment-derived chondrocytes, the here reported biological characteristics are in accordance with our previous studies on this topic [16, 17] and clinical experience for OCD repair of the talus is promising [50]. Thus, we also analyzed the here reported data to uncover potential differences between medial and lateral defect locations. However, our data suggested that defect location did not have a significant effect on the ex vivo mRNA expression profile or the expression profiles after alginate culture, monolayer expansion, or alginate culture after monolayer expansion-induced de-differentiation.

Conclusion

Collectively, human OCD fragment-derived chondrocytes depict chondrogenic but also hypertrophic characteristics, whose re-differentiation with the here described method was effective in modulating hypertrophic characteristics and to a lesser extent chondrogenic characteristics. The here presented data are important for better understanding and ultimately utilizing the clinical potential of human OCD fragment-derived chondrocytes for AC repair.

Acknowledgements
We would like to thank Jana Schömburg und Christine Mollenhauer for their help in sample preparation and Dr. Juergen Mollenhauer for discussing this project. All data were collected at the Orthopaedic Research Laboratories of the University of Jena. We also thank the Deutsche Forschungsgemeinschaft (DFG), the Deutsche Arthrosehilfe e. V., and the Interdisciplinary Center for Clinical Research (IZKF) of the University of Jena for supporting this work.

Funding
This work was supported in part by the Deutsche Forschungsgemeinschaft (DFG 156/6–1), the Deutsche Arthrosehilfe e. V., and the Interdisciplinary Center for Clinical Research (IZKF) (M.A.).

Authors' contributions
MA, GOH, and BR conceived the study, participated in its design, and helped drafting the manuscript. All authors (MA, GOH, FG, BR) interpreted

the data. MA, FG, and BR analyzed the data statistically. MA and BR were major contributors to writing the manuscript. All authors have read and approved the final manuscript. BR is the corresponding author.

Competing interests
The authors declare that they have no competing interests.

Author details
[1]Center for Orthopaedic and Trauma Surgery, Klinikum Mittleres Erzgebirge, Alte Marienberger, Str. 52, 09405 Zschopau, Germany. [2]Department of Trauma, Hand and Reconstructive Surgery, Universitätsklinikum Jena, Erlanger Allee 101, 07747 Jena, Germany. [3]Department of Biochemistry, Rush Medical College, 1735 W. Harrison St, Chicago, IL 60612, USA. [4]G.E.R.N. Tissue Replacement, Regeneration & Neogenesis, Department of Orthopedics and Trauma Surgery, Medical Center - Albert-Ludwigs-University of Freiburg, Faculty of Medicine, Albert-Ludwigs-University of Freiburg, Hugstetter Straße 55, 79106 Freiburg, Germany. [5]Massachusetts Institute of Technology, Center for Biomedical Engineering, 500 Technology Sq, Cambridge, MA 02139, USA.

References
1. Heijink A, Gomoll AH, Madry H, Drobnic M, Filardo G, Espregueira-Mendes J, Van Dijk CN. Biomechanical considerations in the pathogenesis of osteoarthritis of the knee. Knee Surg Sports Traumatol Arthrosc. 2012;20: 423–35. https://doi.org/10.1007/s00167-011-1818-0.
2. Niemeyer P, Albrecht D, Andereya S, Angele P, Ateschrang A, Aurich M, Baumann M, Bosch U, Erggelet C, Fickert S, Gebhard H, Gelse K, Gunther D, Hoburg A, Kasten P, Kolombe T, Madry H, Marlovits S, Meenen NM, Muller PE, Noth U, Petersen JP, Pietschmann M, Richter W, Rolauffs B, Rhunau K, Schewe B, Steinert A, Steinwachs MR, Welsch GH, Zinser W, Fritz J. Autologous chondrocyte implantation (ACI) for cartilage defects of the knee: a guideline by the working group "clinical tissue regeneration" of the German Society of Orthopaedics and Trauma (DGOU). Knee. 2016; https:// doi.org/10.1016/j.knee.2016.02.001.
3. Aurich M, Bedi HS, Smith PJ, Rolauffs B, Muckley T, Clayton J, Blackney M. Arthroscopic treatment of osteochondral lesions of the ankle with matrix-associated chondrocyte implantation: early clinical and magnetic resonance imaging results. Am J Sports Med. 2011;39:311–9. https://doi.org/10.1177/0363546510381575.
4. Ochs BG, Muller-Horvat C, Albrecht D, Schewe B, Weise K, Aicher WK, Rolauffs B. Remodeling of articular cartilage and subchondral bone after bone grafting and matrix-associated autologous chondrocyte implantation for osteochondritis dissecans of the knee. Am J Sports Med. 2011;39:764–73. https://doi.org/10.1177/0363546510388896.
5. Johnstone B, Alini M, Cucchiarini M, Dodge GR, Eglin D, Guilak F, Madry H, Mata A, Mauck RL, Semino CE, Stoddart MJ. Tissue engineering for articular cartilage repair–the state of the art. Eur Cells Mater. 2013;25:248–67.
6. Lin Z, Fitzgerald JB, Xu J, Willers C, Wood D, Grodzinsky AJ, Zheng MH. Gene expression profiles of human chondrocytes during passaged monolayer cultivation. J Orthop Res. 2008;26:1230–7. https://doi.org/10.1002/jor.20523.
7. Aurich M, Hofmann GO, Best N, Rolauffs B. Induced Redifferentiation of human chondrocytes from articular cartilage lesion in alginate bead culture after monolayer dedifferentiation: an alternative cell source for cell-based therapies? Tissue Eng A. 2017; https://doi.org/10.1089/ten.TEA.2016.0505.
8. Stoop R, Albrecht D, Gaissmaier C, Fritz J, Felka T, Rudert M, Aicher WK. Comparison of marker gene expression in chondrocytes from patients receiving autologous chondrocyte transplantation versus osteoarthritis patients. Arthritis Res Ther. 2007;9:R60. https://doi.org/10.1186/ar2218.
9. Cavallo C, Desando G, Facchini A, Grigolo B. Chondrocytes from patients with osteoarthritis express typical extracellular matrix molecules once grown onto a three-dimensional hyaluronan-based scaffold. J Biomed Mater Res A. 2010;93:86–95. https://doi.org/10.1002/jbm.a.32547.
10. Aurich M, Hofmann GO, Rolauffs B. Differences in type II collagen turnover of osteoarthritic human knee and ankle joints. Int Orthop. 2017;41:999–1005. https://doi.org/10.1007/s00264-017-3414-5.
11. Shafiee A, Kabiri M, Langroudi L, Soleimani M, Ai J. Evaluation and comparison of the in vitro characteristics and chondrogenic capacity of four adult stem/progenitor cells for cartilage cell-based repair. J Biomed Mater Res A. 2015; https://doi.org/10.1002/jbm.a.35603.
12. Bianco P, Cao X, Frenette PS, Mao JJ, Robey PG, Simmons PJ, Wang CY. The meaning, the sense and the significance: translating the science of mesenchymal stem cells into medicine. Nat Med. 2013;19:35–42. https://doi.org/10.1038/nm.3028.
13. Aicher WK, Buhring HJ, Hart M, Rolauffs B, Badke A, Klein G. Regeneration of cartilage and bone by defined subsets of mesenchymal stromal cells–potential and pitfalls. Adv Drug Deliv Rev. 2011;63:342–51. https://doi.org/10.1016/j.addr.2010.12.004.
14. Pilz GA, Ulrich C, Ruh M, Abele H, Schafer R, Kluba T, Buhring HJ, Rolauffs B, Aicher WK. Human term placenta-derived mesenchymal stromal cells are less prone to osteogenic differentiation than bone marrow-derived mesenchymal stromal cells. Stem Cells Dev. 2011;20:635–46. https://doi.org/10.1089/scd.2010.0308.
15. Yamashita F, Sakakida K, Suzu F, Takai S. The transplantation of an autogeneic osteochondral fragment for osteochondritis dissecans of the knee. Clin Orthop Relat Res. 1985;(201):43–50.
16. Aurich M, Anders J, Trommer T, Liesaus E, Seifert M, Schomburg J, Rolauffs B, Wagner A, Mollenhauer J. Histological and cell biological characterization of dissected cartilage fragments in human osteochondritis dissecans of the femoral condyle. Arch Orthop Trauma Surg. 2006;126:606–14. https://doi.org/10.1007/s00402-006-0125-6.
17. Aurich M, Hofmann GO, Muckley T, Mollenhauer J, Rolauffs B. In vitro phenotypic modulation of chondrocytes from knees of patients with osteochondritis dissecans: implications for chondrocyte implantation procedures. J Bone Joint Surg Br. 2012;94:62–7. https://doi.org/10.1302/0301-620X.94B1.27528.
18. Hauselmann HJ, Aydelotte MB, Schumacher BL, Kuettner KE, Gitelis SH, Thonar EJ. Synthesis and turnover of proteoglycans by human and bovine adult articular chondrocytes cultured in alginate beads. Matrix. 1992;12:116–29.
19. Brittberg M, Winalski CS. Evaluation of cartilage injuries and repair. J Bone Joint Surg Am. 2003;85-A(Suppl 2):58–69.
20. Niemeyer P, Andereya S, Angele P, Ateschrang A, Aurich M, Baumann M, Behrens P, Bosch U, Erggelet C, Fickert S, Fritz J, Gebhard H, Gelse K, Gunther D, Hoburg A, Kasten P, Kolombe T, Madry H, Marlovits S, Meenen NM, Muller PE, Noth U, Petersen JP, Pietschmann M, Richter W, Rolauffs B, Rhunau K, Schewe B, Steinert A, Steinwachs MR, Welsch GH, Zinser W, Albrecht D. Autologous chondrocyte implantation (ACI) for cartilage defects of the knee: a guideline by the working group "tissue regeneration" of the German Society of Orthopaedic Surgery and Traumatology (DGOU). Z Orthop Unfall. 2013;151:38–47. https://doi.org/10.1055/s-0032-1328207.
21. Marlovits S, Zeller P, Singer P, Resinger C, Vecsei V. Cartilage repair: generations of autologous chondrocyte transplantation. Eur J Radiol. 2006; 57:24–31. https://doi.org/10.1016/j.ejrad.2005.08.009.
22. Guo JF, Jourdian GW, MacCallum DK. Culture and growth characteristics of chondrocytes encapsulated in alginate beads. Connect Tissue Res. 1989;19: 277–97. https://doi.org/10.3109/03008208909043901.
23. Aurich M, Hofmann GO, Best N, Rolauffs B. Induced Redifferentiation of human chondrocytes from articular cartilage lesion in alginate bead culture after monolayer dedifferentiation: an alternative cell source for cell-based therapies? Tissue Eng A. 2018;24:275–86. https://doi.org/10.1089/ten.TEA.2016.0505.
24. Correia C, Pereira AL, Duarte AR, Frias AM, Pedro AJ, Oliveira JT, Sousa RA, Reis RL. Dynamic culturing of cartilage tissue: the significance of hydrostatic pressure. Tissue Eng A. 2012;18:1979–91. https://doi.org/10.1089/ten.TEA.2012.0083.
25. Caron MM, Emans PJ, Coolsen MM, Voss L, Surtel DA, Cremers A, van Rhijn LW, Welting TJ. Redifferentiation of dedifferentiated human articular chondrocytes: comparison of 2D and 3D cultures. Osteoarthr Cartil. 2012;20: 1170–8. https://doi.org/10.1016/j.joca.2012.06.016
26. Hsieh-Bonassera ND, Wu I, Lin JK, Schumacher BL, Chen AC, Masuda K, Bugbee WD, Sah RL. Expansion and redifferentiation of chondrocytes from osteoarthritic cartilage: cells for human cartilage tissue engineering. Tissue Eng A. 2009;15:3513–23. https://doi.org/10.1089/ten.TEA.2008.0628.
27. Babur BK, Ghanavi P, Levett P, Lott WB, Klein T, Cooper-White JJ, Crawford R, Doran MR. The interplay between chondrocyte redifferentiation pellet size and oxygen concentration. PLoS One. 2013;8:e58865. https://doi.org/10.1371/journal.pone.0058865.
28. Meretoja VV, Dahlin RL, Wright S, Kasper FK, Mikos AG. Articular chondrocyte redifferentiation in 3D co-cultures with mesenchymal stem cells. Tissue Eng

Part C Methods. 2014;20:514–23. https://doi.org/10.1089/ten.tec.2013.0532.

29. Schuh E, Hofmann S, Stok K, Notbohm H, Muller R, Rotter N. Chondrocyte redifferentiation in 3D: the effect of adhesion site density and substrate elasticity. J Biomed Mater Res A. 2012;100:38–47. https://doi.org/10.1002/jbm.a.33226.

30. Levett PA, Melchels FP, Schrobback K, Hutmacher DW, Malda J, Klein TJ. Chondrocyte redifferentiation and construct mechanical property development in single-component photocrosslinkable hydrogels. J Biomed Mater Res A. 2014;102:2544–53. https://doi.org/10.1002/jbm.a.34924.

31. Jimenez G, Lopez-Ruiz E, Kwiatkowski W, Montanez E, Arrebola F, Carrillo E, Gray PC, Izpisua Belmonte JC, Choe S, Peran M, Marchal JA. Activin a/BMP2 chimera AB235 drives efficient redifferentiation of long term cultured autologous chondrocytes. Sci Rep. 2015;5:16400. https://doi.org/10.1038/srep16400.

32. Guillen-Garcia P, Rodriguez-Inigo E, Guillen-Vicente I, Guillen-Vicente M, Fernandez-Jaen T, Concejero V, Val D, Maestro A, Abelow S, Lopez-Alcorocho JM. Viability of pathologic cartilage fragments as a source for autologous chondrocyte cultures. Cartilage. 2016;7:149–56. https://doi.org/10.1177/1947603515621998.

33. Pascual-Garrido C, Tanoira I, Muscolo DL, Ayerza MA, Makino A. Viability of loose body fragments in osteochondritis dissecans of the knee. A series of cases. Int Orthop. 2010;34:827–31. https://doi.org/10.1007/s00264-010-0951-6.

34. McCulloch RS, Ashwell MS, O'Nan AT, Mente PL. Identification of stable normalization genes for quantitative real-time PCR in porcine articular cartilage. J Anim Sci Biotechnol. 2012;3:36. https://doi.org/10.1186/2049-1891-3-36.

35. Pombo-Suarez M, Calaza M, Gomez-Reino JJ, Gonzalez A. Reference genes for normalization of gene expression studies in human osteoarthritic articular cartilage. BMC Mol Biol. 2008;9:17. https://doi.org/10.1186/1471-2199-9-17.

36. Al-Sabah A, Stadnik P, Gilbert SJ, Duance VC, Blain EJ. Importance of reference gene selection for articular cartilage mechanobiology studies. Osteoarthr Cartil. 2016;24:719–30. https://doi.org/10.1016/j.joca.2015.11.007.

37. Bustin SA, Benes V, Garson JA, Hellemans J, Huggett J, Kubista M, Mueller R, Nolan T, Pfaffl MW, Shipley GL, Vandesompele J, Wittwer CT. The MIQE guidelines: minimum information for publication of quantitative real-time PCR experiments. Clin Chem. 2009;55:611–22. https://doi.org/10.1373/clinchem.2008.112797.

38. Aurich M, Hofmann GO, Rolauffs B. Tissue engineering-relevant characteristics of ex vivo and monolayer-expanded chondrocytes from the notch versus trochlea of human knee joints. Int Orthop. 2017;41:2327–35. https://doi.org/10.1007/s00264-017-3615-y.

39. Cao H, Shockey JM. Comparison of TaqMan and SYBR green qPCR methods for quantitative gene expression in tung tree tissues. J Agric Food Chem. 2012;60:12296 303. https://doi.org/10.1021/jf304690e

40. Von Der Mark K, Gauss V, Von Der Mark H, MÜLler P. Relationship between cell shape and type of collagen synthesised as chondrocytes lose their cartilage phenotype in culture. Nature. 1977;267:531. https://doi.org/10.1038/267531a0.

41. Foldager CB, Gomoll AH, Lind M, Spector M. Cell seeding densities in autologous chondrocyte implantation techniques for cartilage repair. Cartilage. 2012;3:108–17. https://doi.org/10.1177/1947603511435522.

42. Pietschmann MF, Horng A, Niethammer T, Pagenstert I, Sievers B, Jansson V, Glaser C, Muller PE. Cell quality affects clinical outcome after MACI procedure for cartilage injury of the knee. Knee Surg Sports Traumatol Arthrosc. 2009;17:1305–11. https://doi.org/10.1007/s00167-009-0828-7.

43. Aurich M, Squires GR, Reiner A, Mollenhauer JA, Kuettner KE, Poole AR, Cole AA. Differential matrix degradation and turnover in early cartilage lesions of human knee and ankle joints. Arthritis Rheum. 2005;52:112–9.

44. Rolauffs B, Williams JM, Grodzinsky AJ, Kuettner KE, Cole AA. Distinct horizontal patterns in the spatial organization of superficial zone chondrocytes of human joints. J Struct Biol. 2008;162:335–44. https://doi.org/10.1016/j.jsb.2008.01.010.

45. Aicher WK, Rolauffs B. The spatial organisation of joint surface chondrocytes: review of its potential roles in tissue functioning, disease and early, preclinical diagnosis of osteoarthritis. Ann Rheum Dis. 2014;73:645–53. https://doi.org/10.1136/annrheumdis-2013-204308.

46. Felka T, Rothdiener M, Bast S, Uynuk-Ool T, Zouhair S, Ochs BG, De Zwart P, Stoeckle U, Aicher WK, Hart ML, Shiozawa T, Grodzinsky AJ, Schenke-Layland K, Venkatesan JK, Cucchiarini M, Madry H, Kurz B, Rolauffs B. Loss of spatial organization and destruction of the pericellular matrix in early osteoarthritis in vivo and in a novel in vitro methodology. Osteoarthr Cartil. 2016;24: 1200–9. https://doi.org/10.1016/j.joca.2016.02.001.

47. Jackson DW, Simon TM. Chondrocyte transplantation. Arthroscopy. 1996;12:732–8.

48. Bekkers JE, Saris DB, Tsuchida AI, van Rijen MH, Dhert WJ, Creemers LB. Chondrogenic potential of articular chondrocytes depends on their original location. Tissue Eng A. 2014;20:663–71. https://doi.org/10.1089/ten.TEA.2012.0673.

49. Malicev E, Barlic A, Kregar-Velikonja N, Strazar K, Drobnic M. Cartilage from the edge of a debrided articular defect is inferior to that from a standard donor site when used for autologous chondrocyte cultivation. J Bone Joint Surg Br. 2011;93:421–6. https://doi.org/10.1302/0301-620X.93B3.25675.

50. Giannini S, Buda R, Grigolo B, Vannini F, De Franceschi L, Facchini A. The detached osteochondral fragment as a source of cells for autologous chondrocyte implantation (ACI) in the ankle joint. Osteoarthr Cartil. 2005;13: 601–7. https://doi.org/10.1016/j.joca.2005.02.010.

9

Risk factors for progression of radiographic knee osteoarthritis in elderly community residents in Korea

Jong Jin Yoo[1], Dong Hyun Kim[2] and Hyun Ah Kim[3*]

Abstract

Background: Knee osteoarthritis (OA) is the most common form of arthritis affecting the elderly. Understanding the risk factors for knee OA has been derived from cross sectional studies. There have been few longitudinal studies of risk factors for knee OA among Asian populations. The purpose of this study was to evaluate the risk factors for knee OA in elderly Korean community residents.

Methods: This prospective, population-based study was conducted on residents over 50 years of age in Chuncheon who participated in the Hallym Aging Study. Standardized weight-bearing semi-flexed knee anteroposterior radiographs were obtained in 2007 and in 2010. Of 504 participants at baseline, 322 participants (male: female = 150:172) underwent follow-up knee radiographs. Radiographic knee OA was defined as Kellgren/Lawrence (K-L) grade of ≥ 2. Risk factors assessed at baseline were tested for their association with incidence, progression, and worsening of radiographic knee OA by logistic regression analysis.

Results: The median age of these participants at follow-up was 71 years (interquartile range 66–75 years). Incident OA was observed in 33 (10.2%) and progression of OA (defined as an increase of Kellgren-Lawrence (K-L) grade at follow-up, from grades 2 or 3 at baseline) in 43 (13.55%) participants. In multivariate logistic regression analysis, only females were significantly associated with the progression of radiographic knee OA (odds ratio [OR] = 4.41, 95% confidence interval [CI] 1.32–14.77).

Conclusions: In this 3-year longitudinal study, the yearly incidence and progression of knee OA was higher than those previously reported in Western populations.

Keywords: Osteoarthritis, Knee, Risk factors, Progression

Background

Knee osteoarthritis (OA) is the most common form of arthritis affecting the elderly and is a growing public health concern as the population ages. In the US, in 2004, approximately 431,485 primary knee replacements were performed [1]. This was a 53% increase in primary knee replacements, compared with data from 2000. From 2002 to 2005, 103,601 total knee replacement (TKR) surgeries were performed in South Korea, and approximately 83% of these were associated with knee OA [2]. The rate of TKR increased over the 4 years of the

study and was much higher in women than in men. In rapidly aging societies such as in Korea, the increasing prevalence of knee OA may present serious new health issues. Previous studies have reported various risk factors associated with knee OA such as older age, female sex, hypertension, raised glucose, obesity, history of knee injury, varus/valgus malalignment, quadriceps muscle strength, and physical workload [3–12]. However most of these studies for risk factors of knee OA have been performed in persons of European origin, so the results cannot be extrapolated to Asian populations. There have only been a few longitudinal studies of risk factors for knee OA among Asian peoples [13, 14]. We have previously examined the prevalence of radiographic knee OA (ROA) and symptomatic OA in a 2007 cross-sectional

* Correspondence: kimha@hallym.ac.kr
[3]Rheumatology Division, Department of Internal Medicine, Hallym University Sacred Heart Hospital, 896, Pyongchondong, Dongan-gu, Anyang, Kyunggi-do 431-070, South Korea
Full list of author information is available at the end of the article

study, using the standardized radiographic protocol, and the prevalence was 37.3% and 24.2%, respectively. The presence of hypertension, having a manual occupation and a lower level of education were significantly associated with the presence of ROA [15]. However, cross-sectional studies can neither show how risk factors affect the progression of knee OA, nor define the cause and effect relationship. Therefore, longitudinal studies are needed to clarify the risk factors for the incidence or the progression of knee OA. The objective of the present study was to assess the incidence, progression, and worsening of radiographic knee OA in elderly Korean community residents during a 3-year follow-up period and, furthermore, to evaluate the prospective risk factors for knee OA.

Methods
Participants
The participants in this study were recruited in the Hallym Aging Study (HAS), which commenced in 2004 and involved follow-up examinations at 3-year intervals. The HAS is a prospective cohort of residents aged 50 years or older (70% older than 65 years) in Chuncheon, a city in the northeast area of South Korea. Details of the cohort profile were reported elsewhere [15] and are only briefly described here. The city was divided into 1408 areas based on the Korean National Census conducted in 2000, and 200 areas were randomly selected [16]. Nine hundred eighteen of the 1489 participants completed face to-face interviews at baseline in 2004. Of the 918 participants, 702 participated in the 2007 survey, excluding 216 of them who died, moved, refused participation, or could not be contacted. Among the 702 participants, 504 who underwent knee radiography participated in the 2007 OA study cohort. After 3 years, 182 patients were lost to follow-up and 322 completed the survey, including radiographs, and constituted our present 2010 study cohort. The Hallym University's institutional review board approved the study protocol, and informed consent was obtained from all the study participants.

Data collection
Demographic information, such as educational level, marital status, income, occupation, regular exercise, and comorbidities was collected through face-to-face interviews by trained interviewers. Educational levels were classified as < 10 or ≥10 years. Income was divided into 11 categories, and low income was defined as < 500,000 Korean Won (1000 Korean won is approximately 1.00 US dollars) per month. Occupations were categorized as follows: none, mostly sedentary work, work demanding some walking, work demanding physical exertion, and work demanding heavy physical exertion. Manual work was defined as work demanding physical or heavy physical exertion. Exercise status was self-reported, and

answers were classified as < 3 times/week or ≥3 times/week. Smoking was defined as more than 20 packs of cigarettes smoked during the participants' lifetime. Alcohol consumption was defined as the drinking of any alcoholic beverage more than once per month. Comorbidity health information was also self-reported and recorded using 29 predefined diagnostic categories, which included hypertension, diabetes mellitus, arthritis, stroke, and osteoporosis. Body mass indexes (BMIs) were calculated as the body weight divided by the height squared (kg/m^2).

Radiographic assessment
All the participants underwent radiographic examination of both knees in a weight-bearing anteroposterior view with a semi-flexed knee position. A Plexiglas frame (SYNARC, San Francisco, CA, USA) was used to standardize the knee positions. Details of the study protocol were described elsewhere [15]. Knee OA severity was classified as grade 0–4 according to the Kellgren/Lawrence (K-L) grading system. Radiographic OA was defined as a K-L grade of ≥ 2, and severe radiographic OA was defined as a K-L grade of 3 or 4. Radiographs were read twice by one reader, an academically-based rheumatologist of 17 years of experience (HAK). The reproducibility of the intra-reader assessments was high (for OA vs. no OA, κ = 0.89). Films that allocated different K-L grades at the two readings were adjudicated through consensus between the original reader and a second reader (David Hunter at the University of Sydney).

Statistical analysis
The participants were divided into 4 age groups, namely, 50–59 (29 participants), 60–69 (88 participants), 70–79 (178 participants), and 80–89 years (27 participants). Due to the inherent limitations of complete case analysis, a post hoc available-case analysis was performed, when possible, to check for dropout bias. The age-specific prevalence of 3-year incidence, progression, and worsening of radiographic knee OA were calculated. The incidence of radiographic knee OA was defined as having a K-L grade of 0 or 1 at baseline and a grade of ≥ 2 (radiographic OA) at follow-up. Progression was defined as an increase of the K-L grade at follow-up from grades 2 or 3 at baseline. Worsening was defined as an increase in the K-L grade at follow-up from any other grade (including grades 0 and 1). The group with worsening knee OA essentially included incident cases. The annual cumulative incidence, progression, and worsening were calculated by dividing them with the number of years under observation. To compare participants with/without OA, continuous variables were tested using the Mann-Whitney U test, and categorical variables were tested using Fisher's exact test. Crude odds ratios (OR)

for risk factors for incidence, progression, and worsening of radiographic knee OA were calculated using 95% confidence intervals (CI). Adjusted ORs were calculated using logistic regression analysis after adjusting for the factors significantly associated with incidence, progression, and worsening of knee OA in univariate analysis. Data were analyzed using SPSS version 15. Data are presented as median and interquartile ranges (IQR) or as percentages. P values < 0.05 (2-tailed) were considered statistically significant.

Results

Characteristics of the study participants

Of the 504 participants who underwent knee radiographs in the 2007 survey, 322 completed the survey, including radiographs, and constituted our 2010 study cohort. There was no significant difference in age and sex between the complete follow-up group and the group lost to follow-up (Table 1). The median

Table 1 Baseline characteristics of the entire cohort, participants with complete follow-up, and participants lost to follow-up

[a]Characteristics	Entire cohort (n = 504)	Complete follow-up (n = 322)	Lost to follow-up (n = 182)
Age, median (IQR) years	71 (66.0–75.0)	71.0 (66.0–75.0)	72 (65.0–76.0)
Women	54.4	53.4	56.0
BMI, median (IQR) kg/m²	24.7 (22.4–26.7)	24.6 (22.4–26.5)	25.2 (22.4–27.0)
Lower level of education	78.0	75.5	82.4
Low income	24.4	22.0	28.6
Exercise (≥ 3 times/week)	26.0	28.3	22.0
Previous or current smoker	40.5	40.7	40.1
Previous or current alcohol consumption	41.5	39.4	45.1
Manual occupation	19.8	21.4	17
K/L grade in worst knee			
Grade 3	9.7	9.6	9.9
Grade 4	9.3	8.4	11.0
Diabetes mellitus	10.1	9.0	12.1
Osteoporosis	19.2	19.3	19.2

IQR interquartile range, BMI body mass index, K-L Kellgren-Lawrence, TKR total knee replacement

[a]Except where indicated otherwise, values are written as percentages. Levels of education were classified as < 10 years or ≥ 10 years. Income was divided into 11 categories and low income was defined as < 500,000 Korean won per month. Exercise status was self-reported and responses were classified as < 3 times/week or ≥ 3 times/week. Smoking was defined as more than 20 packs of cigarettes having ever been smoked during the participants' lifetime. Alcohol consumption was defined as the drinking of any alcoholic beverage more than once per month. Manual work was defined as work demanding physical or heavy physical exertion. Co-morbidity health information was also self-reported, and was recorded using 29 pre-defined diagnostic categories. Diabetes mellitus was defined as either a fasting glucose level ≥ 126 mg/dL or a 2-h glucose level of ≥200 mg/dL after 75-g oral glucose loading, or treatment for previously diagnosed diabetes mellitus

participant age was 71.0 years, and 53.4% were women in the complete follow-up group. Fifty-eight participants (18%) had moderate to severe OA, defined as a K-L grade of ≥ 3. The characteristics of the 504 participants at baseline in this study are shown in Table 1. The median age of subjects with knee OA was higher than those without knee OA (72.64: 68.62 years) (Table 2).

Participants who were not obese (BMI < 25 kg/m²) were more likely to have no knee OA (67.4%). The characteristics of the subjects with/without knee OA at baseline are shown in Table 2.

Prevalence of incidence, progression and worsening of radiographic knee OA

The incidence of radiographic knee OA was observed in 33 (10.2%, male: female [M: F] = 9.3%: 11%) participants (7[2.17%], bilateral), and progression in 43 (13.55%, M: F = 3.33%: 22.09%) participants (15[4.66%], bilateral). The worsening of radiographic knee OA was observed in 126 (39.1%, M: F = 29.3%: 47.7%). The rates of incidence, progression, and worsening were the highest in the 70–79 age groups (6.2%, 8.39%, 23.6%, respectively), and leveled off afterwards. Women tended to have higher rates of progression and worsening in all age groups. The prevalence of incidence, progression, and worsening of radiographic knee OA in respect of age and sex are summarized in Figs. 1, 2, and 3.

Longitudinal risk factors for radiographic knee OA

We analyzed the data to determine risk factors for the progression of radiographic knee OA (Table 3). In the univariate analysis, sex, smoking, alcohol consumption, manual occupation, marriage, education level and osteoporosis were significantly associated with the progression of radiographic knee OA. However, in the multivariate logistic regression analysis, only women were significantly associated with the progression of radiographic knee OA (OR = 4.41, 95% CI 1.32–14.77). We next performed an analysis to determine the risk factors for worsening of radiographic knee OA (Table 3). Being female (OR = 1.41, 95% CI 1.02–1.95), and having a lower level of education (OR = 0.52, 95% CI 0.35–0.77) were significantly associated with a worsening of radiographic knee OA in the univariate analysis. In the multivariate logistic regression analysis, only a lower level of education was significantly associated with worsening of radiographic knee OA (OR = 0.56, 95% CI 0.37–0.86). In the incidence analysis of radiographic knee OA, we could not find any correlating risk factor.

Discussion

In this prospective 3-year follow-up study of 504 Chuncheon city residents aged 50 years and older, 322 participants (male: female = 150: 172) underwent a 3-

Table 2 Baseline characteristics of the subjects with/without knee osteoarthritis

[a]Characteristics	No. of subjects	No knee osteoarthritis (n = 307, 60.9%)	Knee osteoarthritis (n = 197, 39.1%)	P value
Age, median (IQR) years		68.62 (67.70–69.53)	72.64 (71.67–73.62)	< 0.001
Sex				< 0.001
Men	230	84.3	15.7	
Women	274	41.2	58.8	
BMI kg/m^2				0.001
< 25	264	67.4	32.6	
≥ 25	239	53.6	46.4	
Lower level of education	393	53.4	46.6	< 0.001
Low income	123	49.6	50.4	< 0.001
Exercise (≥ 3 times/week)	131	75.6	24.4	< 0.001
Previous or current smoker	204	81.9	18.1	< 0.001
Previous or current alcohol consumption	209	76.1	23.9	< 0.001
Manual occupation	100	32	68	< 0.001
Marriage (living without spouse)	157	36.3	63.7	< 0.001
Diabetes mellitus	51	60.8	39.2	0.984
Osteoporosis	97	44.3	55.7	< 0.001

IQR interquartile range, *BMI* body mass index

[a]Except where indicated otherwise, values are written as percentages. Levels of education were classified as < 10 years or ≥10 years. Income was divided into 11 categories and low income was defined as < 500,000 Korean won per month. Exercise status was self-reported and responses were classified as < 3 times/week or ≥3 times/week. Smoking was defined as more than 20 packs of cigarettes having ever been smoked during the participants' lifetime. Alcohol consumption was defined as the drinking of any alcoholic beverage more than once per month. Manual work was defined as work demanding physical or heavy physical exertion. Co-morbidity health information was also self-reported, and was recorded using 29 pre-defined diagnostic categories. Diabetes mellitus was defined as either a fasting glucose level ≥ 126 mg/dL or a 2-h glucose level of ≥200 mg/dL after 75-g oral glucose loading, or treatment for previously diagnosed diabetes mellitus

year follow-up knee radiograph. Incidence, progression, and worsening of knee OA were observed in a significant number of participants at the 3-year follow-up. In the multivariate logistic regression analysis, only women were significantly associated with the progression of radiographic knee OA and a lower level of education

was significantly associated with the worsening of radiographic knee OA.

A limited number of population-based studies have examined the incidence or progression of radiographic knee OA [8, 13, 14, 17, 18] and only two have reported on Asian populations [13, 14]. In the US Framingham

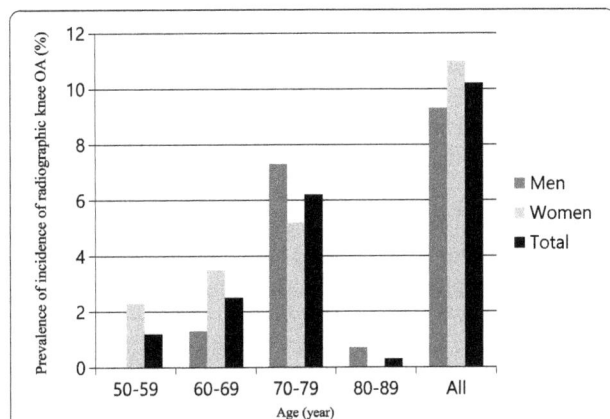

Fig. 1 Prevalence of incidence of radiographic knee OA, according to age and sex. Incidence of radiographic knee OA was defined as having a K-L grade of 0 or 1 at baseline and a grade of ≥ 2 at follow-up

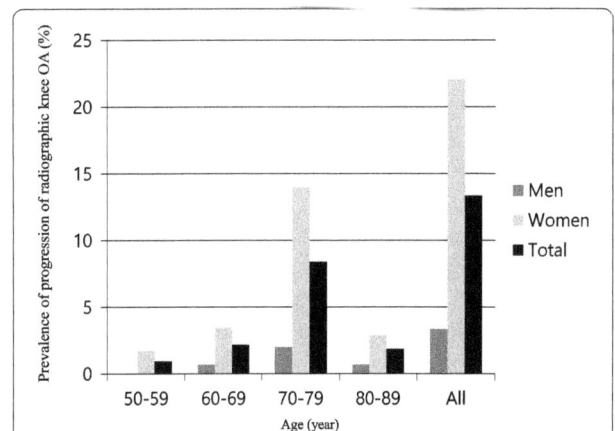

Fig. 2 Prevalence of the progression of radiographic knee OA, according to age and sex. Progression of radiographic knee OA was defined as an increase of the K-L grade at follow-up, from grades of 2 and 3 at baseline

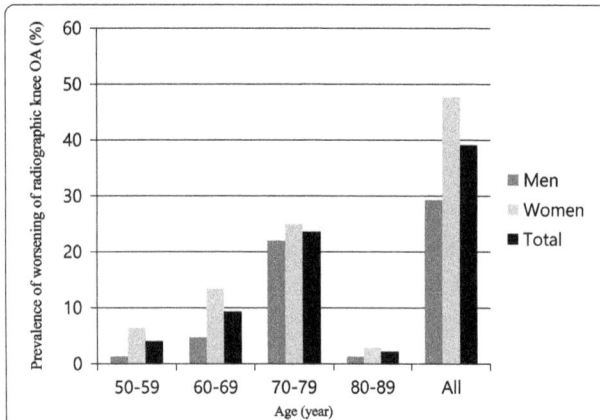

Fig. 3 Prevalence of radiographic knee OA worsening, according to age and sex. Worsening of radiographic knee OA was defined as an increase of the K-L grade at follow-up, from any baseline grade

Osteoarthritis Study which involved follow-up after a mean 8.1-year interval, the progression of radiographic knee OA, defined as having a K-L grade of ≥ 2 at baseline and showing an increase of at least one K-L grade at follow-up, was 24.2% and 31.8% (3.0% and 3.9% per year) in men and women, respectively [17]. In the Chingford Women's Study, a UK community-based cohort were followed-up for more than 14 years, and the annual rates of disease progression and worsening were 2.8% and 3.0%, respectively [18]. In the present study, the annual rate of knee OA progression, and worsening was 7.36%, and 15.9% in women, respectively, which is much higher than that of previous studies in the US and UK [8, 17, 18], implying that progression, and worsening of knee OA is higher among Korean women than in those of European origin. In the Japanese population-based 3-year follow-up ROAD study, the progression rate of knee OA was 6.3% per year in women [14]. The higher progression rate of radiographic knee OA in Korean and Japanese women might be due to lifestyle factors, such as sitting with legs crossed, sitting with knees and feet together on the floor, or genetic factors.

In the Framingham Osteoarthritis Study, the incidence of radiographic knee OA was 1.4% and 2.2% per year, in men and women, respectively [17]. In the Chingford Women's Study, the incidence was 2.3% per year in women [18]. In the ROAD study, the incidence was 2.0% and 3.7% per year, in Japanese men and women, respectively [14]. In the present study, we also examined the incidence of knee OA, and found that the incidence rate of knee OA was 3.1% and 3.7% per year, in Korean men and women, respectively, which was also higher than that of other previous epidemiologic studies in the US, and the UK [17, 18]. We could not find any risk factors

for the incidence of knee OA, which may be attributable to the rather small sample size of the present study.

In this study, only women were significantly associated with the progression of radiographic knee OA after adjustment for covariates including age, BMI, education, income, exercise, smoking, alcohol consumption, manual occupation, marriage, baseline K-L grade, DM, and osteoporosis. Being female has previously been reported as a risk factor for knee OA [6, 13, 14]. Only a low education level was significantly associated with the worsening of radiographic knee OA while being female was significant only in the univariate analysis. The level of education correlates with sex in this study cohort, which suggests that multicollinearity would have been the cause of this discrepancy. Although smoking was negatively associated with the progression of OA in the univariate analysis, it is intuitively improbable that it actually protects against OA progression. In addition, it was strongly correlated with sex; therefore, we excluded smoking in the multivariate analysis. A lower level of education, which was significantly associated with the worsening of radiographic knee OA, has been associated with the increased prevalence, morbidity and mortality of many chronic diseases. Several previous studies have examined the relationship between formal education levels, and hip and knee OA, showing results consistent with our study [19–21]. In the National Health and Nutrition Examination Survey of the USA, adjustment for age, knee injury, ethnicity, obesity, occupation, and low educational attainment were associated with a high prevalence of knee OA in both men and women, [19]. After adjustment for known risk factors, educational attainment, as an indicator of socioeconomic status, is associated with symptomatic knee OA in both men and women and with radiographic knee OA in US women [20]. In a USA study of African-American and European-American men and women aged ≥ 45 years, pain and disability were significantly associated with low educational attainment in radiographic and symptomatic hip OA, after adjusting for covariates included age, sex, ethnicity, BMI, and the presence of knee symptoms [21].

Our study had strengths and limitations. To the best of our knowledge, the present study is the first longitudinal study to evaluate the progression, incidence, and risk factors of radiographic knee OA, using standardized radiographs and a recognized grading system in Korea. However, despite its prospective design, which is rare in Asian population studies, 3 years is a rather short time to evaluate the progression of OA. Our study contains a relatively small sample size, and the previously known risk factors of knee OA may not be statistically significant. The study area included only Chuncheon, a city in South Korea, reducing the representativeness of the study sample.

Table 3 Risk factors for progression and worsening of radiographic knee osteoarthritis in elderly community residents

	Progression of knee OA		Worsening of knee OA	
	Crude OR (95% CI)	Adjusted OR (95% CI)	Crude OR (95% CI)	Adjusted OR (95% CI)
Age	1.04 (0.99–1.09)		0.99 (0.98–1.02)	
Sex				
Men	1.0	1.0	1.0	1.0
Women	7.25 (2.80–18.74)	4.41 (1.32–14.77)	1.41 (1.02–1.95)	1.21 (0.85–1.71)
BMI, kg/m²				
< 25	1.0		1.0	
≥ 25	1.44 (0.77–2.70)		1.32 (0.95–1.82)	
Education (year)				
< 10	1.0	1.0	1.0	1.0
≥ 10	0.24 (0.07–0.81)	0.59 (0.16–2.10)	0.52 (0.35–0.77)	0.56 (0.37–0.86)
Income (10,000 won/month)				
< 50	1.0		1.0	
50–149	0.85 (0.37–1.94)		0.73 (0.48–1.14)	
≥ 150	0.43 (0.16–1.12)		0.72 (0.47–1.13)	
Exercise				
No	1.0		1.0	
Yes	0.44 (0.18–1.06)		0.71 (0.49–1.03)	
[a]Smoking				
No	1.0		1.0	
Yes (ex-, current)	0.26 (0.11–0.59)		0.79 (0.58–1.11)	
Alcohol consumption				
No	1.0	1.0	1.0	
Yes (ex-, current)	0.29 (0.13–0.65)	0.78 (0.30–2.04)	1.12 (0.81–1.56)	
Manual occupation				
No	1.0	1.0	1.0	
Yes	2.66 (1.37–5.16)	1.74 (0.84–3.58)	0.95 (0.63–1.42)	
Marriage				
Yes (living with spouse)	1.0	1.0	1.0	
No	2.53 (1.35–4.75)	1.11 (0.55–2.26)	1.25 (0.88–1.77)	
Baseline K-L grade				
0	1.0		1.0	
1	1.00 (< 0.001– > 999.99)		0.96 (0.62–1.49)	
2	> 999.9 (< 0.001– > 999.9)		1.21 (0.72–2.03)	
3	> 999.9 (< 0.001– > 999.9)		1.23 (0.66–2.31)	
Diabetes mellitus				
No	1.0		1.0	
Yes	1.19 (0.45–3.17)		1.23 (0.72–2.11)	
Osteoporosis				
No	1.0	1.0	1.0	
Yes	2.48 (1.27–4.84)	1.18 (0.58–2.41)	1.17 (0.77–1.76)	

[a]Most of the women were non-smokers (male: female = 27.3%: 93.6%). Smoking was removed from the multivariate analysis because of the multicollinearity problem with sex

OR odds ratio, 95% CI 95% confidence interval, BMI body mass index, K-L Kellgren-Lawrence

Conclusions

The incidence, progression, and worsening of radiographic knee OA were observed in a significant number of participants at 3-year follow-up. Being female was a risk factor for the progression of radiographic knee OA, and having a lower level of education was a risk factor for the worsening of radiographic knee OA in this longitudinal study. Understanding the risk factors for knee OA may provide insights into preventative measures and therapeutic strategies for knee OA.

Abbreviations

BMI: Body mass index; CI: Confidence interval; DM: Diabetes mellitus; IQR: Interquartile range; K-L: Kellgren/Lawrence; OA: Osteoarthritis; OR: Odds ratio; ROA: Radiographic knee OA; TKR: Total knee replacement

Acknowledgements

Not applicable.

Funding

Funded by the Ministry of Health & Welfare, Republic of Korea (grant number: HI16C0287).

Authors' contributions

Research conception and design: HAK and JJY. Data acquisition: DH K and HAK. Statistical analysis: HAK and JJY. Drafting of the manuscript: JJY and HAK. Critical revision of the manuscript: JJY and HAK. Approval of the final manuscript: all the above-listed authors.

Consent for publication

Not applicable.

Competing interests

The authors declare that they have no competing interests.

Author details

[1]Department of Internal Medicine, Kangdong Sacred Heart Hospital, Seoul, South Korea. [2]Department of Social and Preventive Medicine, Hallym University College of Medicine, Chuncheon, South Korea. [3]Rheumatology Division, Department of Internal Medicine, Hallym University Sacred Heart Hospital, 896, Pyongchondong, Dongan-gu, Anyang, Kyunggi-do 431-070, South Korea.

References

1. Kim S. Changes in surgical loads and economic burden of hip and knee replacements in the US: 1997-2004. Arthritis Rheum. 2008;59:481–8.
2. Kim HA, Kim S, Seo YI, Choi HJ, Seong SC, Song YW, Hunter D, Zhang Y. The epidemiology of total knee replacement in South Korea: national registry data. Rheumatology. 2008;47:88–91.
3. Davis MA, Ettinger WH, Neuhaus JN, Cho SA, Hauck WW. The association of knee injury and obesity with unilateral and bilateral osteoarthritis of the knee. Am J Epidemiol. 1989;130:278–88.
4. Hart DJ, Doyle DV, Spector TD. The association between metabolic factors and knee osteoarthritis in women: the Chingford study. J Rheumatol. 1995;22:1118–23.
5. Felson DT, Zhang Y, Hannan MT, Naimark A, Weissman B, Aliabadi P, Levy D. Risk factors for incident radiographic knee osteoarthritis in the elderly: the Framingham study. Arthritis Rheum. 1997;40:728–33.
6. Slemenda C, Heilman DK, Brandt KD, Katz BP, Mazzuca SA, Braunstein EM, Byrd D. Reduced quadriceps strength relative to body weight: a risk factor for knee osteoarthritis in women? Arthritis Rheum. 1998;41:1951 9.
7. McAlindon TE, Wilson PW, Aliabadi P, Weissman B, Felson DT. Level of physical activity and the risk of radiographic and symptomatic knee osteoarthritis in the elderly: the Framingham study. Am J Med. 1999;106:151–7.
8. Cooper C, Snow S, McAlindon TE, Kellingray S, Stuart B, Coggon D, Dieppe PA. Risk factors for the incidence and progression of radiographic knee osteoarthritis. Arthritis Rheum. 2000;43:995–1000.
9. Wilder FV, Hall BJ, Barrett JP Jr, Lemrow NB. History of acute knee injury and osteoarthritis of the knee: a prospective epidemiological assessment. The Clearwater Osteoarthritis Study Osteoarthritis Cartilage. 2002;10:611–6.
10. Cerejo R, Dunlop DD, Cahue S, Channin D, Song J, Sharma L. The influence of alignment on risk of knee osteoarthritis progression according to baseline stage of disease. Arthritis Rheum. 2002;46:2632–6.
11. Reijman M, Pols HA, Bergink AP, Hazes JM, Belo JN, Lievense AM, Bierma-Zeinstra SM. Body mass index associated with onset and progression of osteoarthritis of the knee but not of the hip: the Rotterdam study. Ann Rheum Dis. 2007;66:158–62.
12. Bastick AN, Runhaar J, Belo JN, Bierma-Zeinstra SM. Prognostic factors for progression of clinical osteoarthritis of the knee: a systematic review of observational studies. Arthritis Res Ther. 2015;17:152.
13. Nishimura A, Hasegawa M, Kato K, Yamada T, Uchida A, Sudo A. Risk factors for the incidence and progression of radiographic osteoarthritis of the knee among Japanese. Int Orthop. 2011;35:839–43.
14. Muraki S, Akune T, Oka H, Ishimoto Y, Nagata K, Yoshida M, Tokimura F, Nakamura K, Kawaguchi H, Yoshimura N. Incidence and risk factors for radiographic knee osteoarthritis and knee pain in Japanese men and women: a longitudinal population-based cohort study. Arthritis Rheum. 2012;64:1447–56.
15. Kim I, Kim HA, Seo YI, Song YW, Jeong JY, Kim DH. The prevalence of knee osteoarthritis in elderly community residents in Korea. J Korean Med Sci. 2010;25:293–8.
16. Korean Statistical Office, The Republic of Korean Government. Korean census. 2000. http://kosis.kr/index/index.jsp. Accessed 21 Nov 2017.
17. Felson DT, Zhang Y, Hannan MT, Naimark A, Weissman BN, Aliabadi P, Levy D. The incidence and natural history of knee osteoarthritis in the elderly. The Framingham osteoarthritis study. Arthritis Rheum. 1995;38:1500–5.
18. Leyland KM, Hart DJ, Javaid MK, Judge A, Kiran A, Soni A, Goulston LM, Cooper C, Spector TD, Arden NK. The natural history of radiographic knee osteoarthritis: a fourteen-year population-based cohort study. Arthritis Rheum. 2012;64:2243–51.
19. Hannan MT, Anderson JJ, Pincus T, Felson DT. Educational attainment and osteoarthritis: differential associations with radiographic changes and symptom reporting. J Clin Epidemiol. 1992;45:139–47.
20. Callahan LF, Shreffler J, Siaton BC, Helmick CG, Schoster B, Schwartz TA, Chen JC, Renner JB, Jordan JM. Limited educational attainment and radiographic and symptomatic knee osteoarthritis: a cross-sectional analysis using data from the Johnston County (North Carolina) osteoarthritis project. Arthritis Res Ther. 2010;12:R46.
21. Knight JB, Callahan LF, Luong ML, Shreffler J, Schoster B, Renner JB, Jordan JM. The association of disability and pain with individual and community socioeconomic status in people with hip osteoarthritis. Open Rheumatol J. 2011;5:51–8.

10

Modified Lemaire extra-articular stabilisation of the knee for the treatment of anterolateral instability combined with diffuse pigmented villonodular synovitis

Cliodhna Farthing*[iD], Gernot Lang, Matthias J. Feucht, Norbert P. Südkamp and Kaywan Izadpanah

Abstract

Background: Diffuse pigmented villonodular synovitis (PVNS) of the knee is a rare proliferative joint disease associated with high recurrence rates following surgical treatment. Intra-articular joint instability in conjunction with PVNS implies complex reconstructive strategies due to the destructive nature of the disease.

Case presentation: Here, we present the case of a young patient with refractory PVNS and a chronic ipsilateral anterior cruciate ligament (ACL) rupture. Clinically, the patient presented with a grade 3 pivot shift phenomenon, indicating anterolateral rotational instability. Usually, PVNS implies a contraindication for ACL reconstruction due to the degenerative and pro-inflammatory joint microenvironment that is induced and maintained by PVNS. Therefore, we have performed a modified Lemaire extra-articular stabilization resulting in significant clinical improvement and subjective joint stability. In the latest follow-up examination at 12 months, the patient reported subjective joint stability and no swelling. In the clinical examination, the patient showed dynamic joint stability during walking. Additionally, the patient presented with grade 0 in pivot-shifting compared to the contralateral knee. The Lachman test exhibited no increased side-to-side difference and a firm endpoint.

Conclusions: Extra-articular anterolateral stabilisation of the knee in patients having anterolateral knee instability combined with PVNS is a safe and efficient surgical treatment option yielding significant clinical improvement as well as subjective joint stability.

Keywords: PVNS, Tenodesis, Anterolateral instability, Lemaire procedure

Background

Diffuse pigmented villonodular synovitis (PVNS) is a rare proliferative disease (prevalence of 1.8 cases per 1 million) with recurrence rates as high as 48% after surgical procedures [1]). PVNS mainly affects patients between 20 and 40 years of age with a slight female predilection [1, 2]. However, there is no difference between the genders considering age distribution [2]. Current research suggests the knee being the most commonly affected site for PVNS in 50–75% of cases [2–4]. Common symptoms of diffuse PVNS are slowly progressive soft tissue swelling surrounding the joint, impaired range of motion and recurring joint locking. As PVNS frequently presents with a refractory pattern, its long term management can be difficult, since it often includes complicated and demanding courses of disease as well as a high socioeconomic burden.

Chronic progressive tissue degeneration (cartilage, ligaments etc.) can be a pattern of PVNS due to the chronic proinflammatory and catabolic microenvironment within the joint [4, 5]. Therefore, in addition to synovectomy, reconstructive surgery may also have to be

* Correspondence: cliodhna.farthing@uniklinik-freiburg.de
Department of Orthopedic and Trauma Surgery, Medical Center - Albert-Ludwigs-University of Freiburg, Faculty of Medicine, Albert-Ludwigs-University of Freiburg, Freiburg im Breisgau, Germany

carried out to preserve the structural integrity of the knee [6, 7]. However, due to impaired fibrous healing of intra-articular transplants, conventional ACL reconstructive techniques are mostly contraindicated [8]. Therefore, alternative approaches such as the Lemaire procedure have recently gained interest, since these novel techniques might help to overcome current limitations in ACL reconstruction in PVNS [7, 9], which include impaired graft healing and graft failure [8, 10]. Biomechanically, lateral extra-articular tenodeses can reduce rotatory laxity of the knee [11]. Therefore, this technique may be considered to restore native joint kinematics in a subset of patients after careful consideration of chances and risks.

As far as we are aware, we describe the first case of a young patient with diffuse PVNS and chronic anterolateral instability to undergo an isolated modified Lemaire extra-articular stabilisation of the knee.

Case presentation

A 21-year-old patient, amateur basketball player, presented initially in 2014 with a diffuse swelling of the knee. The swelling occurred intermittently over approximately two months without an obvious trigger. Furthermore, the patient reported pain after extended basketball training sessions. Magnetic resonance imaging (MRI) of the knee revealed significant articular effusion and villous synovial proliferation. A histological biopsy was taken which revealed chronic synovialitis, villous hyperplasia and hemosiderin stained giant cells. Arthroscopic findings (Fig. 1) confirmed the diagnosis of diffuse PVNS of the knee and an intact ACL. Subsequently, an arthroscopic total synovectomy was performed in order to slow down the progression of cartilage degeneration as

well as to restore range-of-motion, reduce pain, and joint instability.

After 6 asymptomatic months, the patient started suffering repeated knee distortions due to persistent anterolateral instability in his knee joint. A follow-up MRI confirmed the recurrent PVNS and an ipsilateral ACL rupture (Figs. 2 and 3). At this point, the patient opted for intensive physical therapy to stabilise the joint. During this time, he described an acute rotational trauma while exiting his car resulting in a small bucket handle tear in the white-white zone of the medial meniscus of the ipsilateral knee. Owing to coexisting degenerative changes of the dislocated fragment of the medial meniscus, anatomical reduction of the meniscus was not reasonable. Therefore, a re-synovectomy with a partial meniscectomy was conducted. 7 months later a similar mechanism of injury caused a re-rupture of the medial meniscus. Again a bucket handle tear was present, this time at the basis of the meniscus running from the pars intermedia to the posterior horn. Under the intention of restoring the structural integrity of this young patient's knee another synovectomy and meniscus repair was undertaken. However, the patient suffered persistent giving away phenomena and was not able to further perform sports or properly work as an electrician.

The remaining therapeutic options to address the patient's persisting anterolateral instability were re-assessed within a multidisciplinary consultation with oncologists, radiologists and orthopaedic surgeons. Due to the chronic intra-articular effusion and synovitis, an extra-articular stabilisation of the knee was suggested.

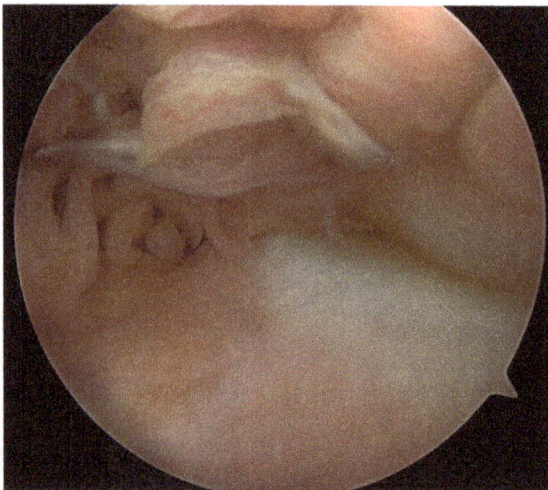

Fig. 1 Diagnostic arthroscopy showing exhuberant intra-articular synovial proliferation, synovial inflammation and papillary projections, which are typical of diffuse PVNS

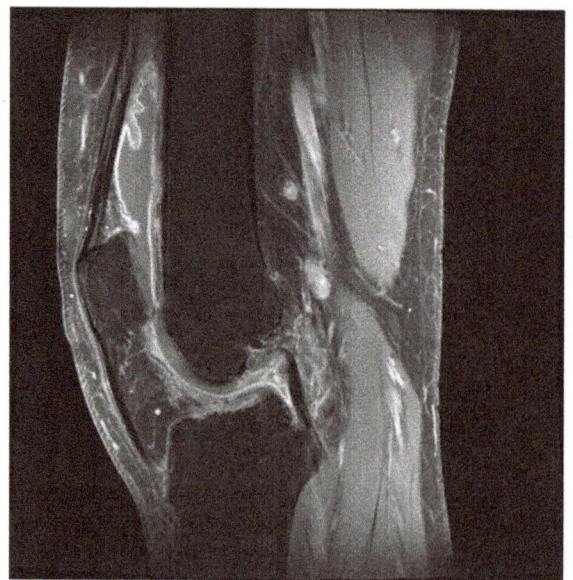

Fig. 2 Saggital T2 MRI of the knee with fat saturation showing extensive intra-articular inflamed synovia and a ruptured ACL

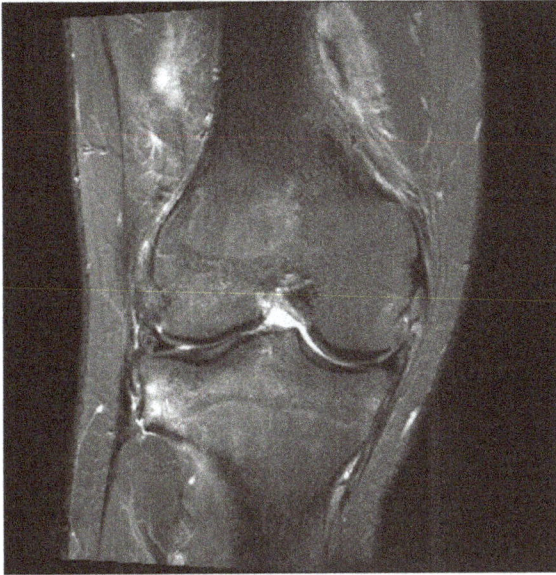

Fig. 3 Coronal T2 MRI of the knee with fat saturation showing a ruptured ACL and high intensity signalling in the notch

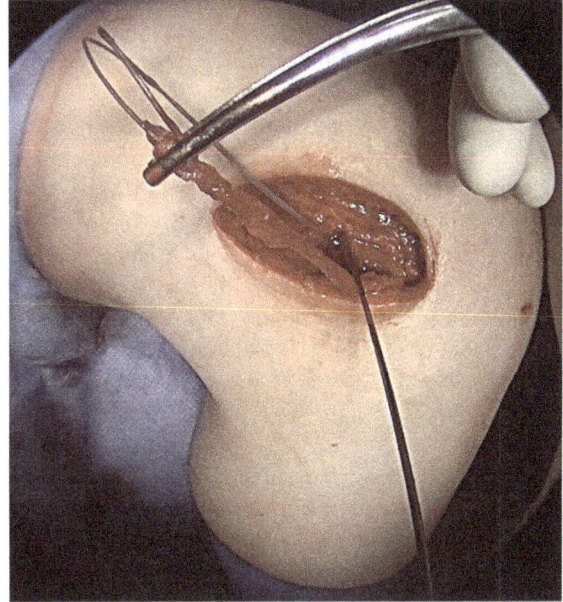

Fig. 4 First intra-operative image. The tractus band transplant was inserted underneath the LCL and pulled into the socket

Pre-operative clinical examination of the right knee revealed minimal muscular atrophy and a considerable joint effusion compared to the healthy knee. The patient reported tenderness during palpation over the medial joint line. His active range of motion was unrestricted. During the Lachman test the knee exhibited greater anterior translation than the contralateral knee without a firm endpoint. The knee presented a grade 3 pivot shift. There was no posterior drawer effect. The valgus and varus stress tests were negative at 0° and 30° degrees flexion. Steinmann I was discretely positive for the medial meniscus.

After conventional pre-operative preparations, surgery was performed. Briefly, a renewed medial meniscus suturing was performed arthroscopically, as again a complex tear of the posterior horn was present. All-inside suturing using a meniscus suturing device was carried out. Successively, the tractus iliotibialis was exposed and the lateral epicondyle was identified through palpation. The tractus was exised 0.5 cm dorsal of the lateral epicondyle, followed by its split parallel to the direction of the fibres, until yielding slightly proximal of Gerdy's tubercle. A 10x1cm strip was separated and armed with a Fiberwire with a baseball-stitch technique. The lateral collateral ligament (LCL) was exposed underneath the tractus iliotibialis. A 6 mm socket was made proximal and slightly posterior to the origin of the LCL. The tractus band transplant was inserted underneath the LCL and pulled into the socket (Fig. 4). The lower leg was secured in 70° flexion and neutral position to ensure the optimal tension of the transplant during the anchoring. Finally, the transplant was tensed gradually from 20 N, 30 N to finally 40 N until the pivot

shift was suspended and was subsequently fixated with an interference screw (Fig. 5).

Post-operatively, the clinical examination revealed a grade 0 pivot-shift test compared to the contralateral side. The Lachman test exhibited no increased side-to-side difference. The patient was compliant with

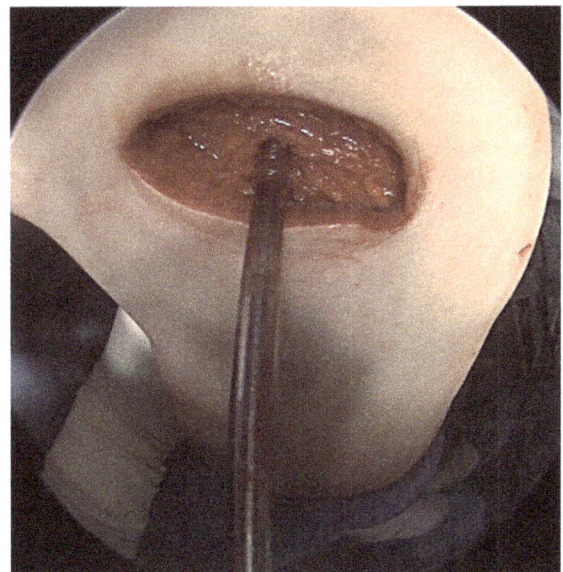

Fig. 5 Second intra-operative image. The lower leg was secured in 70° flexion and neutral position to ensure the optimal tension of the transplant during the anchoring. Finally, the transplant was tensed gradually until the pivot shift was suspended and was subsequently fixated with an interference screw at 40 N

the standard functional aftercare for meniscal suturing (range-of-motion limitation of 45° flexion for 3 weeks, followed by a limit of 90° flexion for further 3 weeks). In the latest follow-up examination at 12 months, the patient reported no further subjective instability and no swelling. He was able to perform moderate sports such as jogging and fully returned to work. In the clinical examination the patient showed dynamic joint stability during walking. The patient showed a grade 0 pivot-shift test compared to the contralateral knee. The Lachman test exhibited little increased side-to-side difference (Grade 1). Clinically, the patient showed no signs of progression of structural damage in the knee.

Discussion

In this case, we conducted an extra-articular reconstruction resulting in a clinical and functional improvement in the condition of the patient's knee. Usually, an intra-articular ACL reconstruction is contraindicated in patients with degenerative and pro-inflammatory intra-articular joint diseases such as PVNS. This condition was compounded by the patient describing chronic anterolateral instability with multiple distortions, causing additional structural damage to the knee. Therefore, this report suggests that isolated extra-articular anterolateral stabilisation of the knee in patients having anterolateral knee instability combined with PVNS presents a safe and efficient surgical treatment yielding in clinical improvement as well as subjective joint stability.

Extra-articular anterolateral reconstruction can be performed as an isolated surgery or to augment an intra-articular reconstruction [7, 12]. Combined extra- and intra-articular reconstruction may protect the intra-articular graft during the healing process and providing secondary restraint to the pivot-shift phenomenon [12–14]. Historically, most isolated extra-articular procedures performed in the 1970s–1980s were shown to provide restraint to the pivot-shift and Lachman manoeuvres. However, they were liable to stretch out in the long-term [15]. Additionally, these procedures were not able to address increased anterior tibial translation [9, 16]. With the recent resurgence of interest in extra-articular ACL reconstruction procedures, current literature suggests isolated extra-articular reconstruction may be performed in a small subset of patients with high-grade rotational laxity and an increased risk of failure with ACL reconstruction, such as revision cases [17–19].

The Lemaire procedure was first described in 1967 to treat ACL deficient knees with chronic instability. A long graft of fascia lata still attached to Gerdy's tubercle was passed below the LCL [13, 20], and then attached through a femoral bone tunnel. In the following, the graft was reinserted under the LCL before being attached at another bony tunnel under Gerdy's tubercle [9, 17]. This process has been simplified by securing the graft in the femur utilizing an interference screw as described by M. Wagner and A. Weiler [7]. Great care should be taken to perform pre-operative examination under anaesthesia before securing a tourniquet since the pressure of the tourniquet causes tension of the iliotibial tract which can stabilise the pivot-shift, therefore, causing a false-negative test [7].

Recent literature examining the biomechanics of extra-articular tenodesis suggests graft tension exceeding 20 N may increase lateral contact pressures and lead to overconstraint in internal rotation [21–23]. Specifically, one study by Inderhaug E. et al. comparing anterolateral procedures in combination with ACL reconstruction shows that grafts with 20 N of tension best restore native knee kinematics. In this case, an isolated anterolateral tenodesis was carried out in absence of an anterior cruciate ligament. During surgery tensioning was carried out using a spring scale. The pivot-shift was reduced at 20 N, however was still present. At 40 N the pivot-shift was suspended completely. In this set-up suspension of the pivot-shift was given higher priority compared to possible overconstraint of the knee in deep flexion degrees, as persistent instability might cause secondary damage to cartilage and menisci of the knee. In this case, our patient currently does not exhibit symptoms of overconstrained internal rotation or increased lateral tibiofemoral pressures.

The pivot-shift phenomenon is considered to have a multi-factorial pathogenic background in many cases. Contributing factors may include ligamentous laxity, altered bone morphology, and other soft tissue injuries [24–26]. Succeeding careful consideration of these factors, the pivot-shift test can be considered a reliable examination to evaluate rotational laxity. An increase in the grade of pivot-shift has been noted in injuries of the lateral structures in the ACL- deficient knee [24]. Additionally, some studies have shown the pivot-shift test can remain positive after intra-articular ACL reconstruction in a subset of patients, since even successful ACL reconstruction may fail to restore native knee functionality in regards to rotational abnormalities [17, 27, 28].

It is well established that timely ACL reconstruction reduces the risk of medial meniscal ruptures [29]. In the present case, PVNS presented a contraindication for ACL reconstruction due to the locally destructive and inflammatory nature of the disease. The pro-inflammatory joint microenvironment maintained by PVNS may have impaired the graft healing and increased the risk of graft failure [8, 10]. Additionally, the patient presented a high-grade anterolateral rotational instability. We presume that this chronic instability caused the recurrent medial meniscal tears over the course of the disease [29].

Therefore, despite the limitations which are historically described in isolated extra-articular reconstruction, in this case, a modified Lemaire extra-articular stabilisation of the knee was the most suitable procedure to restore knee kinematics and provide joint stability. In the future, it would be interesting to see studies showing the influence of isolated extra-articular stabilisation or combined intra- and extra-articular reconstruction on meniscal pathologies [13].

Conclusion

Extra-articular anterolateral reconstruction of the knee is a feasible alternative for patients with anterolateral knee instability combined with PVNS yielding in clinical improvement and subjective joint stability. Diffuse PVNS of the knee can be a complex disease which can be associated with a long-drawn-out clinical course with multiple complications. In the present case, the objective of the treatment was to prevent further recurrence and restore the structural integrity of the patient's knee. Especially in light of the patient's young age, the long-term goal was to forestall the indication for knee arthroplasty.

Summary

The present manuscript describes the case of a young patient with diffuse PVNS of the knee. We hereby show that an extra-articular stabilisation of the knee can be utilized for managing patients who imply contraindications for intra-articular reconstruction.

Abbreviations
ACL: Anterior cruciate ligament; LCL: Lateral collateral ligament; PVNS: Pigmented villonodular synovitis

Authors' contributions
KI and NPS treated the patient. CF collected the data and wrote the manuscript. GL and MJF were major contributors in writing the manuscript. All authors read and approved the final manuscript.

Consent for publication
We confirm that written patient consent was obtained for the publication of this case report and the figures included in this article.

Competing interests
Gernot Lang, M.D. has the following financial disclosures:
Educational grants: DePuy-Synthes
Travel grants: GSK Foundation, DePuy-Synthes

References
1. Patel KH, Gikas PD, Pollock RC, Carrington RW, Cannon SR, Skinner JA, et al. Pigmented villonodular synovitis of the knee: a retrospective analysis of 214 cases at a UK tertiary referral centre. Knee. 2017;24:808–15.
2. Xie G, Jiang N, Liang C, Zeng J, Chen Z, Xu Q, et al. Pigmented villonodular synovitis: a retrospective multicenter study of 237 cases. PLoS One. 2015;10: e0121451.
3. Mukhopadhyay K, Smith M, Hughes PM. Multifocal PVNS in a child – followed over 25 years. Skelet Radiol. 2006;35:539–42.
4. Darling JM, Glimcher LH, Shortkroff S, Albano B, Gravallese EM. Expression of metalloproteinases in pigmented villonodular synovitis. Hum Pathol. 1994;25:825–30.
5. Uchibori M, Nishida Y, Tabata I, Sugiura H, Nakashima H, Yamada Y, et al. Expression of matrix metalloproteinases and tissue inhibitors of metalloproteinases in pigmented villonodular synovitis suggests their potential role for joint destruction. J Rheumatol. 2004;31:110–9.
6. Imhoff AB. Pigmentierte villonoduläre Synovialitis (PVNS). In: Orthopädie und Orthopädische Chirurgie: Knie; 2005. p. 207–9.
7. Wagner M, Weiler A. Anterolaterale Stabilisierung. Arthroskopie. 2014;27:198–201.
8. Rajani R, Ogden L, Matthews CJ, Gibbs CP. Diffuse pigmented villonodular synovitis as a rare cause of graft failure following anterior cruciate ligament reconstruction. Orthopedics. 2018;41:e142–4.
9. Lemaire M, Combelles F. Plastic repair with fascia lata for old tears of the anterior cruciate ligament (author's transl). Rev Chir Orthop Reparatrice Appar Mot. 1980;66:523–5.
10. Deehan DJ, Cawston TE. The biology of integration of the anterior cruciate ligament. J Bone Joint Surg Br Vol. 2005;87-B:889–95.
11. Schon JM, Moatshe G, Brady AW, Serra Cruz R, Chahla J, Dornan GJ, et al. Anatomic anterolateral ligament reconstruction of the knee leads to overconstraint at any fixation angle. Am J Sports Med. 2016;44:2546–56.
12. Engebretsen L, Lew WD, Lewis JL, Hunter RE. The effect of an iliotibial tenodesis on intraarticular graft forces and knee joint motion. Am J Sports Med. 1990;18:169–76.
13. Vincent J-P, Magnussen RA, Gezmez F, Uguen A, Jacobi M, Weppe F, et al. The anterolateral ligament of the human knee: an anatomic and histologic study. Knee Surg Sports Traumatol Arthrosc. 2012;20:147–52.
14. Williams A, Ball S, Stephen J, White N, Jones M, Amis A. The scientific rationale for lateral tenodesis augmentation of intra-articular ACL reconstruction using a modified 'Lemaire' procedure. Knee Surg Sports Traumatol Arthrosc. 2017;25:1339–44.
15. Kennedy JC, Stewart R, Walker DM. Anterolateral rotatory instability of the knee joint. An early analysis of the Ellison procedure. J Bone Joint Surg Am. 1978;60:1031–9.
16. Schindler OS. Surgery for anterior cruciate ligament deficiency: a historical perspective. Knee Surg Sports Traumatol Arthrosc. 2012;20:5–47.
17. Dodds AL, Gupte CM, Neyret P, Williams AM, Amis AA. Extra-articular techniques in anterior cruciate ligament reconstruction: a literature review. J Bone Joint Surg Br. 2011;93:1440–8.
18. Lording TD, Lustig S, Servien E, Neyret P. Lateral reinforcement in anterior cruciate ligament reconstruction. Asia-Pac J Sports Med Arthrosc Rehabil Technol. 2014;1:3–10.
19. Noyes FR, Huser LE, Jurgensmeier D, Walsh J, Levy MS. Is an anterolateral ligament reconstruction required in ACL-reconstructed knees with associated injury to the anterolateral structures? A robotic analysis of rotational knee stability. Am J Sports Med. 2017;45:1018–27.
20. der Watt LV, Khan M, Rothrauff BB, Ayeni OR, Musahl V, Getgood A, et al. The structure and function of the anterolateral ligament of the knee: a systematic review. Arthroscopy. 2015;31:569–82. e3
21. Inderhaug E, Stephen JM, El-Daou H, Williams A, Amis AA. The effects of anterolateral tenodesis on tibiofemoral contact pressures and kinematics. Am J Sports Med. 2017;45:3081–8.
22. Inderhaug E, Stephen JM, Williams A, Amis AA. Anterolateral tenodesis or anterolateral ligament complex reconstruction: effect of flexion angle at graft fixation when combined with ACL reconstruction. Am J Sports Med. 2017;45:3089–97.
23. Inderhaug E, Stephen JM, Williams A, Amis AA. Biomechanical comparison of anterolateral procedures combined with anterior cruciate ligament reconstruction. Am J Sports Med. 2017;45:347–54.
24. Tanaka M, Vyas D, Moloney G, Bedi A, Pearle AD, Musahl V. What does it take to have a high-grade pivot shift? Knee Surg Sports Traumatol Arthrosc. 2012;20:737–42.
25. Fu FH, Herbst E. Editorial commentary: the pivot-shift phenomenon is multifactorial. Arthroscopy. 2016;32:1063–4.
26. Herbst E, Albers M, Burnham JM, Shaikh HS, Naendrup J-H, Fu FH, et al. The anterolateral complex of the knee: a pictorial essay. Knee Surg Sports Traumatol Arthrosc. 2017;25:1009–14.

27. Ristanis S, Stergiou N, Patras K, Vasiliadis HS, Giakas G, Georgoulis AD. Excessive tibial rotation during high-demand activities is not restored by anterior cruciate ligament reconstruction. Arthroscopy. 2005;21:1323–9.

28. Woo SL-Y, Kanamori A, Zeminski J, Yagi M, Papageorgiou C, Fu FH. The effectiveness of reconstruction of the anterior cruciate ligament with hamstrings and patellar tendon . A cadaveric study comparing anterior tibial and rotational loads. J Bone Joint Surg Am. 2002;84-A:907–14.

29. Yoo JC, Ahn JH, Lee SH, Yoon YC. Increasing incidence of medial meniscal tears in nonoperatively treated anterior cruciate ligament insufficiency patients documented by serial magnetic resonance imaging studies. Am J Sports Med. 2009;37:1478–83.

11

RHAMM induces progression of rheumatoid arthritis by enhancing the functions of fibroblast-like synoviocytes

Jing Wu, Yuan Qu, Yu-Ping Zhang, Jia-Xin Deng and Qing-Hong Yu*ⓘ

Abstract

Background: Rheumatoid arthritis (RA) is a chronic and refractory autoimmune joint disease. Fibroblast-like synoviocytes (FLS) produce inflammatory cytokines and are involved in the migration and invasion of panuus tissue, which leads to the destruction of joints in RA. Receptor for hyaluronan mediated motility (RHAMM), is known to be one of the important receptors for hyaluronic acid. It has the ability to regulate migration of fibrocytes and infiltration of inflammatory cells. Here,we explored the mechanisms of RHAMM in RAFs.

Methods: Quantitative PCR and western blot were performed to test the expression of RHAMM in synoviocytes of RA patients and osteoarthritis (OA) controls. Collagen antibody-induced arthritis (CAIA) was used to investigate the RHAMM expression in mouse synovial issues. RHAMM siRNA was used to detect the function of RHAMM in FLS.

Results: RA-FLS has a significantly higher expression of RHAMM than OA-FLS. Expression of RHAMM in joint synovial tissue was markedly increased in the CAIA mice compared with the controls. RHAMM silencing using SiRNA was not only decreased the production of IL-6 and IL-8, but also inhibited the migration and invasion of RA-FLS.

Conclusions: RHAMM has an important role in the FLS induced modulation of inflammation and destruction of joints in RA.

Keywords: Receptor for hyaluronan-mediated motility, Rheumatoid arthritis, Synoviocyte, siRNA

Background

Rheumatoid arthritis (RA) is an immune-mediated disorder induced by chronic and refractory autoimmunity in the synovial joints, which leads to the damage of the cartilage and bone. RA affects approximately 1% of the population globally, although its complex pathogenesis is not fully understood.[1, 2] The fibroblast-like synoviocytes (FLS) play a critical role in the progression of RA. These cells normally line the synovium, but in RA they proliferate in an uncontrolled manner and form the pannus tissue, a tumor-like structure that causes significant damage to the joints [3, 4]. In the synovial tissue, FLS secrete cytokines that induce persistent inflammation and degradation of the cartilage and bone[5–7]. Some pro-inflammatory cytokines like IL-6

and IL-8 were proposed as important factors in the pathogenesis of the synovial inflammation[8, 9]. FLS not only invades into the extracellular matrix and thus aggravates the joint damage, but it also promotes disease progression by migrating to the unaffected joints [10, 11]. Although the invasion and migration of FLS are known in RA pathology, the molecular basis of FLS activities is still undefined.

Several similarities have been observed between RA pathogenesis and tumor development, like inflammation, angiogenesis, and cell migration and proliferation. The extracellular matrix, hyaluronan (HA), and its receptor for RHAMM are implicated in the tumor progression [12], however, their role in RA is yet to be explored. RHAMM has an important role in several diseases, such as OA and ocular surface inflammation [13–15]. RHAMM interacts with all the types of cells and their functions, such as cell-cell adhesion, cell migration, cell proliferation, cell differentiation and metastasis [16].

* Correspondence: yuqinghong@smu.edu.cn
Department of Rheumatology and Clinical Immunology, ZhuJiang Hospital, Southern Medical University, 253 Gongye Ave GuangZhou, GuangDong 510282, China

Moreover, RHAMM aggravates the effect of CD44 deficiency on joint inflammation [17], which suggests RHAMM as an essential mediator of cell migration in RA pathogenesis. Hence, we hypothesized that RHAMM decreases the levels of IL-6 and IL-8, and is also involved in the migration of synoviocytes and in the infiltration process of inflammatory cells.

Methods

Human FLS culture

Synovial tissue samples were taken from the knees of three active RA and OA patients. RA patients were diagnosed according to 2010 the Rheumatoid arthritis classification criteria [18]. All OA patients were diagnosed based on American College of Rheumatology Subcommittee Guidelines for Osteoarthritis [19]. Biopsy samples were obtained during the knee joint arthroscopy. Synovial tissues were sectioned into $1-2\,mm^3$ pieces and cultured with DMEM containing 10% fetal calf serum, 100 U/ml of penicillin and 100 μg/mL of streptomycin, and incubated in a humidified incubator containing 5% CO_2. The culture medium was changed every 3–4 days. FLS was maintained as monolayers and serial passages between 3 to 6 were used for experiments described herein.

Quantitative PCR

Total RNA was isolated from RA-FLS and OA-FLS using Trizol reagent (Invitrogen, USA) according to manufacturer's protocols. Reverse transcription was carried out using the first-strand cDNA synthesis kit (TaKaRa, China). To assess the RHAMM mRNA, IL-6 and IL-8 expression, real-time PCR was performed using a SYBR Premix ExTaq kit (TaKaRa, China). The primers for RHAMM are listed as follows: Forward-CAGGTCACCCAAAGGAGTCTCG, Reverse-CAAGCTCATCCAGTGTTTGC, IL-6: Forward-CCGGGAACGAAAGAGAAGCT, Reverse-GCGCTTGT GGAGAAGGAGTT, IL-8: Forward-ATGACTCAGATG TGCTCTCAAAGG and Reverse-GCTTGCATCATGTC AGAGGAAATTC, β-actin: Forward-AACTACCTTCAA CTCCATCA, Reverse-GCCAGACTCGTCATACTC.

Western blot

Proteins were extracted from RA-FLS and OA-FLS with an extraction buffer. The samples were loaded on 8% polyacrylamide Tris/glycine gels and separated at 90 V for 1 h, then transferred to a nitrocellulose membrane at a setting of 90 V for 1 h. After blocking, the membrane was incubated over-night with primary Rabbit antibodies specific to RHAMM (1:10000, Santa Cruz, USA) or Mouse anti-β-actin (1:5000, Santa Cruz, USA) at 4 °C for overnight, and then incubated with Goat-anti-Rabbit HRP (1:5000, Santa Cruz, USA) or Equine-anti-Mouse HRP (1:10000, Santa Cruz, USA) respectively. After chemiluminescent staining and fixing, gel images were scanned and analyzed using image processing software (Image J).

Collagen antibody-induced arthritis

Ten weeks-old C57BL/6 mice were obtained from the animal laboratory of Southern Medical University, Guangzhou,China. The mice were housed in a standard environment (25 °C and 12 h light/dark cycle), and the mice were fed with standard food and water ad libitum. All the animal treatments were conducted in accordance with the ethical guidelines of the National Institutes of Health Guide for the Care and Use of Laboratory Animals [20]. Experiments were approved by the Ethics Committee of Southern Medical University (license no.SCXK 2011–0015). Mice were randomly divided into two groups ($n = 5$/group), CAIA and control groups. In the CAIA group mice were injected intravenously with 150 μL (1.5 mg) of five anti-type II collagen monoclonal antibodies at day 0, and 70 μL (35 μg) LPS after 3 days. Every mouse in the control group was injected intravenously with 150 μL of 0.9% saline and 70 μL of 0.9% saline after 3 days.

Arthritis scores

Mice were scored for arthritis from days 0 to 12 by using 5-point scale scoring system: 0 = no arthritis; 1 = mild joint deformity and swelling; 2 = moderate joint deformity and swelling; 3 = severe swelling in the toe, foot and ankle and 4 = severe inflammation.

Histology

On day 12, all the mice were sacrificed by decapitation, and their ankle, lung and kidney tissues were collected and fixed in 4% paraformaldehyde at room temperature for 6 h, dehydrated, embedded in paraffin and sectioned. Paraffin sections were HE stained for the evaluating the morphology of the joint. After heat-mediated antigen retrieval, sections were incubated with primary antibody for RHAMM (1:50) at 4 °C for 12 h, and then with secondary antibody (1:50) at room temperature for 30 min. For antigen visualization, the sections were immersed in 3-amino-9-ethylcarbazole+substrate-chromogen for 30 min, and counter-stained with Gill's haematoxylin for 30 min.

The RNA interference assay

In this assay, the small interfering RNA (siRNA) for against RHAMM (AM16708, Invitrogen) and the no-target control siRNA (AM4611, Invitrogen) were used. FLS were transiently transfected with the indicated combinations of the siRNAs using Lipofectamine™ 2000 transfection reagent (Invitrogen, USA) according to the manufacturer's recommendations. The efficiency of siRNA-mediated gene silencing was assessed using real-time quantitative PCR and Western blot.

Enzyme linked immunosorbent assay

After treatement with RHAMM siRNA, 2×10^4 RA-FLS or OA-FLS were stimulated in 24 wells using human IL-1 alpha (10 ng/ml, Invitrogen, USA) for 24 h, supernatant was collected and used for the detection of IL-6 and IL-8 levels by ELISA (Thermo Fisher Scientific, USA). The optical density (OD) of each sample was measured at 450 nm. Recombinant IL-6 and IL-8 cytokines were used as standards.

Migration and invasion assay of FLS

Wound scratch assay

To demonstrate the effects of siRNA on the migratory capacity of FLS, wound scratch assay was performed. After treatment with RHAMM siRNA, 2×10^4 RA-FLS and OA-FLS were seeded in 24-well plates. After serum starvation for 24 h, 200 µL pipette tip was used to make a perforation. FLS were viewed for 0–24 h. The rate of migration was calculated by measuring the distance of the wound after scratching as follows: rate of migration in % = [distance moved (migrating cell front)/total distance (wound margin)] × 100.

Transwell migration and invasion assay

The directed chemotaxis assay was performed using transwell chambers with 8 µm pores (Corning, BD Biosciences) coated with bovine serum albumin (BSA). Briefly, 10% fetal bovine serum (FBS)/DMEM as a chemoattractant was placed in the lower chambers. A total of 2×10^4 FLS were suspended in serum-free DMEM in the upper chambers for 48 h. After non-migrated cells were removed with a cotton swab, the membranes were fixed with 4% paraformaldehyde for 30 min and then stained with 0.1% crystal violet. Migration was quantified by using an optical microscope and counting the stained cells that migrated to the lower side of the filter. The number of migrated cells was presented as the migration index, and this value was calculated by normalizing relative to the media control,. For the invasion assay, similar experiments were performed using inserts coated with a Matrigel membrane matrix. Briefly, the FLS were seeded at a density of 2×10^4 and grown in DMEM for 48 h. Cells that invaded through the matrix to the basolateral side of the membrane were fixed and stained. For further calculations, means values of the number of invading cells from six field-of-view images normalized relative to the control were used.

Statistical analysis

Data are presented as the mean ± standard deviation. The Mann–Whitney U and the Kruskal-Wallis statistic tests using GraphPad Prism 5 were used to analyze the differences between groups. Differences were considered to be statistically significant when $p < 0.05$ at 95% confidence interval.

Results

Expression of RHAMM mRNA and protein in FLS

The RHAMM mRNA and protein expressions in the FLS of RA group were significantly higher ($p < 0.05$) compared with OA group (Fig. 1).

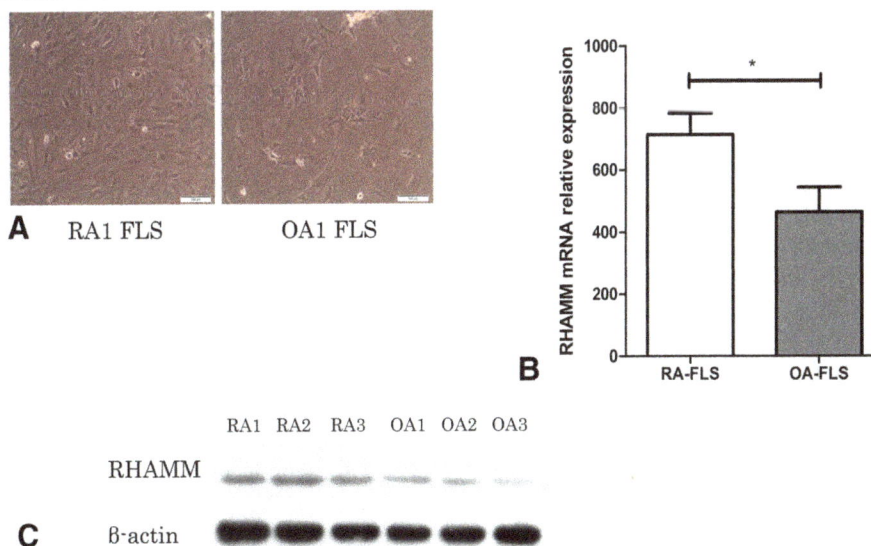

Fig. 1 a RA-FLS and OA-FLS culture ($n = 3$). Each sample was analyzed twice; (b) FLS mRNA and (c) protein expressions from active RA patients were higher than OA patients. *$p < 0.05$, Mann–Whitney U test.

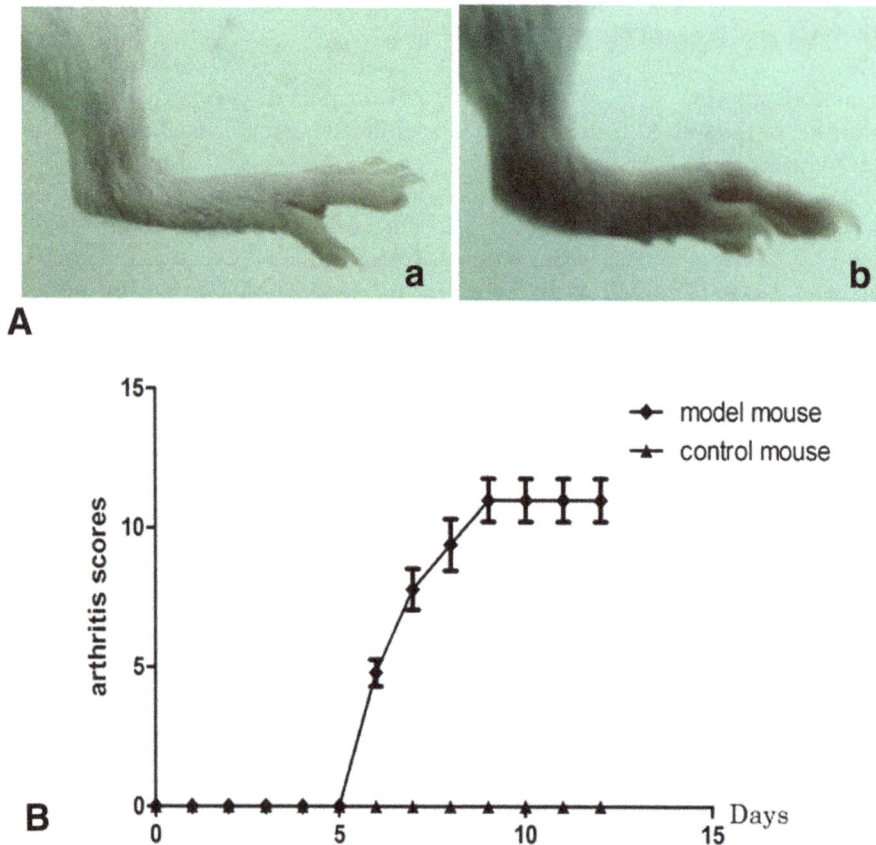

Fig. 2 Joint swelling (a) and arthritis scores (b) in CAIA and control mice (n = 5/group). a: normal joint in the control mouse; b: joint swelling and inflammation of CAIA mouse on 7th day.

Collagen antibody induced arthritis (CAIA) experiments
After injection with five anti-type II collagen monoclonal antibodies and stimulated with LPS, the arthritis scores of the control and CAIA mice were 0 points on days 1 to 5 (Fig. 2). The arthritis scores of the CAIA mice increased from days 6 to 12. The ankles of the control mice didn't show any damage on H/E staining (Fig. 3 A: a and b). On the contrary, destruction of the cartilage and bone, synovial hyperplasia, visible articular cartilage surface roughness, local infiltration of inflammatory cells, synovial hyperplasia were observed in the CAIA mice (Fig. 3 A: c and d). Immunohistochemical analysis of the ankles exhibited increased expression of RHAMM in the CAIA mice compared with the control mice, especially in the cartilage, bone and synovial membrane (Fig. 3 A: e, f and g, h).Expression of RHAMM was different in joints tissues, particularly in synovial tissues both in CAIA induced and control mice. Accordingly, elevated RHAMM expression was observed in cartilage, bone and synovial tissues compared to that in other tissues.

Assessment of siRNA-mediated RHAMM gene silencing
To evaluate the efficacy of RNA interference assay and efficacy of siRNA against RHAMM gene, RT-PCR and

western blot were performed. Results showed that RHAMM expression was successfully-suppressed as a result of siRNA interference. (Fig. 4 A and B).

Expression of IL-6 and IL-8 in synovial cells
The pro-inflammatory cytokines IL-6 and IL-8 are known key markers for FLS. We assessed the expression of IL-6 and IL-8 in the synovial cells. Both IL-6 and IL-8 levels were observed to be significantly decreased in the synovial cell culture medium (Fig. 4 C and D). In additionFurthermore, RT-PCR results showed that after interfering with the RHAMM expression, the levels of IL-6 and IL-8 were significantly decreased (Fig. 4. E and F).

Migration and invasion
Our results demonstrate that migration and invasion of FLS were significantly affected after the inhibition of RHAMM. In the wound scratch assay, migration ability of the RHAMM-siRNA group was decreased compared to that of the control group (Fig. 5: A). In the migration and invasion test, cell number was significantly decreased in the RHAMM-siRNA group (Fig. 5: B and C),

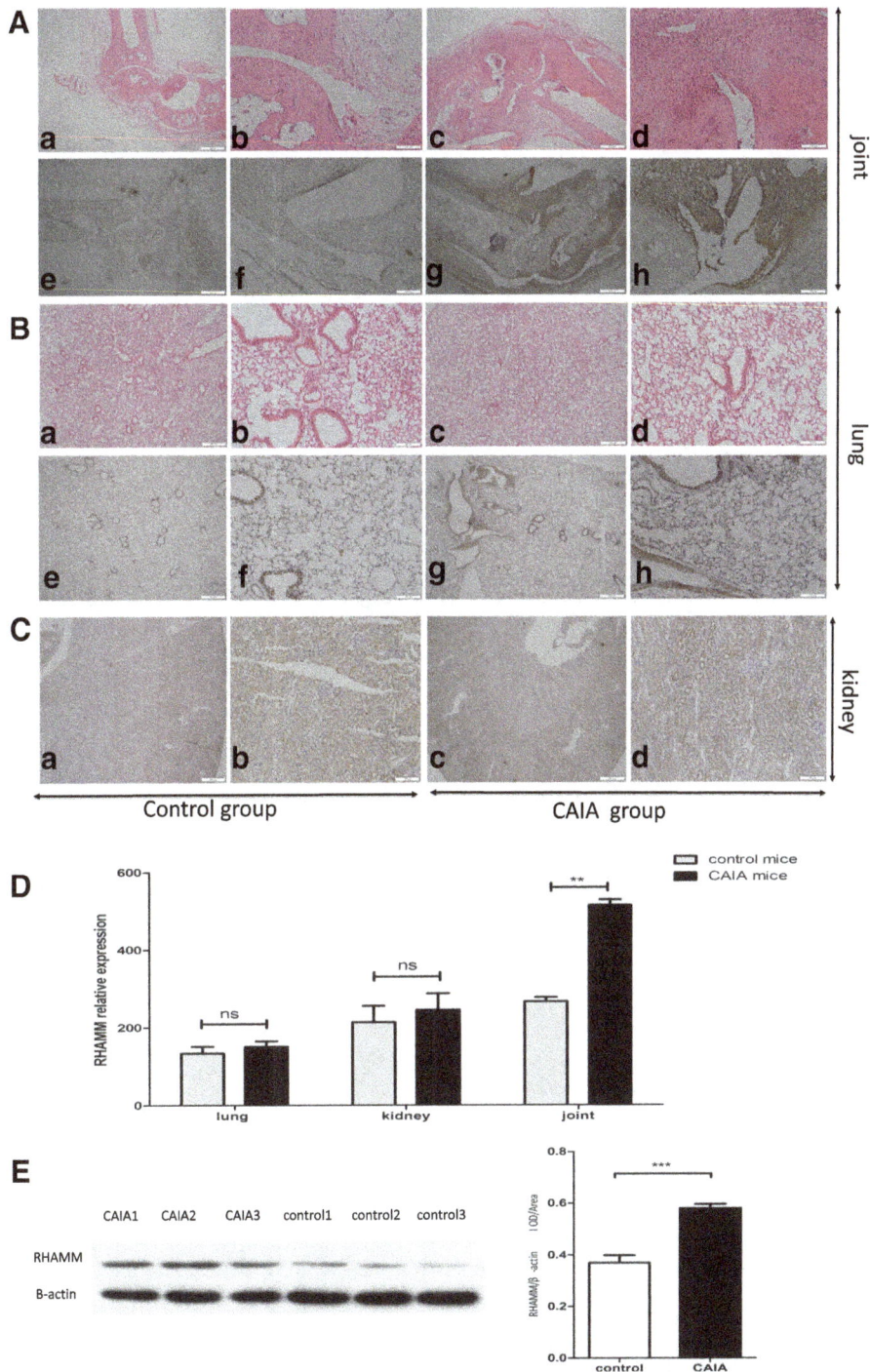

Fig. 3 a HE/ Immunohistochemistry staining of joints of control mice (a, b, e, f) compared with CAIA mice (c, d, g, h). Control mice have no obvious hyperplasia of the synovial tissue and synovial tissue probably made up of 3 to 4 layers of synovial cells, low level expression of RHAMM (arrows in b and f); CAIA mice, had synovial hyperplasia and articular cartilage surface roughness, local inflammatory cell infiltration, part of synovial cells infiltrating the cartilage and bone tissue, high level expression of RHAMM (arrows in d and h). **b** No significant differences in the staining of lungs between control (a, b, e, f) and CAIA mice (c, d, g, h). **c** Immunohistochemistry staining of kidneys, control mice (a, b) compared to CAIA mice (c, d), no significant difference of RNAMM expression. **d** RT-PCR results of RHAMM expression in lung, kidney and joint sections. RHAMM was expressed in CAIA mice joints at higher levels. **e** Quantitative analyses of western-blot of joint proteins from CAIA and control mice. RHAMM was expressed higher in CAIA mice joints than control mice. ** $p < 0.01$, *** $p < 0.001$, Mann–Whitney U test.

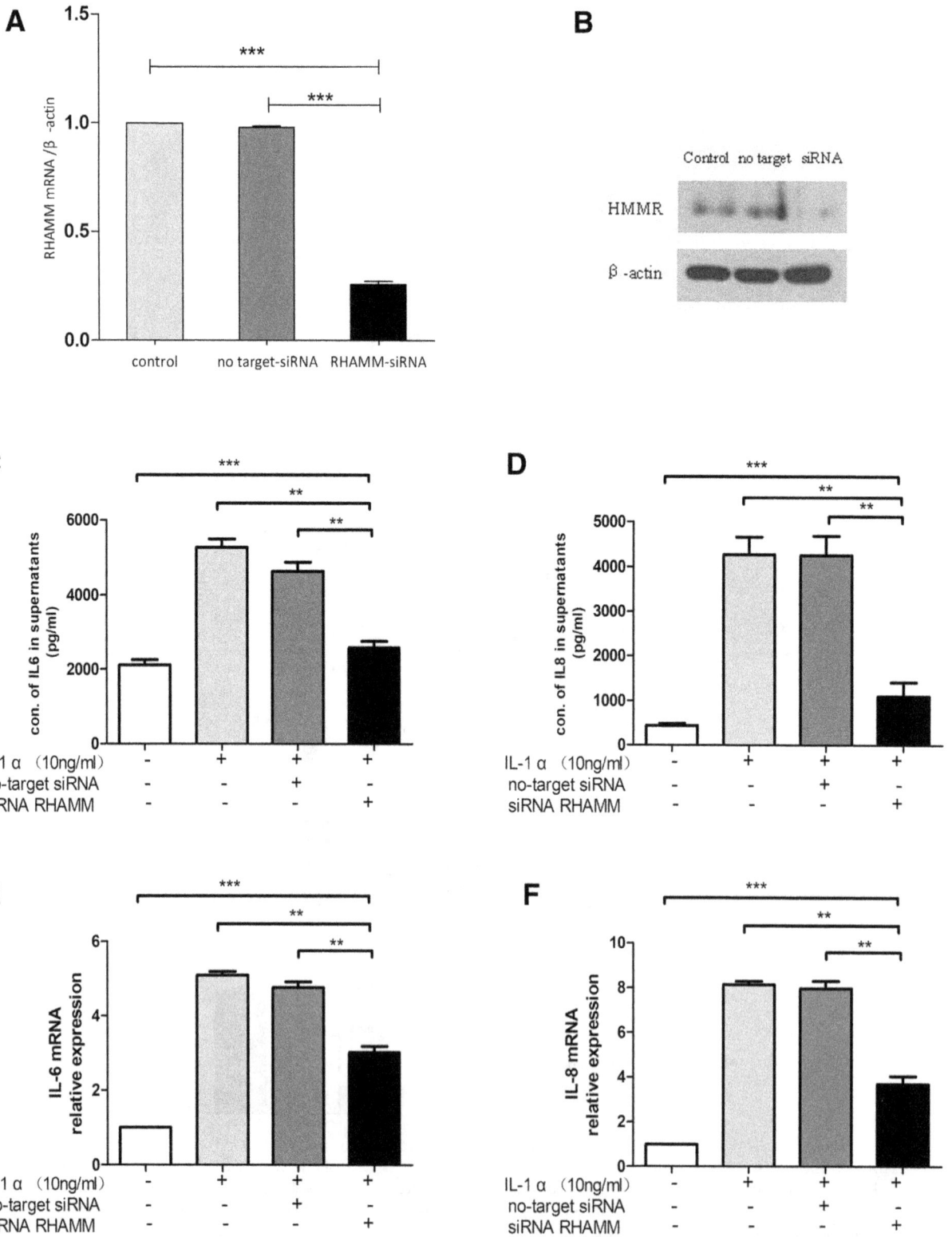

Fig. 4 a Low levels of RHAMM mRNA and (**b**) protein in FLS after siRNA interference ($n = 3$). Each sample was analyzed twice; (**c**) IL-6 and (**d**) IL-8 secretions were low in siRNA treated RHAMM FLS; (**e**) Quantitative RT-PCR amplified IL-6, and (**f**) IL-8 gene expressions were lower in siRNA treated RHAMM FLS. ** $p < 0.01$, *** $p < 0.001$, Mann–Whitney U test (two groups) or Kruskal-Wallis test (more than two groups).

while no obvious difference was observed in the control group and no-target interference groups.

Discussion

The pathogenesis of RA remains to be completely elucidated, but it is well known that FLS play a key role in it. Normally,synovial fibroblasts line the joints, but in RA they are increased in numbers as part of the pannus, a tumor-like structure that causes significant joint destruction. Despite their invasive potential, not much is known about the factors and processes that mediate the invasion of FLS. HA is a ubiquitous extracellular matrix polysaccharide that belongs to the glycosaminoglycan family, which is characterized by repeating hexosamines and uronic acid units [21–23]. Low molecular weight HA is speculated to exacerbate inflammation in RA. In this context, variations in quantity and functions of HA receptors would affect the severity of inflammation in FLS, and play critical roles in maintaining the hyperplasia of synovium, pannus formation and the destruction of cartilage in RA. RHAMM is thought to be involved in the reorganization of cytoskeletal structures and movement, the essential components of the inflammatory response. Although in recent years, many studies have shown that RHAMM is involved in the migration of malignant cells and hence has an important role in immune-related diseases, so far very few data available demonstrating the role of RHAMM in RA pathogenesis. Role of RHAMM in the mechanisms of OA but not in RA was reported earlier [15]. CD44, another hyaluronan receptor, regulates cell adhesion, homing and trans endothelial migration. Most of the CD44 splice variants are more strongly expressed in the synovial membrane of RA but not OA patients [24]. Both these proteins are involved in the wound repair process and their aberrant regulation contributes to a variety of diseases including arthritis [25]. CD44 and RHAMM influence their functions reciprocally in collagen-induced arthritis. and blocking CD44 function attenuates arthritis [17]. Genetic deletion of CD44 increases arthritis severity, but blocking RHAMM function attenuates arthritis suggesting that RHAMM possibly compensates for genetic loss of CD44. Here we demonstrate higher expression of RHAMM FLS from RA patients compared with OA patients. This finding implies that RHAMM has a key role in the pathogenesis of RA.

This assumption was further validated by animal experiments. In an earlier study, visible roughness of the cartilage surface, infiltration of inflammatory cells and bone erosions were observed in the joints of CAIA mice as reported earlier [26, 27]. Immunohistochemistry results showed that RHAMM was expressed highly in the joints of CAIA mice compared to the joints of control mice. Interestingly, RHAMM is expressed in the thickened synovial membrane, cartilage and bone of the articular joints. Both RT-PCR and Western blot analyses confirm that RHAMM is indeed essential in the pathological process of RA. In RA patients, sometimes lung and kidney damages are known to be present, but in our experiments, lung and kidney damages were not observed. Our results also demonstrate organ-specificity of RHAMM in RA because of its expression in synovial tissue markedly increased compared to that in lung and kidney tissues. This specific expression pattern suggests presence of RHAMM in the synovial cells could be part of RA pathogenesis, in which RHAMM possibly regulates behavioral and functional aspects of FLS. To our knowledge, for the first time we are report that RHAMM plays an important role in the regulation of inflammation and biological behaviour of FLS isolated from RA patients. In order to investigate the functions of RHAMM, siRNA was successfully used to knock down its expression in RA-FLS resulting in decreased production of IL-6 and IL-8 cytokines, and a strong inhibitory effect on the migration and invasion of FLS.

RAFs produce IL-6 and IL-8, which are pro-inflammatory cytokines that play crucial roles in the pathophysiology of RA, and contribute to the inflammation and joint damage [28–32]. These inflammatory cytokines have been observed to degrade cartilage and bone in human patients and mouse models. Accordingly, treatment using anti-IL-6 receptor has significantly improved the clinical scores and laboratory indicators in RA patients [33, 34]. In addition, IL-6-deficient mice did not develop arthritis symptoms or joint destructions [35]. Furthermore, therapeutic targeting of cytokines in RA suggests that IL-8 may have pathogenic importance in RA [36] and IL-8 expression in RA synovial tissue associated with disease activity [37]. Decreased levels of IL-6 and IL-8 because of RHAMM expression suggests thier involvement in the modulation of FLS induced joint inflammation.

Migration and invasion of synoviocytes contribute greatly to the pathogenesis of RA [10]. Synoviocyte migration to cartilage and bone is a crucial process in aggravating of cartilage destruction in RA. FLS can invade into the extracellular matrix leading to a further aggravation of joint damage, and promote disease progression by migrating to the unaffected joints [11]. In our study, RHAMM silencing of RHAMM gene using siRNA has decreased the production of IL-6 and IL-8, and had a strong inhibitory effect on the migration and invasion of FLS. This suggests RHAMM's ability in the modulation of joint destruction induced by RA-FLS.

Conclusions

Our results provide important evidence for RHAMM involvement in the modulation of inflammation and joint

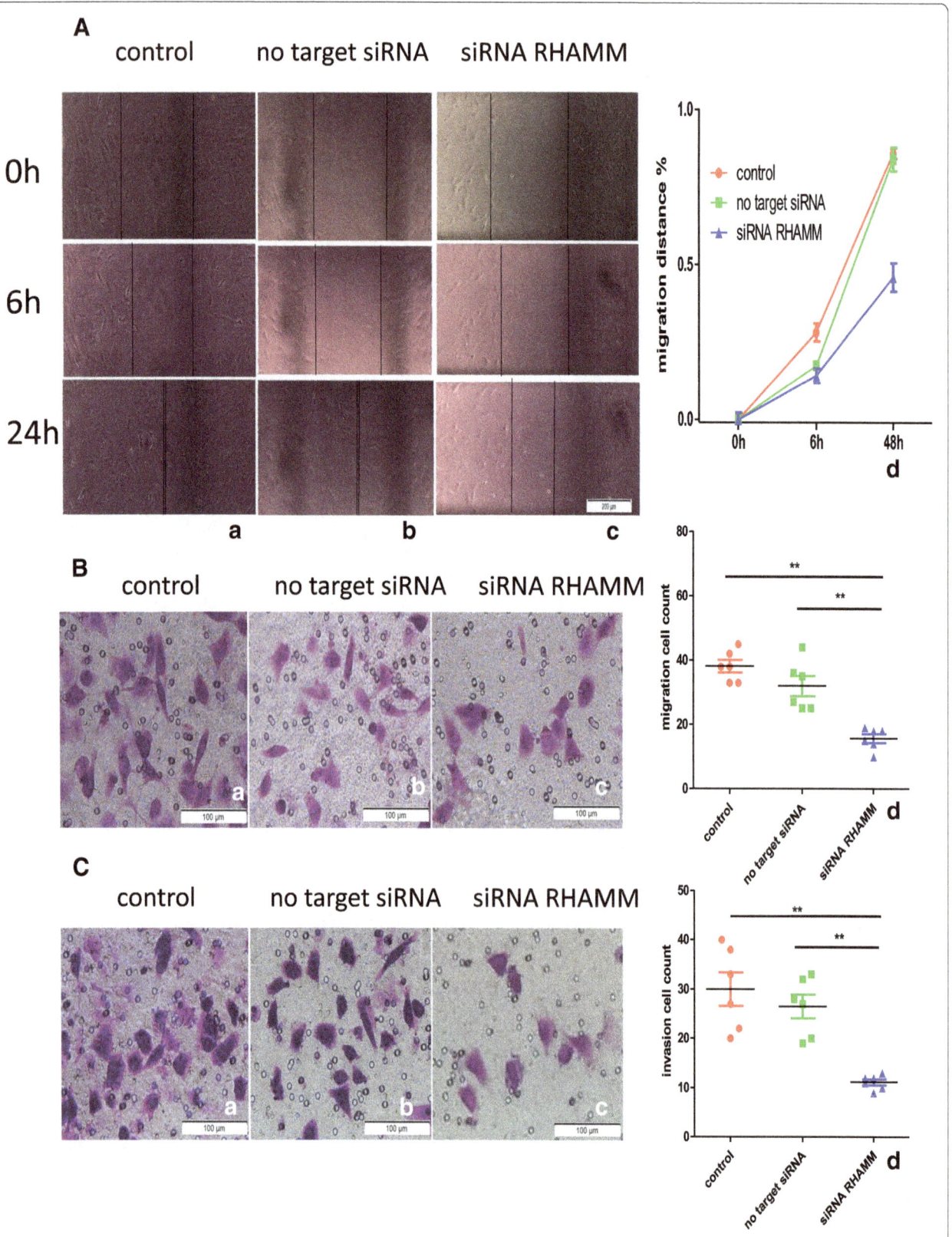

Fig. 5 Migration and invasion results (*n* = 3). Each sample was analysed twice.(a: control group; b: no target control group; c: RHAMM siRNA group; d: statistics results). **a** Migration ability of RHAMM-siRNA group was significantly decreased compared with the control group; FLS migration cell numbers, (**b**) control and (**c**) RHAMM siRNA interference groups; ** *p* < 0.01, Mann–Whitney U test (two groups) or Kruskal-Wallis test (more than two groups).

destruction caused by RA-FLS. RHAMM controls the secretion of pro-inflammatory factors, like IL-6 and IL-8, but the exact mechanisms remain to be investigated. RHAMM is well-known for its role in the hyaluronan mediated motility pathway, which affects the functions of the immune system. Here, we observed high level expression of RHAMM in RA-FLS. RHAMM controls the invasion and migration of FLS and also modulates the secretion of IL-6 and IL-8 from FLS. Therefore, we propose involvement of RHAMM in the enhancement of inflammation and subsequent deterioration of RA.

Abbreviations

CAIA: Collagen antibody-induced arthritis; FLS: Fibroblast-like synoviocytes; OA: Osteoarthritis; RA: Rheumatoid arthritis; RHAMM: Receptor for hyaluronan mediated motility

Acknowledgements

The authors would like to thank Prof. Kutty Selva Nandakumar and Dr. Bibo Liang for their help in reviewing the manuscript for English Language.

Funding

This study was supported by the National Natural Science Foundation of China (No. 81601397).

Authors' contributions

JW and QHY were major contributors in the planning and designing of the study. YPZ: Data analysis, statistical analysis, results and discussion. YQ and JXD: Data collection, data analysis and critical review. JW performed the statistical analysis and drafted the manuscript. All the authors read and approved the final manuscript.

Consent for publication

Not applicable.

Competing interests

All the authors declare that they have no competing interests.

References

1. Firestein GS. Evolving concepts of rheumatoid arthritis. Nature. 2003;423: 356–61.
2. Scott DL, Wolfe F, Huizinga TW. Rheumatoid arthritis. Lancet. 2010;376: 1094–108.
3. Bottini N, Firestein GS. Duality of fibroblast-like synoviocytes in RA: passive responders and imprinted aggressors. Nat Rev Rheumatol. 2013;9:24–33.
4. Filer A. The fibroblast as a therapeutic target in rheumatoid arthritis. Curr Opin Pharmacol. 2013;13:413–9.
5. McInnes IB, Schett G. The pathogenesis of rheumatoid arthritis. N Engl J Med. 2011;365:2205–19.
6. Huber LC, Distler O, Tarner I, Gay RE, Gay S, Pap T. Synovial fibroblasts: key players in rheumatoid arthritis. Rheumatology (Oxford). 2006;45:669–75.
7. Noss EH, Brenner MB. The role and therapeutic implications of fibroblast-like synoviocytes in inflammation and cartilage erosion in rheumatoid arthritis. Immunol Rev. 2008;223:252–70.
8. Feldmann M, Brennan FM, Maini RN. Rheumatoid arthritis. Cell. 1996;85:307–10.
9. Terenzi R, Romano E, Manetti M, Peruzzi F, Nacci F, Matucci-Cerinic M, et al. Neuropeptides activate TRPV1 in rheumatoid arthritis fibroblast-like synoviocytes and foster IL-6 and IL-8 production. Ann Rheum Dis. 2013;72: 1107–9.
10. Bartok B, Firestein GS. Fibroblast-like synoviocytes: key effector cells in rheumatoid arthritis. Immunol Rev. 2010;233:233–55.
11. Lefevre S, Knedla A, Tennie C, Kampmann A, Wunrau C, Dinser R, et al. Synovial fibroblasts spread rheumatoid arthritis to unaffected joints. Nat Med. 2009;15:1414–20.
12. Gust KM, Hofer MD, Perner SR, Kim R, Chinnaiyan AM, Varambally S, et al. RHAMM (CD168) is overexpressed at the protein level and may constitute an immunogenic antigen in advanced prostate cancer disease. Neoplasia. 2009;11:956–63.
13. Naor D, Nedvetzki S, Walmsley M, Yayon A, Turley EA, Golan I, et al. CD44 involvement in autoimmune inflammations: the lesson to be learned from CD44-targeting by antibody or from knockout mice. Ann N Y Acad Sci. 2007;1110:233–47.
14. Garcia-Posadas L, Contreras-Ruiz L, Arranz-Valsero I, Lopez-Garcia A, Calonge M, Diebold Y. CD44 and RHAMM hyaluronan receptors in human ocular surface inflammation. Graefes Arch Clin Exp Ophthalmol. 2014;252:1289–95.
15. Dunn S, Kolomytkin OV, Waddell DD, Marino AA. Hyaluronan-binding receptors: possible involvement in osteoarthritis. Mod Rheumatol. 2009;19:151–5.
16. Savani RC, Cao G, Pooler PM, Zaman A, Zhou Z, DeLisser HM. Differential involvement of the hyaluronan (HA) receptors CD44 and receptor for HA-mediated motility in endothelial cell function and angiogenesis. J Biol Chem. 2001;276:36770–8.
17. Nedvetzki S, Gonen E, Assayag N, Reich R, Williams RO, Thurmond RL, et al. RHAMM, a receptor for hyaluronan-mediated motility, compensates for CD44 in inflamed CD44-knockout mice: a different interpretation of redundancy. Proc Natl Acad Sci U S A. 2004;101:18081–6.
18. Aletaha D, Neogi T, Silman AJ, Funovits J, Felson DT, Bingham CO, 3rd, et al. 2010 rheumatoid arthritis classification criteria: an American College of Rheumatology/European league against rheumatism collaborative initiative. Arthritis Rheum 2010; 62:2569–2581.
19. Recommendations for the medical management of osteoarthritis of the hip and knee: 2000 update. American College of Rheumatology Subcommittee on Osteoarthritis Guidelines Arthritis Rheum. 2000;43:1905–15.
20. Institute of Laboratory Animal Resources (U.S.). Committee on Care and Use of Laboratory Animals.: Guide for the care and use of laboratory animals. In: NIH publication. Bethesda, Md.: U.S. Dept. of Health and Human Services, Public Health Service: v.
21. Ballard PL, Gonzales LW, Godinez RI, Godinez MH, Savani RC, McCurnin DC, et al. Surfactant composition and function in a primate model of infant chronic lung disease: effects of inhaled nitric oxide. Pediatr Res. 2006;59: 157–62.
22. Khan F, Ahmad SR. Polysaccharides and their derivatives for versatile tissue engineering application. Macromol Biosci. 2013;13:395–421.
23. Breitkreutz D, Koxholt I, Thiemann K, Nischt R. Skin basement membrane: the foundation of epidermal integrity--BM functions and diverse roles of bridging molecules nidogen and perlecan. Biomed Res Int. 2013;2013: 179784.
24. Grisar J, Munk M, Steiner CW, Amoyo-Minar L, Tohidast-Akrad M, Zenz P, et al. Expression patterns of CD44 and CD44 splice variants in patients with rheumatoid arthritis. Clin Exp Rheumatol. 2012;30:64–72.
25. Turley EA, Naor D. RHAMM and CD44 peptides-analytic tools and potential drugs. Front Biosci (Landmark Ed). 2012;17:1775–94.
26. Croxford AM, Whittingham S, McNaughton D, Nandakumar KS, Holmdahl R, Rowley MJ. Type II collagen-specific antibodies induce cartilage damage in mice independent of inflammation. Arthritis Rheum. 2013;65:650–9.
27. Nandakumar KS, Holmdahl R. Collagen antibody induced arthritis. Methods Mol Med. 2007;136:215–23.
28. Miyazawa K, Mori A, Yamamoto K, Okudaira H. Constitutive transcription of the human interleukin-6 gene by rheumatoid synoviocytes: spontaneous activation of NF-kappaB and CBF1. Am J Pathol. 1998;152:793–803.
29. Tan PL, Farmiloe S, Yeoman S, Watson JD. Expression of the interleukin 6 gene in rheumatoid synovial fibroblasts. J Rheumatol. 1990;17:1608–12.
30. Georganas C, Liu HT, Perlman H, Hoffmann A, Thimmapaya B, Pope RM. Regulation of IL-6 and IL-8 expression in rheumatoid arthritis synovial fibroblasts: the dominant role for NF-kappa B but not C/EBP beta or c-Jun. J Immunol. 2000;165:7199–206.
31. Nanki T, Nagasaka K, Hayashida K, Saita Y, Miyasaka N. Chemokines regulate IL-6 and IL-8 production by fibroblast-like synoviocytes from patients with rheumatoid arthritis. J Immunol. 2001a;167:5381–5.

32. Nanki T, Nagasaka K, Hayashida K, Saita Y, Miyasaka N. Chemokines regulate IL-6 and IL-8 production by fibroblast-like synoviocytes from patients with rheumatoid arthritis. J Immunol. 2001b;167:5381–5.
33. Genovese MC, McKay JD, Nasonov EL, Mysler EF, da Silva NA, Alecock E, et al. Interleukin-6 receptor inhibition with tocilizumab reduces disease activity in rheumatoid arthritis with inadequate response to disease-modifying antirheumatic drugs: the tocilizumab in combination with traditional disease-modifying antirheumatic drug therapy study. Arthritis Rheum. 2008;58:2968–80.
34. Nishimoto N, Yoshizaki K, Miyasaka N, Yamamoto K, Kawai S, Takeuchi T, et al. Treatment of rheumatoid arthritis with humanized anti-interleukin-6 receptor antibody: a multicenter, double-blind, placebo-controlled trial. Arthritis Rheum. 2004;50:1761–9.
35. Yokota K, Miyazaki T, Hirano M, Akiyama Y, Mimura T. Simvastatin inhibits production of interleukin 6 (IL-6) and IL-8 and cell proliferation induced by tumor necrosis factor-alpha in fibroblast-like synoviocytes from patients with rheumatoid arthritis. J Rheumatol. 2006;33:463–71.
36. Koch AE, Kunkel SL, Burrows JC, Evanoff HL, Haines GK, Pope RM, et al. Synovial tissue macrophage as a source of the chemotactic cytokine IL-8. J Immunol. 1991;147:2187–95.
37. Kraan MC, Patel DD, Haringman JJ, Smith MD, Weedon H, Ahern MJ, et al. The development of clinical signs of rheumatoid synovial inflammation is associated with increased synthesis of the chemokine CXCL8 (interleukin-8). Arthritis Res. 2001;3:65–71.

12

The influence of radio frequency ablation on intra-articular fluid temperature in the ankle joint

Philipp Ahrens[1,2†], Dirk Mueller[3†], Sebastian Siebenlist[1*], Andreas Lenich[1,4], Ulrich Stoeckle[5] and Gunther H. Sandmann[5,6]

Abstract

Background: Radio frequency ablation devices have found a widespread application in arthroscopic surgery. However, recent publications report about elevated temperatures, which may cause damage to the capsular tissue and especially to chondrocytes. The purpose of this study was the investigation of the maximum temperatures that occur in the ankle joint with the use of a commercially available radio frequency ablation device.

Methods: Six formalin-fixed cadaver ankle specimens were used for this study. The radio frequency device was applied for 120 s to remove tissue. Intra-articular temperatures were logged every second for 120 s at a distance of 3, 5 and 10 mm from the tip of the radio frequency device. The irrigation fluid flow was controlled by setting the inflow pressure to 10 mmHg, 25 mmHg, 50 mmHg and 100 mmHg, respectively. The controller unit voltage setting was set to 1, 5 and 9.

Results: Maximum temperatures exceeding 50 °C/122 °F were observed for all combinations of parameters, except for those with a pressure of 100 mmHg pressure. The main critical variable is the pressure setting, which is highly significant. The controller unit voltage setting showed no effect on the temperature measurements. The highest temperature was 102.7 °C/215.6 °F measured for an irrigation flow of 10 mmHg. The shortest time span to exceed 50 °C/122 °F was 3 s.

Conclusion: In order to avoid temperatures exceeding 50 °C/122 °F in the use of radio frequency devices in arthroscopic surgeries of the ankle joint, it is recommended to use a high irrigation flow by setting the pressure difference across the ankle joint as high as feasible. Even short intervals of a low irrigation flow may lead to critical temperatures above 50 °C/122 °F.

Level of Evidence: Level II, diagnostic study.

Keywords: Ankle joint, Radio frequency, Ablation, Thermal damage, Chondrocytes

Background

Arthroscopic surgery of the ankle joint is widespread and tissue ablation is one of the main indications in the "Soccer's Ankle" or anterior impingement. In this condition, fibrous tissue causes pain above the anterior aspect of the ankle joint and the removal of this tissue is an

adequate therapy to provide pain-free motion. Most of these devices use electromagnetic energy for shrinking, coagulation or ablation of tissue [3, 4]. In contrast, we used a bipolar device in which the energy comes from a plasma layer at the tip of the wand. Radio frequency (RF) ablation devices are widely used to remove soft tissue in arthroscopic surgery. The basic idea of a RF device is to destroy soft tissue by electrolyte plasmarization with the side effect of increased heating of the irrigation fluid. To avoid intraarticular heat, the RF device has vents that are inset at the tip to increase the outflow of the arthroscopic irrigation fluid. Unfortunately, some

* Correspondence: Sebastian.siebenlist@mri.tum.de

†Philipp Ahrens and Dirk Mueller contributed equally to this work.

[1]Department of Orthopaedic Sports Medicine, Klinikum rechts der Isar, Technische Universitaet Muenchen, Germany, Ismanninger, Str. 22, D- 81675 Muenchen, Germany

Full list of author information is available at the end of the article

hot water, gas and denatured material may escape into the joint cavity where it might lead to unwanted increased local temperatures. Recent publications have shown dermal burns of patients due to hot water spilling originating from the RF ablation process and there are also some cases of glenohumeral chondrolysis after labral repair in hip arthroscopy [1–7]. Different reports investigated safety limits and found that chondrocyte damage may occur at temperatures as low as 45 °C/113 ° F. Evaluations of the ability of the chondrocytes to recover showed a sharp increase of chondrocyte death between 50 to 55 °C (122 to 131 °F) [8, 9]. Thus, in recent publications on temperatures in shoulder joints [10] and hip joints [11], a 50 °C/122 °F criterion was used as limit for safe temperatures. Both publications report temperatures exceeding the critical point of 50 °C, which can easily be reached by RF ablation in the shoulder and hip joints depending on the flow of the irrigation fluid and their extraction. Until now, only limited data exists on the effects of RF ablation in the ankle joint, where especially the resection of hypertrophic synovia is useful and frequently used [12].

Anatomically, the capsular volume of the hip (2.5–10 ml) [13] is comparable to the volume of the ankle joint (6–10 ml) [14]. We therefore hypothesized that temperatures exceeding 50 °C/ (122 °F) may be reached by RF ablation. In our study, we wanted to investigate the impact of the irrigation flow rate, the controller unit voltage setting and the distance from the heat source on maximum temperatures, mean temperatures, time to reach the 50 ° C/122 °F limit and – in view of the fact that the results of thermo-fluid dynamics experiments may vary substantially – the percentage of experimental runs exceeding 50 °C/122 °F with the same parameter settings.

Methods

A controlled laboratory study was designed using six formalin-fixed human cadaver ankle joints. All human specimen enrolled in this study were post-mortem donors to the Anatomical Institute of the University of Munich. The use of donated post-mortem specimens for scientific investigations is in accordance with the Declaration of Helsinki and was approved by the ethical committee of the University of Munich. Surrounding soft tissue around the ankle was preserved. The experiments were performed at room temperature using an antero-medial and antero-lateral portal. The irrigation inflow was placed in the antero-medial portal, while the bipolar RF device "Ambient Super Turbo Vac 90 IFS" with the Quantum II controller (Arthocare Corporation, Austin, Texas, USA) was placed via the antero-lateral portal (Fig. 1). The device uses a physical bipolar radio frequency process to stimulate electrolytes in the conductive natrium chloride solution. The energized particles in the plasma denaturize organic molecular bonds and dissolve tissue at temperatures between 40 °C and 70 °C/104 ° F and 158 °F, a current does not pass through the tissue. The result is volumetric removal of the target tissue with marginal collateral tissue damage. The RF device has vents at the tip, which are the outlets for the arthroscopic fluid. The Quantum II controller measures the temperature at the vents and cuts the power supply when temperatures exceed 40 °C/104 °F. Different voltage levels are possible, allowing a potential adaption according to the tissue treated.

All measurements were performed under direct arthroscopic vision, providing a free and unobstructed flow path for the irrigation fluid. To measure the temperature inside the ankle joint, three thermoprobes (TP) were placed 3, 5 and 10 mm off the tip (Fig. 2). Continuous temperature

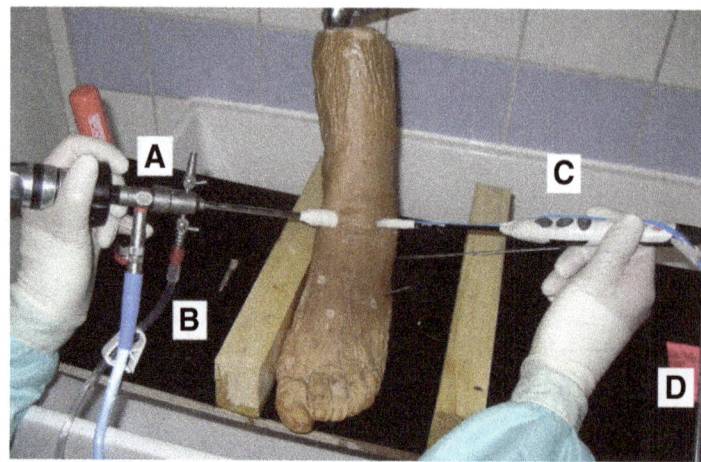

Fig. 1 The laboratory setup used in this study with the arthroscope (A) and the irrigation hose (B) on the left side in the antero-medial portal and the bipolar radiofrequency device (C) in the antero-lateral portal. The thermometer probes are attached to the device. The radio frequency device was moved during the ablation process

measurement was performed by a multichannel fiberoptical thermometer unit, which is sensitive enough to detect temperature changes of 0.01 °C. Temperatures were recorded and analyzed each second, while a measurement cycle took 120 s. In our view, the flow is the key parameter to excess heat in arthroscopy (Fig. 3). In order to vary the plasma power inside the cavity, the voltage was set from 1 to 5 and 9 at the end (minimum, medium and maximum level). The irrigation flow was controlled using the inlet pressures with 10, 25, 50 and 100 mmHg. The experiments started at room and irrigation fluid temperature of 20 °C/68 °F. During the 120 s, there is very little conductive heat flow from the cavity to the surrounding tissue and the heat capacity of the fluid in the ankle joint cavity is small (5–10 ml) (1). The experiments show that the heat escaping from the RF device leads to a heat build-up within 20 s at low coolant flow conditions. This clearly indicates that using 37 °C/98.6 °F instead of 20 °C/68 °F does not affect the maximum temperatures, but only reduces the time span before the stationary conditions are reached by a few seconds.

After having run four experiments for each combination as mentioned above, we analyzed our material and found that all experiments with the 100 mmHg pressure setting did not exceed the 50 °C/122 °F criterion, while the criterion was exceeded at least in one experiment for the other parameter combinations. However, we found no detectable effect of the voltage settings. Thus, the experiments with the same pressure setting are statistically in the same group, which means that we had 12 experiments for each pressure setting, which is sufficient for a meaningful statistical evaluation.

Statistical analysis

Statistical analysis was performed using the software package SPSS™ (Version 19, IBM® Corporation, Somers, New York, USA) and the software EXCEL from Microsoft Office 2010 Professional. The temperature time histories were assessed and evaluated with EXCEL. Also, bounding curves and maxima and mean values were calculated with EXCEL. Linear regression analysis of the maximum and mean values was performed with both programs, SPSS and EXCEL. For the evaluation of the data, a p-value of 0.05 was assumed.

Results

Low, medium and high pressure temperature curves

In order to eliminate random effects, bounding curves were calculated for maximum temperatures for each pair of parameter settings for voltage and pressure position by averaging the TP positions and the four experimental runs. It was found that the maximum curves can be divided into three groups: low pressure (10 mmHg), medium pressure (25 and 50 mmHg) and high pressure (100 mmHg).

Figure 4 shows the resulting maximum curves for the low pressure setting. Without doubt, it is obvious that low pressure is not an option for ankle joint RF ablation - independent of the voltage setting.

Figure 5 shows the resulting maximum curves for the medium pressure setting (25 and 500 mmHg). All curves show strong fluctuations and an overall upward tendency. All curves exceeded the 50 °C/122 °F criterion, for curves with 50 mmHg pressure, it takes some seconds longer. It is worse that the 50 °C/122 °F criterion is exceeded in all curves, if the time span is longer than 50 s in all cases. This means that an improved and more realistic version of the 50 °C/122 °F criterion is not feasible, e.g. a criterion like "surpassing the 50 °C/122 °F for a time span for less than 10 seconds", in which no damage can be done because the time span is too short for a substantial heat build-up of the tissue.

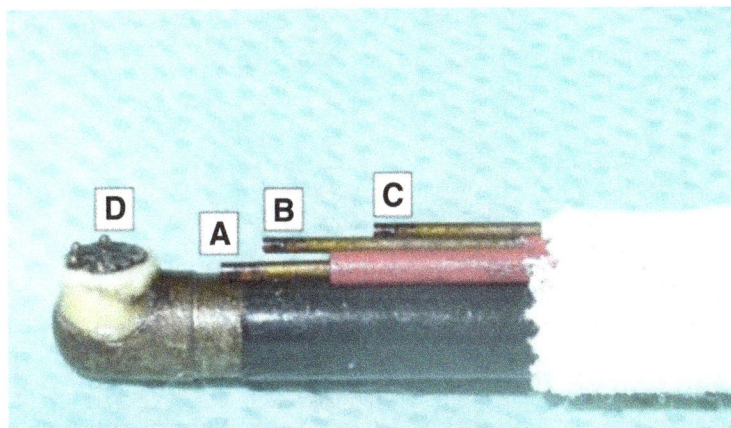

Fig. 2 Three fiberoptical thermometer probes were attached to the radio frequency ablation device at 3 mm (A), 5 mm (B) and 10 mm (C) from the electrode plate with four ball electrodes where the heat is generated. The suction inlet consists of six triangular holes in this plate (D)

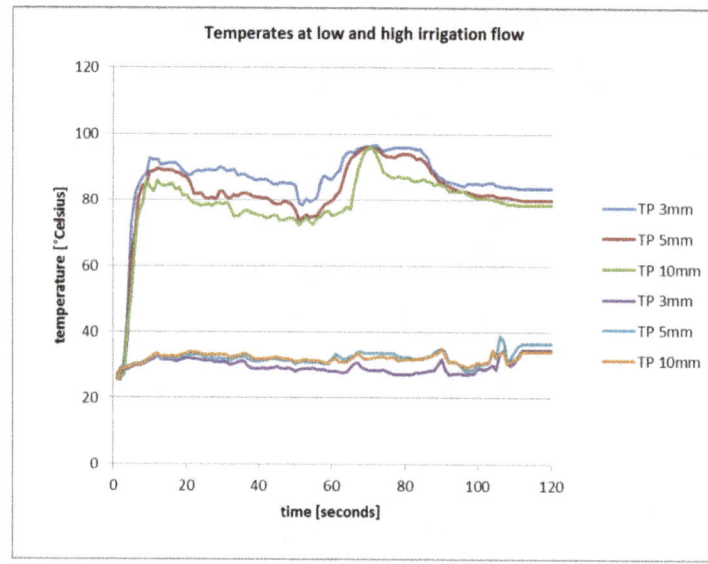

Fig. 3 This figure shows temperature plots for an experiment with a pressure setting of 10 mmHg (three curves on the top) and with 100 mmHg (three bottom curves) for three thermometer probes at 3, 5 and 10 mm distance. For 10 mmHg, a rapid heat build-up is observed within the first 10 s. After the heat build-up, the temperature curves fluctuate around the average temperature. For 10 mmHg, the temperature fluctuations are more rapid and have smaller amplitudes than for 100 mmHg

Figure 6 shows the resulting maximum curves for the high pressure setting (100 mmHg). These stay clearly below the 50 °C/122 °F criterion, show a stationary mean and only small fluctuation amplitudes. This indicates that using RF ablation with 100 mmHg is safe.

Figure 7 shows the mean temperatures for all voltage settings (1, 5 and 9) and all pressures (10, 25, 50 and 100 mmHg). The mean temperatures for the low pressure setting are substantially higher than the medium and high pressures. The range of mean temperatures at high pressure is marked by dotted lines forming a rectangle. Some of the temperatures at medium pressures stay within the dotted lines for some time and then rise above the upper boundary, while others are clearly above this range most of the time. The overall behavior of the mean temperatures is similar to the overall behavior of the maximum temperatures as far as the influence of the different pressure settings is concerned.

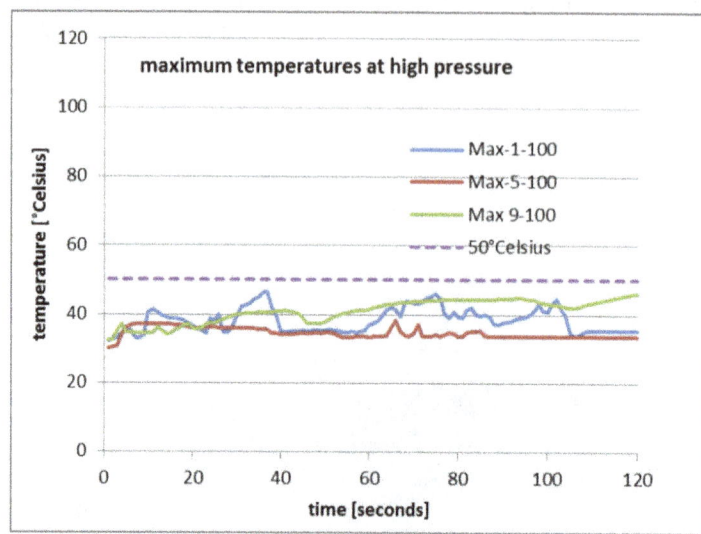

Fig. 4 All maximum temperature curves for the different voltage settings 1, 5 and 9 and at low pressure of 10 mmHg are similar. Within a few seconds, the 50 °C criterion is exceeded and the temperature remains at high values of about 90 °C for the rest of the time

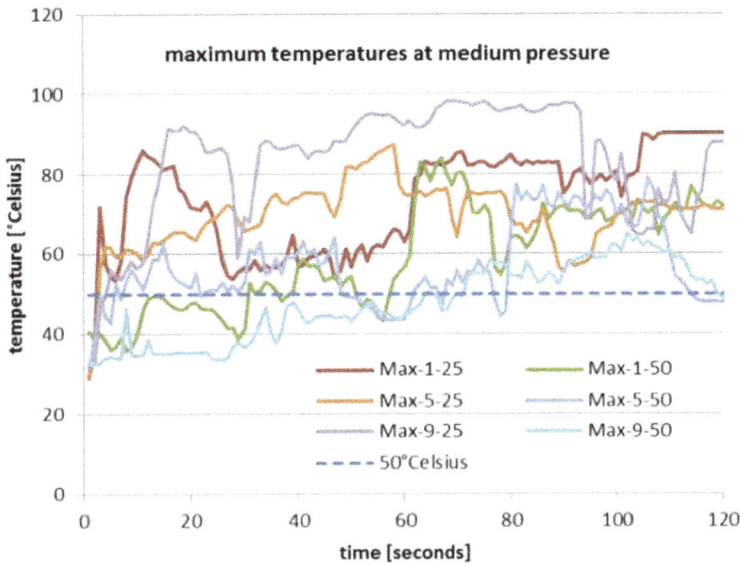

Fig. 5 Maximum temperatures for voltage settings 1, 5 and 9 at medium pressure (25 and 50 mmHg). The curves show a strong oscillatory behavior and an upward tendency. All curves exceed the 50 °C criterion, lasting some seconds longer for curves with 50 mmHg

Regression analysis

In order to substantiate the expectations from a "quick look" analysis of the data and the physical interpretation of the process, regression analysis of the overall maximum and mean temperatures was carried out starting with the three parameters: voltage setting, square root of pressure and TP distance. Then, the parameter, which had the least effect was eliminated in two additional steps: in the second step, the voltage setting was eliminated and in the third step the TP distance. In a linear regression analysis, a multi-linear response surface is constructed that minimizes the distance of the measured data from the surface. The parameter R-squared is the proportion of variance of the maximum or mean temperature, respectively, which can be explained by the independent variables pressure, TP distance and voltage setting. We found that about 80% of the variances can be explained by the two variables pressure and TP distance. The p-value for the pressure is highly significant ($p < 0.001$), while the p-value for the TP distance is 0.011 for the mean temperature and 0.039 for the maximum temperature. This finding is in good compliance

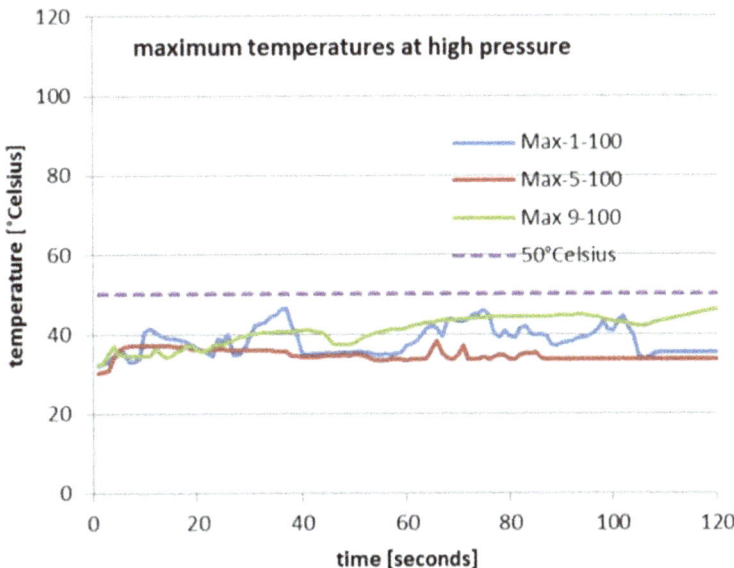

Fig. 6 Maximum temperature for voltage settings 1, 5 and 9 at high pressure (100 mmHg). All curves remain below the 50 °C criterion

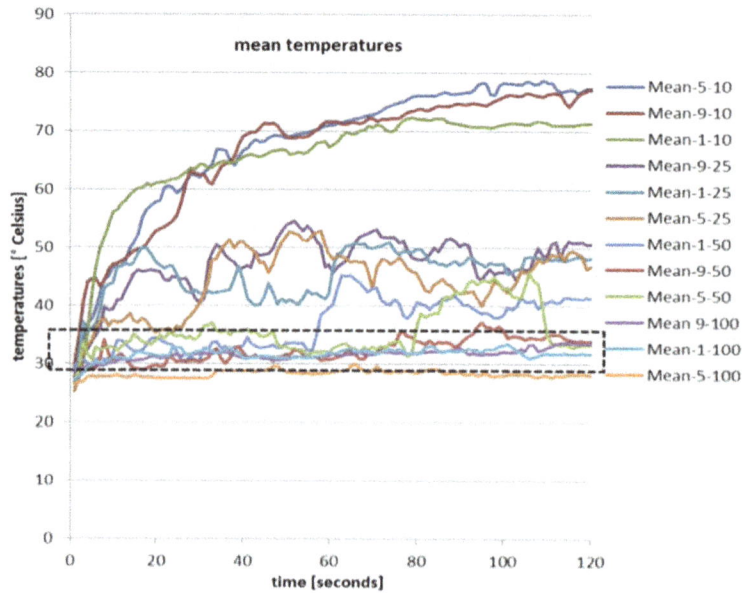

Fig. 7 Mean temperatures for all voltage settings (1, 5 and 9) and all tested pressures (10, 25, 50 and 100 mmHg). The mean temperatures for the low pressure are substantially higher than the medium and high pressures. The range of mean temperatures at high pressure is marked by the dotted rectangle. Some of the temperatures at medium pressures stay within this rectangle for a limited amount of time, while others are clearly above this range all the time

with the temperature fluctuations due to thermal convection, which may lead to a situation where the most distant TP sees higher temperatures than the TPs closer to the RF device with a certain probability. The p-value for the voltage setting is 0.856 for the mean and 0.818 for the maximum temperature, which means that any connection of the mean and maximum temperatures with the voltage setting is random. In summary, voltage setting did not have any impact on the maximum and mean temperatures and the key parameter to control the temperatures is pressure.

Specific findings on individual experimental runs

Until now, we have presented findings on maximum and mean temperatures calculated by averaging the experimental runs. Next, the specifics of the individual runs will be addressed. It is characteristic for experiments in thermo-fluid dynamics in which some turbulence is generated that the temperature-time functions vary substantially from one experimental run to the next due to the dynamics of flow patterns and fluctuations. Running the same experiment with the parameters kept constant may result in temperature curves that differ substantially and fundamental aspects can only be identified by averaging various runs. A closer view on the individual violations of the 50 °C criterion illustrates this issue. In 100% of the low pressure experiments, the criterion was violated. In the medium pressure range for the 25 mmHg experiments, it was found that 66% of the experimental runs violated the criterion, while for the 50 mmHg runs only

38% violated the criterion. In the high pressure experiment, no violation was observed. Table 1 shows more details on the individual findings [11].

The main findings presented in this table are

1) The shortest time span in which 50 °C/122 °F were reached was 2 s.
2) The highest maximum temperature was 102.7 °C (exceeding the boiling point of the saline fluid used as irrigation fluid) in experiments with low pressure and 32.4 °C/89.6 °F in experiments with high pressure.

3) The percentage of runs that exceed the criterion is an almost exact linear function of the square root of pressure.
4) The mean temperature ranges from 77.0 °C/170.6 °F at low pressure to 27.1 °C/80.6 °F at high pressure.

Discussion

The purpose of this study was to investigate the effect of RF use in the ankle joint and how the three parameters irrigation fluid pressure, thermometer probe distance from the wand tip and the voltage setting of the controller affect the maximum temperatures in the ankle joint. The purpose was also to derive recommendations for the safe use of RF in the ankle joint.

Table 1 Incidence of damaging temperatures reached Column 1 to 3 give the independent parameters. Column 4 lists the time needed to achieve temperatures above 50 °C. Column 5 lists the maximum temperatures observed in an individual experimental run

Parameters			Individual		Mean	
controller voltage setting	flow pressure [mm Hg]	Thermometer probe distance [mm]	first time $\geq 50\,°C$ [$_s$]	T_{max} [°C]	Percentage of runs with $T_{max} \geq 50\,°C$	Average Temp [°C] of all runs
1	10	3	4	96,5	100%	72,3
		5	5	96,0	75%	66,4
		10	5	95,8	75%	58,4
1	25	3	3	90,0	75%	52,7
		5	3	88,5	75%	47,6
		10	7	74,7	25%	36,6
1	50	3	31	47,6	40%	38,2
		5	58	48,2	40%	37,0
		10	58	46,4	20%	35,6
1	100	3	XX	46,6	0%	33,4
		5	XX	37,8	0%	31,9
		10	XX	38,5	0%	30,0
5	10	3	4	102,7	100%	77,0
		5	8	98,6	100%	65,7
		10	8	96,5	100%	60,3
5	25	3	3	87,2	0%	53,1
		5	30	87,4	25%	42,7
		10	37	74,2	50%	37,3
5	50	3	3	78,9	50%	39,6
		5	23	69,6	50%	36,9
		10	91	57,9	50%	30,8
5	100	3	XX	37,2	0%	29,6
		5	XX	38,3	0%	28,4
		10	XX	37,2	0%	27,1
9	10	3	2	99,6	100%	72,4
		5	3	100,5	75%	67,5
		10	20	92,3	75%	60,2
9	25	3	5	98,2	75%	55,6
		5	13	95,2	75%	49,8
		10	104	80,5	50%	36,2
9	50	3	72	58,6	25%	32,9
		5	64	46,2	25%	33,8
		10	XX	35,9	0%	30,5
9	100	3	XX	46,1	0%	33,1
		5	XX	40,4	0%	32,1
		10	XX	32,4	0%	29,9

There have been several reports about the deleterious effects of thermal damage to chondrocytes in shoulder arthroscopy resulting in chondrolysis [15, 16] and other papers indicate that a 50 °C/122 °F criterion should be observed since only temperatures below 50 °C/122 °F seem to be safe [9]. Two papers on the effect of RF use in the hip joint [11] and the shoulder joint [10] were published recently. Both papers found that temperatures in the joint, which exceed the criterion of 50 °C/122 °F, can be measured under no flow or low flow of irrigation fluid. From the analysis of the physical problem, it follows that the power output of the RF wand and the amount of irrigation flow are the key parameters, which influences the thermo-fluid dynamics. A typical phenomenon in thermo-fluid dynamics is temperature fluctuation. To measure these fluctuations close to the tip of the wand, three TPs were attached to the wand. From the physical analysis, it is also clear that there are many other parameters which may influence the temperature and which are not controlled in the experiment and therefore provide a random contribution to the data.

As the ankle joint volume (6–10 ml) is similar to the volume of the hip joint cavity (2.5–10 ml), we expected findings similar to those in the paper [10]. The regression analysis of the maximum temperatures (absolute maximum) and the mean temperatures (averaged over time) showed that 80% of the variances can be explained by the square root of the pressure ($p < 0.001$) and by the TP distance, which is also statistically significant ($p < 0.05$).

The effect of the voltage setting of the controller was random, which is hard to understand if one assumes that the voltage setting is relevant for the power output of the RF device. The maximum temperatures of the 12 runs at 100 mmHg were well below the 50 °C criterion, but for all other pressure settings, some or all runs clearly exceeded the criterion. It has to be concluded that high pressure has to be applied for safe temperatures. The physical analysis indicates that only the pressure difference across the cavity is relevant, thus an additional vacuum at the wand could be used to obtain the same thermo-fluid dynamics in the cavity with lower inlet pressure. The disadvantage of high pressures in the cavity is that water causes edema in the surrounding tissue. The situation can be improved by applying additional suction vacuum to reach the required pressure difference.

One option to reduce maximum temperatures in the ankle joint is the use of a turbulence-generating inflow opening at the arthroscope, which improves thermal mixing.

In addition, two issues were analyzed that might lead to even higher temperatures compared to those observed in this study: Hot non-condensable bubbles and outflow plugging. As the heat capacity of a non-condensable gas is lower than the heat capacity of water or tissue by orders of magnitude, it has to be concluded that hot non-condensable bubbles do not represent a potential hazard. As the RF device emits energized particles that break the molecular bounds within the tissue causing the tissue to dissolve, the ablation process generates more or less vapor and not particles, which might lead to plugging. Nevertheless, plugging cannot be ruled out as tissue may be cut loose and may be sucked into the RF device opening in the ablation process. Comparing the data found in our study and the studies on hip [10] and shoulder ablation [9], we could find similar temperature levels and no significant effect of the joint volume in view of the fact that the glenohumeral joint volume is more than twice the volume of the hip or the ankle joint [13, 14, 17].

Finally, the 50 °C/122 °F criterion is rather strict and does not reflect the chondrocyte damage mechanism. Obviously, a short contact with 50 °C will do no harm. Therefore, a better criterion that is based on more sophisticated and in-depth studies should be developed.

We deem the experimental settings of the study to be comparable to the surgical setting. We simulated the use of a RF device and were able to measure temperatures at the tip of the device directly. Although continuous use of the RF device for 60 s might be extreme, even a shorter time period (2 s) is able to cause cartilage damage. Therefore, it is tremendously important to ensure the correct irrigation and thereby diminish the risk of cartilage damage significantly.

In this context, it is crucial to keep in mind that not only high temperatures can have deleterious effects on the surrounding tissue, but also the use of increased water pressure. There have been reports about compartment syndromes of the lower leg after knee arthroscopy with injury to the posterior capsule [18] and of the anterior compartment after ankle arthroscopy in Maisonneuve fractures [19]. Mc Brayer et al. [20] could find an increase of swelling and deltoid muscle pressure during shoulder arthroscopy of 9 mmHg - particularly in operations lasting more than 90 min. Fortunately, they could not find a negative effect on the outcome in their study group.

Still, one has to think of the negative effects of increased pump pressures and what is more, Ross et al. [21] showed in their study that the operative field fluid pressure and the pressure readout might differ considerably.

There are limitations in this study: first, the use of cadaveric specimens leads to a different distraction of the ankle joint and the ankle joint cavity will differ in volume and shape affecting the flow pattern and fluctuations inside the cavity. Six cadaveric specimens cannot represent the full range of variability of human anatomy. Second, the procedure in this study with continuous ablation for more than 60 s may not reproduce the typical clinical scenario. Third, the cadaveric specimens were evaluated at room temperature and not at normal body temperature. Normal blood flow might work as a heat sink and dissipate heat. However, temperatures above the criterion of 50 °C/122 °F might be reached even faster at normal body temperature.

Conclusions

This study investigated the temperatures in the ankle joint during RF ablation. It showed that the key parameter to guaranty temperatures below the 50 °C/122 °F criterion is irrigation pressure. At pressures of 100 mmHg, temperatures in the ankle joint were found to remain well below this criterion. At lower pressure levels, temperatures clearly exceeding 50 °C/122 °F were reached in some or all experiments. Until a more sophisticated in-depth study reveals more detailed information on the effect of RF ablation on the temperatures in the ankle joint and potential hazard for chondrocytes, the authors recommend to keep the pressure difference across the ankle joint as high as feasible, the ablation time short and the temperature of the irrigation fluid low.

Abbreviations
RF: Radiofrequency; TP: Thermoprobe

Funding
No funding was obtained for this study.

Authors' contributions
All authors contributed in a significant way in the steps of processing the patient history as well as writing and editing the manuscript. GHS and PA conceived the idea for the study/publication and engaged in writing the first draft. DM, SS and AL provided research support, gave advice throughout the project and were involved in the experiments and the review of the manuscript. AL, US and GHS gave research advice and reviewed the manuscript. All authors read and approved the final manuscript.

Competing interest
PA is a member of the Editorial Board of BMC Muskuloskeletal Disorders. The other authors have no competing interests.

Consent for publication
Not applicable.

Author details
[1]Department of Orthopaedic Sports Medicine, Klinikum rechts der Isar, Technische Universitaet Muenchen, Germany, Ismanninger, Str. 22, D- 81675 Muenchen, Germany. [2]Sportklinik Stuttgart, Taubenheimstraße 8, D-70372 Stuttgart, Germany. [3]Schön Klinik Harthausen, Dr.-Wilhelm-Knarr- Weg 1-3, D-83043 Bad Aibling, Germany. [4]Helios Klinikum München West, Steinerweg 5, D- 81241 Muenchen, Germany. [5]BG Unfallklinik Tuebingen, Schnarrenbergstraße 95, 72076 Tuebingen, Germany. [6]Sportklinik Ravensburg, Bachstraße 57, 88214 Ravensburg, Germany.

References
1. Kouk SN, Zoric B, Stetson WB. Complication of the use of a radiofrequency device in arthroscopic shoulder surgery: second-degree burn of the shoulder girdle. Arthroscopy. 2011;27:136–41.
2. Troxell CR, Morgan CD, Rajan S, Leitman EH, Bartolozzi AR. Dermal burns associated with bipolar radiofrequency ablation in the subacromial space. Arthroscopy. 2011;27:142–4.
3. Petty DH, Jazrawi LM, Estrada LS, Andrews JR. Glenohumeral chondrolysis after shoulder arthrosocpy: case reports and review of the literature. Am J Sports Med. 2004;32:509–15.
4. Jerosch J, Aldawoudy AM. Chondrolysis of the glenohumeral joint following arthroscopic capsular release for adhesive capsulitis: a case report. Knee Surg Sports Traumatol Arthrosc. 2007;15:292–4.
5. Good CR, Shindle MK, Kelly BT, Wanich T, Warren RF. Glenohumeral chondrolysis after shoulder arthroscopy with thermal capsulorrhaphy. Arthroscopy 2007;23:797 e791–795.
6. Rapley JH, Beavis RC, Barber FA. Glenohumeral chondrolysis after shoulder arthroscopy associated with continuous bupivacaine infusion. Arthroscopy. 2009;25:1367–73.
7. Rehan Ul H, Yang HK, Park KS, Lee KB, Yoon TR. An unusual case of chondrolysis of the hip following excision of a torn acetabular labrum. Arch Orthop Trauma Surg. 2010;130:65–70.
8. Horstman CL, McLaughlin RM. The use of radiofrequency energy during arthroscopic surgery and its effects on intraarticular tissues. Vet Comp Orthop Traumatol. 2006;19:65–71.
9. Voss JR, Lu Y, Edwards RB, Bogdanske JJ, Markel MD. Effects of thermal energy on chondrocyte viability. Am J Vet Res. 2006;67:1708–12.
10. Zoric BB, Horn N, Braun S, Millett PJ. Factors influencing intra-articular fluid temperature profiles with radiofrequency ablation. J Bone Joint Sur Am Volume. 2009;91:2448–54.
11. McCormick F, Alpaugh K, Nwachukwu BU, Xu S, Martin SD. Effect of radiofrequency use on hip arthroscopy irrigation fluid temperature. Arthroscopy. 2013;29(2):336–42.
12. Arnold H. Posttraumatic impingement syndrome of the ankle--indication and results of arthroscopic therapy. Foot and ankle surgery. 2011;17:85–8.
13. Luke TA, Rovner AD, Karas SG, Hawkins RJ, Plancher KD. Volumetric change in the shoulder capsule after open inferior capsular shift versus arthroscopic thermal capsular shrinkage: a cadaveric model. J Shoulder and Elbow Surg. 2004;13:146–9.
14. Draeger RW, Singh B, Parekh SG. Quantifying normal ankle joint volume: an anatomic study. Indian journal of orthopaedics. 2009;43:72–5.
15. Lu Y, Edwards RB 3rd, Nho S, Heiner JP, Cole BJ, Markel MD. Thermal chondroplasty with bipolar and monopolar radiofrequency energy. effect of treatment time on chondrocyte death and surface contouring Arthroscopy. 2002;18:779–88.
16. Lu Y, Edwards RB 3rd, Nho S, Cole BJ, Markel MD. Lavage solution temperature influences depth of chondrocyte death and surface contouring during thermal chondroplasty with temperature-controlled monopolar radiofrequency energy. Am J Sports Med. 2002;30:667–73.
17. Yen CH, Leung HB, Tse PY. Effects of hip joint position and intra-capsular volume on hip joint intra-capsular pressure: a human cadaveric model. J Orthop Surg Res. 2009;4:8.
18. Keskinbora M, Yalcin S, Oltulu I, Erdil ME, Örmeci T. Compartment syndrome following arthroscopic removal of a bullet in the knee joint after a low-velocity gunshot injury. Clin Orthop Surg. 2016;8(1):115–8.
19. Imade S, Takao M, Miyamoto W, Hishi H, Uchio Y. Leg anterior compartment syndrome following ankle arthroscopy after Maisonneuve fracture. Arthroscopy. 2009;25(2):215–8.
20. McBrayer DE, Debelak BP, Femicola PJ, Tu R, Baker CL Jr. Deltoid muscle pressures during arthroscopic rotator cuff repair. Orthopedics 2013; 36(1): 33–37.
21. Ross JA, Marland JD, Payne B, Whiting DR, West HS. Do arthroscopic fluid pumps display true surgical site pressure during hip arthrosocpy? Arthroscopy. 2018;34(1):126–32.

13

A comparison of outcome measures used to report clubfoot treatment with the Ponseti method: results from a cohort in Harare, Zimbabwe

Tracey Smythe[1]*, Maxman Gova[2], Rumbidzai Muzarurwi[3], Allen Foster[1] and Christopher Lavy[4]

Abstract

Background: There are various established scoring systems to assess the outcome of clubfoot treatment after correction with the Ponseti method. We used five measures to compare the results in a cohort of children followed up for between 3.5 to 5 years.

Methods: In January 2017 two experienced physiotherapists assessed children who had started treatment between 2011 and 2013 in one clinic in Harare, Zimbabwe. The length of time in treatment was documented. The Roye score, Bangla clubfoot assessment tool, the Assessing Clubfoot Treatment (ACT) tool, proportion of relapsed and of plantigrade feet were used to assess the outcome of treatment in the cohort. Inter-observer variation was calculated for the two physiotherapists. A comparative analysis of the entire cohort, the children who had completed casting and the children who completed more than two years of bracing was undertaken. Diagnostic accuracy was calculated for the five measures and compared to full clinical assessment (gold standard) and whether referral for further intervention was required for re-casting or surgical review.

Results: 31% (68/218) of the cohort attended for examination and were assessed. Of the children who were assessed, 24 (35%) had attended clinic reviews for 4–5 years, and 30 (44%) for less than 2 years. There was good inter-observer agreement between the two expert physiotherapists on all assessment tools. Overall success of treatment varied between 56 and 93% using the different outcome measures. The relapse assessment had the highest unnecessary referrals (19.1%), and the Roye score the highest proportion of missed referrals (22.7%). The ACT and Bangla score missed the fewest number of referrals (7.4%). The Bangla score demonstrated 79.2% (95%CI: 57.8–92.9%) sensitivity and 79.5% (95%CI: 64.7–90.2%) specificity and the ACT score had 79.2% (95%CI: 57.8–92.9%) sensitivity and 100% (95%CI: 92–100%) specificity in predicting the need for referral.

Conclusion: At three to five years of follow up, the Ponseti method has a good success rate that improves if the child has completed casting and at least two years of bracing. The ACT score demonstrates good diagnostic accuracy for the need for referral for further intervention (specialist opinion or further casting). All tools demonstrated good reliability.

Keywords: Clubfoot, CTEV, Measurement, Quality, Ponseti, Evaluate, Indicator, Low resource, Tool

* Correspondence: tracey.smythe@lshtm.ac.uk
[1]International Centre for Evidence in Disability, London School of Hygiene & Tropical Medicine, Keppel Street, London WC1E7HT, UK
Full list of author information is available at the end of the article

Background

Clubfoot, or congenital talipes equinovarus, is a condition that is present at birth in which the foot is in a rigid turned-in position. Corrective treatment of a high quality remains a key requirement for reducing disability and improving function related to the deformity. Over the past decades there has been an increase in the use of the Ponseti method to correct clubfoot [1]. This method involves the simultaneous correction of three components of the clubfoot deformity through manipulation and serial casting. The equinus (downward pointing of the foot) is corrected last, often with a percutaneous achilles tenotomy. This is followed by long term use of a foot abduction brace at night to maintain the foot position [2]. Despite the global trend toward increased use of the Ponseti method, there remains variation in how success of clubfoot treatment is measured [3, 4].

The Ponseti method is administered by locally trained therapists in resource constrained settings in Africa [5]. These clubfoot therapists often work alone and have no specialised physiotherapy or surgical support present in the clinics or nearby. It is important that they have a user friendly assessment system with agreed criteria for when treatment is not working and referral to a specialist for further management is indicated.

No globally accepted outcome scoring system exists to inform locally trained clubfoot therapists of the need for referral for further intervention. The most frequently used approach to measuring whether the Ponseti method has been successful (or not) is clinical assessment. In sub-Saharan Africa 68 to 98% of cases are reported to have a successful outcome with the Ponseti method [4]. This study aims to compare the results of the Ponseti method of clubfoot management at three to five years from initial correction using five different outcome measures. We explore the diagnostic accuracy of the outcome measures, which is the ability of the assessments to discriminate between the need for referral for further intervention and a successful outcome [6]. For methodology review, outcome score results in this study are compared with a reference standard of 'true' treatment success status (defined by full clinical assessment). The results are categorised as true positive, false positive (referred but not needed), true negative, and false negative (should have been referred but was missed) [7]. Sensitivity of the scoring system relates to the proportion of the children who need referral for further intervention and who are correctly classified by the outcome measure as requiring referral. Specificity is the proportion of children who do not need referral and who are correctly classified as not requiring referral by the outcome measure. Positive predictive value and negative predictive value are useful to understand the probability that a child with a given positive or negative outcome

score result has the need for referral for further intervention and are therefore correctly classified.

Methods

Study design and population

This study was conducted and reported according to established STARD (Standards for Reporting of Diagnostic Accuracy Studies) guidelines [8] (Additional file 1). A cohort study of 218 children with idiopathic clubfoot was conducted in 2016. The children were managed with manipulation and casting at Parirenyatwa Hospital, Harare and the results are published elsewhere [9]. All children with a diagnosis of unilateral or bilateral idiopathic clubfoot who started treatment with the Ponseti method at the study hospital between 22nd March 2011 and 23rd April 2013 (25 months) were included in the cohort. The only exclusion criterion was foot conditions other than idiopathic clubfoot, for example clubfoot associated with neural-tube defects such as spina-bifida.

Sampling technique

The phone numbers of all carers of the cohort children were extracted from the clinic records in January 2017 and contact with them was attempted at least three times. Caregivers and their children were invited to attend the study. The children were between 3.5 and 5 years from initial casting.

Ethics, consent and permissions

Ethical approval for this study was granted by the Medical Research Council of Zimbabwe (MRCZ) and the London School of Hygiene & Tropical Medicine (LSHTM) (ref:11132 /RR/4725). All children and their caregivers were read an information sheet about the study and given an opportunity to ask questions. If they agreed to participate, written consent was taken from the caregiver who remained present throughout the assessment as per national requirements. Transport costs were reimbursed and referral services available in Harare were mapped pre-emptively to ensure appropriate onward referral for any children that required further intervention.

Data collection

Two physiotherapists who are experienced in co-ordinating national clubfoot programmes reviewed the assessment tools over three days for contextual relevance. The questionnaires were available in English and Shona and were cognitively tested. We used five outcome methods, three that give a score, and two that give a binary (success/failure) outcome. The Roye score [10] is a self-reported measurement that is used in high income settings. The Bangla clubfoot assessment tool [11] and the Assessing Clubfoot Treatment (ACT) score [12] combine physical assessment and parent reported outcome measures, and have been developed for low resource settings. The Bangla score includes a functional assessment. The two binary outcomes were assessment of a plantigrade foot [5] and the relapse pattern [13]. The study protocol was pilot tested for suitability in July 2016. Children were examined independently in January 2017 by the two physiotherapists and a decision was made if referral for further intervention (re-casting or surgical review) was required. Clinical examination composed observation, physical assessment and functional review; it included assessment of passive and active range of motion (plantiflexion, dorsiflexion, eversion, inversion of the foot, and knee extension), muscle strength tests of the calf and evertors of the foot, heel raises, squatting ability and gait analysis (walking and running).

Data management and analysis strategy

The data were entered into a Microsoft Excel 2000 (Microsoft Inc., Redmond, Washington) software package. Data were analysed using Stata 14.1 (Stata-Corp 4905, Lakeway Drive College Station, Texas 77, 845, USA). Statistical significance was set at the 95% confidence level. The inter-observer variation for the measurement of the physical assessment tools was assessed i.e. Intra-class correlation coefficient (ICC) ≥0.75 [10]. Outcomes of children who had completed casting and ≥ two years of bracing were compared to all of the children who were followed up, and to those who had only completed casting. A two-tailed paired t-test was used to assess the mean difference between the outcome measures of Roye, Bangla and ACT scores. Fisher's exact test of independence was used to assess the difference in proportion of children with an outcome of relapse and plantigrade foot. The five measures were compared against the standard of whether referral for further intervention was required (for re-casting or surgical review) as defined by a

consensus agreement of two expert physiotherapists with experience of managing clubfoot in countries in Africa. Sensitivity, specificity, positive and negative predictive values were calculated for the five measures and compared to full clinical assessment (gold standard). The threshold for diagnostic accuracy was based on previous studies and was defined prior to the study. It was set at 70% for the three scores with continuous scales [14] and positive/negative for the binary outcomes [7].

Results

31% (68/218) of the cohort attended for review and were assessed. 50 (73%) children were boys and 18 (27%) were girls. There were 35 (51%) bilateral and 33 (49%) unilateral clubfeet. Tenotomies had been performed in 52 (76%) cases and the average number of casts to correction was 6.9 (5.9–8.0 casts). The average length of time attending appointments from initial review was 30 months (26 – 35 months). Of the children followed up, 24 (35%) attended clinic reviews for 4–5 years (Fig. 1).

All tools demonstrated good reliability, with an intra-class coefficient (ICC) of ≥0.82 on all criteria (Table 1). An ICC of 1.00 demonstrates perfect correlation.

In the children who were followed up ($n = 68$) the success of treatment with different scores varied between 56 and 89% (Table 2). In the children who completed casting ($n = 63$) it was between 57 and 93%; and in the children who completed casting and at least two years of bracing ($n = 38$) it was from 58 to 97% (Table 3). The individual category calculations for each outcome measurement are in Additional files 2, 3, 4 and 5.

The proportion of children with relapse and the Bangla tool had the lowest good outcome results of 56 and 59% respectively. Figure 2 demonstrates the variation in outcome when compared to full clinical assessment (the gold standard illustrated in the first row of the

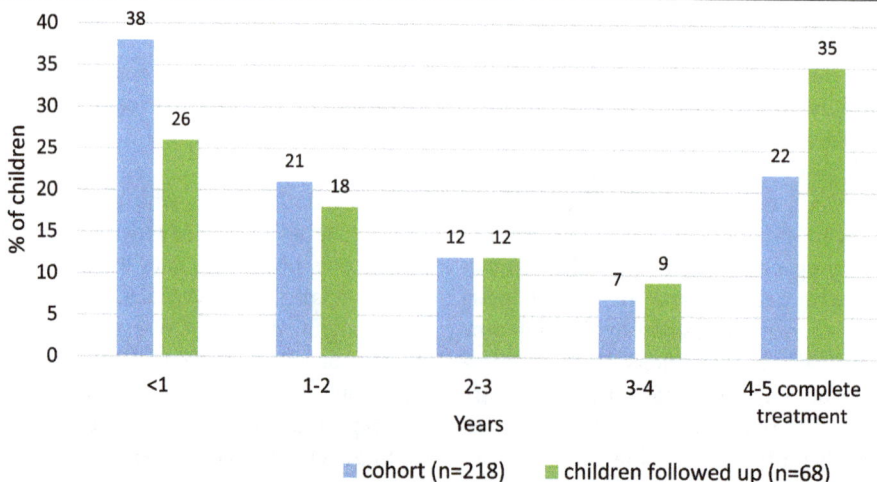

Fig. 1 Length of time child attended clubfoot clinic appointments

Table 1 Inter-observer variation for outcome measures

Outcome Measure	ICC	95%CI
Bangla Score		
1. Happy with child's feet?	0.96	0.94–0.98
2. Recommmend to others?	1.00	1.00
3. Does child play with others?	1.00	1.00
4. Does child wear shoes of choice?	0.97	0.95–0.98
5. Does child have pain?	1.00	1.00
6. Squatting	1.00	1.00
7. Walking	1.00	1.00
8. Running	1.00	1.00
9. Up/down stairs	1.00	1.00
10a. Heel position L	0.94	0.88–0.97
10b. Heel position R	0.98	0.97–0.99
11a. Ankle range L	0.82	0.66–0.90
11b. Ankle range R	0.99	0.98–0.99
Relapse assessment		
1A - reduced DF	0.96	0.93–0.98
2A - fixed equinus	1.00	1.00
1B - dynamic supination, flex add	0.88	0.79–0.93
2B - fixed forefoot add	1.00	1.00
3–2 or more deformities	1.00	1.00
ACT score		
1. Foot is plantigrade	0.99	0.98–0.99
2. Does child complain of pain?	1.00	1.00
3. Can child wear shoes of choice?	0.99	0.99–1.00
4. How satisfied is the carer?	1.00	1.00
Plantigrade foot	0.99	0.98–0.99
Roye score	1.00	1.00

(ICC > 75 = good consistency)

figure). 87% (33/38) children who completed ≥2 years bracing were assessed as successfully treated with full clinical assessment. The scores that demonstrate a higher success (Plantigrade: 97% and Roye score: 94%) miss cases that require further intervention. The scores that demonstrate a lower success (Relapse: 58% and Bangla: 66%) are restrictive in the measurement of success.

There was strong evidence for a difference between the outcomes of the Roye score and the Bangla score ($p < 0.0001$), the Roye and the ACT score ($p = 0.0013$), and the ACT and Bangla score ($p < 0.0001$). It follows that none of these assessments can provide essentially the same estimate of success as the other measures.

There was a difference in the relative proportion of the cohort with relapse and plantigrade foot when assessed with Fischer's exact test ($p = 0.012$). The binary outcomes are therefore not interchangeable.

No adverse events occurred as a result of any of the outcome measures undertaken. When compared to the standard of full clinical assessment and the subsequent decision on the need for referral for further intervention, the Roye score had a sensitivity of 31.8% (95%CI: 13.9–54.9%) and a specificity of 100% (95%CI: 92–100%), with positive and negative predictive values of 100 and 74.6% respectively. The Bangla score demonstrated 79.2% (95%CI: 57.8–92.9%) sensitivity and 79.5% (95%CI: 64.7–90.2%) specificity with 67.9% positive predictive and 87.5% negative predictive values, and the ACT score had 79.2% (95%CI: 57.8–92.9%) sensitivity and 100% (95%CI: 92–100%) specificity in predicting the need for referral, with positive and negative predictive values of 100 and 89.8% respectively. Of the 44 children that did not require referral for further intervention, all achieved plantigrade or more (positive predictive value: 100%) and of those who did require referral ($n = 24$), 14 were identified with the plantigrade assessment (achieved less than

Table 2 Results of cohort of children followed up (n = 68)

Outcome measure	Poor < 49 N (%)	Fair: 50–69 N (%)	Good: 70–84 N (%)	V Good: 85–100 N (%)
Roye[a]	4 (6%)	3 (5%)	20 (30%)	39 (59%)
Total Roye[a]	7 (11%)		59 (89%)	
Bangla	12 (17%)	16 (24%)	15 (22%)	25 (37%)
Total Bangla	28 (41%)		40 (59%)	
ACT score	7 (10%)	12 (18%)	13 (19%)	36 (53%)
Total ACT score	19 (28%)		49 (72%)	
	Cannot achieve plantigrade		Achieved plantigrade or better	
Plantigrade	13 (19%)		55 (81%)	
Any form of relapse	Yes		No	
	30 (44%)		38 (56%)	
Requires referral for further intervention	Yes		No	
	16 (24%)		52 (76%)	

[a]data missing for 2 children

Table 3 Results of cohort of children followed up who completed > 2 years bracing (n = 38)

Outcome measure	Poor < 49 N (%)	Fair: 50–69 N (%)	Good: 70–84 N (%)	V Good:85–100 N (%)
Roye[a]	1 (3%)	1 (3%)	10 (28%)	24 (66%)
Total Roye[a]	2 (6%)		34 (94%)	
Bangla	3 (8%)	10 (26%)	9 (24%)	16 (42%)
Total Bangla	13 (34%)		25 (66%)	
ACT score	1 (3%)	5 (13%)	9 (24%)	23 (60%)
Total ACT score	6 (16%)		32 (84%)	
	cannot achieve plantigrade		Achieved plantigrade or better	
Plantigrade	1 (3%)		37 (97%)	
Any form of relapse	Yes		No	
	16 (42%)		22 (58%)	
Requires referral for further intervention	Yes		No	
	5 (13%)		33 (87%)	

[a]data missing from 2 children

plantigrade). The relapse score was most restrictive in identifying good outcome. False positive and false negative scores are displayed in Table 4.

Discussion

This study found that five scoring systems that are used to report outcomes of clubfoot treatment provided a wide spectrum of success (from 56 to 89% of cases) in a cohort with 3.5–5 years of follow up. When compared with the standard of clinical assessment, missed referrals ranged from 7.4% (the Bangla and ACT scores) to 22.7% (the Roye score). The measurements assess different aspects of clubfoot correction, from parent reported outcome measures (the Roye score) to scores that include

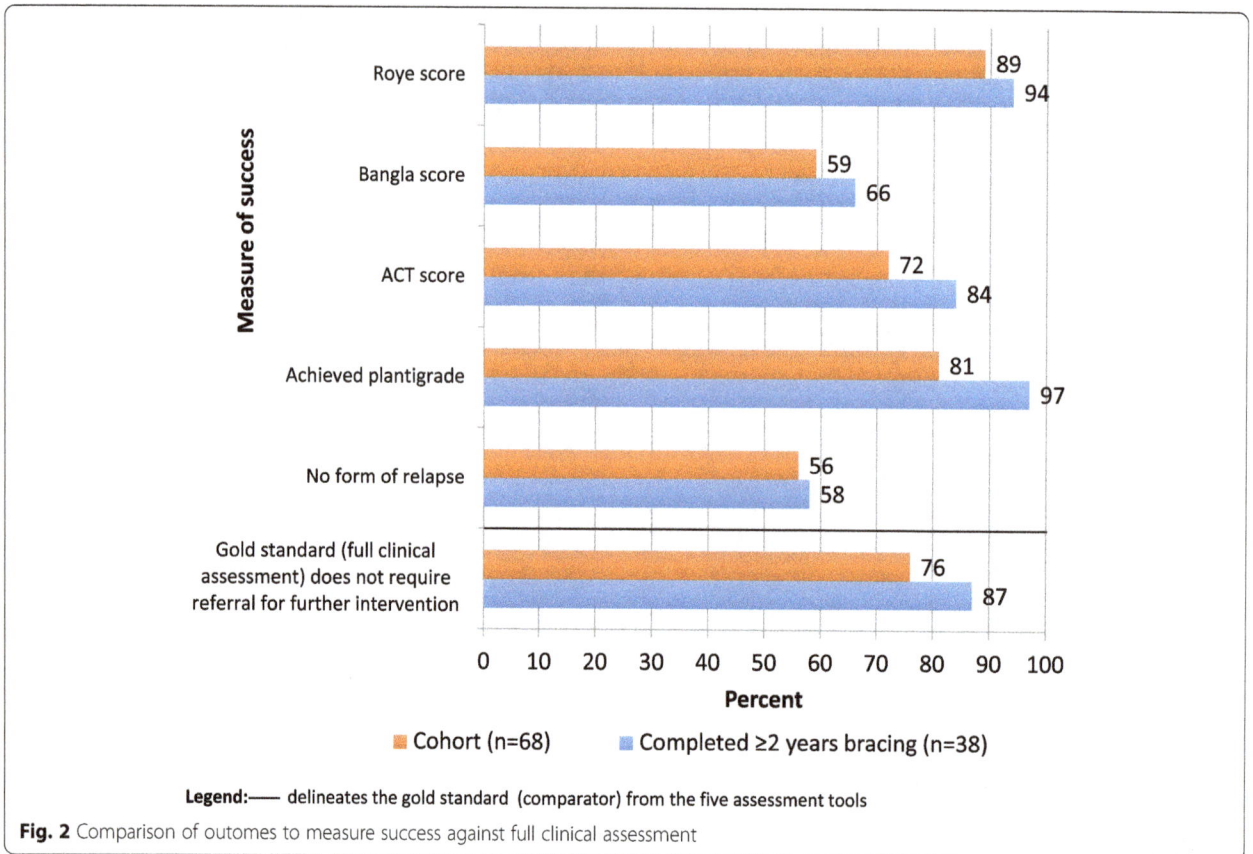

Fig. 2 Comparison of outomes to measure success against full clinical assessment

Table 4 A comparison of measurement methods with the need for referral for further intervention

Method	Unnecessary referral (false positive) n (%)	Missed Referral (false negative) n (%)
Roye (n = 66)	0 (0%)	15 (22.7%)
Bangla (n = 68)	10 (14.7%)	5 (7.4%)
ACT (n = 68)	1 (1.5%)	5 (7.4%)
Plantigrade (n = 68)	0 (0%)	10 (14.7)
Relapse (n = 68)	13 (19.1%)	6 (8.8%)

physical assessment (the Bangla and ACT score) and single measurements (plantigrade foot and evidence of recurrence). Success improves in all measures with the completion of casting and at least two years of bracing.

Comparison to previous studies

There are limited studies that compare measurement tools in the same patient against which to compare our findings. However, success of treatment in this cohort is similar to other studies in sub-Saharan Africa (between 63 and 98% of cases) [9]. Non-adherence and surgical intervention, often defined as failure, are reported to vary from 7 to 61% and 3–39.4% [15] respectively. Ponseti and Laaveg [16] describe a scoring system that rates functional results as satisfactory in 88.5% of feet. Further studies describe success using the Ponseti and Laaveg system as 89.3% [17]. The criteria includes the need for a goniometer and the tool was therefore not included in evaluation of this cohort.

Use of outcome measures

The ease of use and rate of incorrect classification in the tools used to measure success need to be considered when selecting an outcome measure. Single item scales for assessment of individual children require no further calculation and may be easier to use in clinics (such as plantigrade foot or evidence of relapse), however their simplicity may not allow a full assessment of success. Multi-scale items prove difficult to transform into useful statistics without technology and are unlikely to be routinely used in clinics. This study found no clear agreement between the different outcome measurements in use.

All of the assessments used in this study have limitations. The Roye score has been validated in high income settings and parents in our study reported difficulty in answering the question of "How often does your child have problems finding shoes that he or she likes?" as it was understood to be related to the availability of a variety of shoes. The Bangla score took the longest time to transform with statistical analysis. Acceptability and feasibility of the ACT score is needed to be studied in future research. The ACT score is likely easy to teach, however this

is unknown as the examiners were physiotherapists; the time taken for other cadres of health workers to use the ACT tool is also unknown. With regard to the relapse score, Bhaskar et al. (2013) considered ankle dorsiflexion < 15 degrees with knee in extension as grade IA relapse. This may be a reason for the restriction in defining good outcome as an evaluation of 85 normal feet in children found that the mean ankle dorsiflexion was 12.8 degrees with knees in extension [18]. Greater than 15 degrees may therefore be difficult to achieve.

Relationship between the outcome measures and clinical assessment

The Bangla and ACT tool were most helpful in predicting the need for referral for further intervention (specialist opinion or for further manipulation and casting). The five referrals that were missed with the ACT score were children who required review of a mobile curvature of the lateral border of the foot or supination in swing phase, neither of which are assessed with the score. Despite this, the ACT tool demonstrates the best diagnostic accuracy for the need for referral for further intervention.

Strengths and limitations of study

This study reports on five measurements of success in a cohort at 3.5–5 years from initial treatment. Repeat phone calls facilitated assessments when caregivers were initially unavailable. Two independent raters reduced the likelihood of reporting bias and all outcome measures were verified by the reference standard. The threshold for diagnostic accuracy was based on previous studies and was defined prior to the study. There were also study limitations. No distinction between a clubfoot that may not have been fully corrected and a relapsed clubfoot was made, and all cases with elements of the deformity were classified with the relapse score, which may be a source of potential bias that underestimates the accuracy of the relapse score. The tools were chosen based on ease of use in low resource high volume clinics and were not all initially developed to identify need for referral for further intervention.

Implications for practice

Task shifting and task sharing between orthopaedic and non-specialised health workers in some clinics means that outcome measures are even more important as teams expand. As older children are being treated with the principles of the Ponseti method [19], expert guidance on assessment and measurement in these cases is needed. The Roye score is overly optimistic of good outcomes, the Bangla score is restrictive in identifying good outcome, and the ACT score most closely aligns to clinical examination. However, the Bangla, relapse and ACT scores closely agree on false negatives and have the least chance of missing recurrence; the Bangla score and the relapse score over-estimate referral needs compared to the ACT score.

Conclusions

In this small comparative study, missed referrals ranged from 7.4% (the Bangla and ACT scores) to 22.7% (the Roye score) when compared with the standard of clinical assessment. Ease of use and the cost of false positives need to be considered in the selection of a tool. All scores demonstrated good reliability. The Roye score will miss cases and the Bangla and the Relapse tools are restrictive in assessment of successful outcome. We found no clear agreement between the different scores in use. When compared to the normal practice of full clinical assessment, the measurement tool with the best evidence for diagnostic accuracy was the ACT tool.

Additional files

Additional file 1: The STARD 2015 list. Standards for Reporting of Diagnostic Accuracy Studies guidelines.

Additional file 2: Summary of outcomes: Roye score. Individual category calculations for the Roye score.

Additional file 3: Summary of outcomes: Bangla score. Individual category calculations for the Bangla score.

Additional file 4: Summary of outcomes: ACT score. .Individual category calculations for the ACT score.

Additional file 5: Summary of outcomes: Relapse score. Individual category calculations for the Relapse score.

Abbreviations
ACT: Assessing Clubfoot Treatment; ICC: Intra-class correlation coefficient

Acknowledgements
Zimbabwe Ministry of Health and Child Welfare, Parirenyatwa clubfoot clinic staff, Ryan Bathurst ZSCP, Debra Mudariki, Memory Mwadziwana and Mediatrice Mutsambi for data collection.

Funding
The Beit Trust, MiracleFeet, ZANE as scholarship to TS. The funding bodies had no role in the design of the study and collection, analysis, and interpretation of data and in writing the manuscript.

Authors' contributions
TS, CL and AF designed the study. TS, MG and RM designed the study protocol. TS analysed and interpreted the data. TS wrote the first draft of the manuscript. MG, RM, AF and CL reviewed and edited the manuscript. All authors read and approved the final manuscript.

Consent for publication
Not applicable.

Competing interests
The authors declare that they have no competing interests.

Author details
[1]International Centre for Evidence in Disability, London School of Hygiene & Tropical Medicine, Keppel Street, London WC1E7HT, UK. [2]Department of Surgery, Parirenyatwa Group of Hospitals, Harare, Zimbabwe. [3]Rehabilitation Department, Parirenyatwa Group of Hospitals, Harare, Zimbabwe. [4]Nuffield Department of Orthopaedics Rheumatology and Musculoskeletal Science, University of Oxford, Oxford, UK.

References
1. Shabtai L, Specht SC, Herzenberg JE. Worldwide spread of the Ponseti method for clubfoot. World J Orthop. 2014;5(5):585–90.
2. Ponseti IV. The ponseti technique for correction of congenital clubfoot. J Bone Joint Surg Am. 2002;84-A(10):1889–90 author reply 90-1.
3. Ganesan B, Luximon A, Al-Jumaily A, Balasankar SK, Naik GR. Ponseti method in the management of clubfoot under 2 years of age: a systematic review. PLoS One. 2017;12(6):e0178299.
4. Smythe T, Mudariki D, Kuper H, Lavy C, Foster A. Assessment of success of the Ponseti method of clubfoot management in sub-Saharan Africa: a systematic review. BMC Musculoskelet Disord. 2017;18(1):453.
5. Tindall AJ, Steinlechner CWB, Lavy CBD, Mannion S, Mkandawire N. Results of manipulation of idiopathic clubfoot deformity in Malawi by Orthopaedic clinical officers using the Ponseti method: a realistic alternative for the developing world? [article]. J Pediatr Orthop. 2005;25(5):627–9.
6. Šimundić A-M. Measures of diagnostic accuracy: basic definitions. EJIFCC. 2009;19(4):203–11.
7. Mallett S, Halligan S, Thompson M, Collins GS, Altman DG. Interpreting diagnostic accuracy studies for patient care. BMJ. 2012;345:e3999.
8. Cohen JF, Korevaar DA, Altman DG, Bruns DE, Gatsonis CA, Hooft L, et al. STARD 2015 guidelines for reporting diagnostic accuracy studies: explanation and elaboration. BMJ Open. 2016;6(11):e012799.
9. Smythe T, Chandramohan D, Bruce J, Kuper H, Lavy C, Foster A. Results of clubfoot treatment after manipulation and casting using the Ponseti method: experience in Harare, Zimbabwe. Tropical Med Int Health. 2016;21(10):1311–8.
10. Roye BD, Vitale MG, Gelijns AC, Roye DP Jr. Patient-based outcomes after clubfoot surgery. J Pediatr Orthop. 2001;21(1):42–9.
11. Evans AM, Perveen R, Ford-Powell VA, Barker S. The Bangla clubfoot tool: a repeatability study. J Foot Ankle Res. 2014;7(1):27.
12. Smythe T, Wainwright A, Foster A, Lavy C. What is a good result after clubfoot treatment? A Delphi-based consensus on success by regional clubfoot trainers from across Africa. PLoS One. 2017;12(12):e0190056.
13. Bhaskar A, Patni P. Classification of relapse pattern in clubfoot treated with Ponseti technique. Indian J Orthop. 2013;47(4):370–6.
14. Evans AM, Chowdhury MMH, Kabir MH, Rahman MF. Walk for life - the National Clubfoot Project of Bangladesh: the four-year outcomes of 150 congenital clubfoot cases following Ponseti method. Journal of Foot and Ankle Research. 2016;9(1):42.
15. Zhao D, Li H, Zhao L, Liu J, Wu Z, Jin F. Results of clubfoot management using the Ponseti method: do the details matter? A systematic review. Clin Orthop Relat Res. 2014;472(4):1329–36.
16. Laaveg SJ, Ponseti IV. Long-term results of treatment of congenital club foot. J Bone Joint Surg Am. 1980;62(1):23–31.
17. Porecha MM, Parmar DS, Chavda HR. Mid-term results of Ponseti method for the treatment of congenital idiopathic clubfoot--(a study of 67 clubfeet with mean five year follow-up). J Orthop Surg Res. 2011;6:3.
18. Tabrizi P, McIntyre WM, Quesnel MB, Howard AW. Limited dorsiflexion predisposes to injuries of the ankle in children. J Bone Joint Surg Br. 2000;82(8):1103–6.
19. Ayana B, Klungsoyr PJ. Good results after Ponseti treatment for neglected congenital clubfoot in Ethiopia. A prospective study of 22 children (32 feet) from 2 to 10 years of age. Acta Orthop. 2014;85(6):641–5.

14

Can we improve cognitive function among adults with osteoarthritis by increasing moderate-to-vigorous physical activity and reducing sedentary behaviour? Secondary analysis of the MONITOR-OA study

Ryan S. Falck[1], John R. Best[1], Linda C. Li[2], Patrick C. Y. Chan[1], Lynne M. Feehan[2] and Teresa Liu-Ambrose[1*]

Abstract

Background: Preliminary evidence suggests osteoarthritis is a risk factor for cognitive decline. One potential reason is 87% of adults with osteoarthritis are inactive, and low moderate-to-vigorous physical activity and high sedentary behaviour are each risk factors for cognitive decline. Thus, we investigated whether a community-based intervention to increase moderate-to-vigorous physical activity and reduce sedentary behaviour could improve cognitive function among adults with osteoarthritis.

Methods: This was a secondary analysis of a six month, proof-of-concept randomized controlled trial of a community-based, technology-enabled counselling program to increase moderate-to-vigorous physical activity and reduce sedentary behaviour among adults with knee osteoarthritis. The *Immediate Intervention* (n = 30) received a Fitbit® Flex™ and four bi-weekly activity counselling sessions; the *Delayed Intervention* (n = 31) received the same intervention two months later. We assessed episodic memory and working memory using the National Institutes of Health Toolbox Cognition Battery. Between-group differences (Immediate Intervention vs. Delayed Intervention) in cognitive performance were evaluated following the primary intervention (i.e., Baseline – 2 Months) using intention-to-treat.

Results: The intervention did not significantly improve cognitive function; however, we estimated small average improvements in episodic memory for the Immediate Intervention vs. Delayed Intervention (estimated mean difference: 1.27; 95% CI [− 9.27, 11.81]; d = 0.10).

Conclusion: This small study did not show that a short activity promotion intervention improved cognitive health among adults with osteoarthritis. However, the effects of increased moderate-to-vigorous physical activity and reduced sedentary behaviour are likely to be small and thus we recommend subsequent studies use larger sample sizes and measure changes in cognitive function over longer intervals.

Keywords: Physical activity, Sedentary behaviour, Cognitive function, Osteoarthritis

* Correspondence: teresa.ambrose@ubc.ca
[1]Faculty of Medicine, Aging, Mobility and Cognitive Neuroscience Laboratory, Djavad Mowafaghian Centre for Brain Health, Department of Physical Therapy, University of British Columbia, 212-2177 Wesbrook Mall, Vancouver, BC V6T 1Z3, Canada
Full list of author information is available at the end of the article

Background

One new diagnosis of osteoarthritis (OA) occurs every 60 s, such that 9.6% of all men and 18.0% of all women over age 60 have symptomatic OA [1, 2]. Of those living with OA, 80% will have limitations in movement and 25% cannot perform their major daily activities of life [2]. The pain of OA is associated with 1) reduced physical function and mobility [3]; and 2) increased frailty and falls risk [4]. While total knee replacement is effective for end-stage OA [5], it does not uniformly restore joint function, and 20% of patients continue to experience pain [6].

Preliminary evidence also suggests OA is associated with an increased risk of cognitive decline and dementia [7]. Although the association between OA and dementia is still under investigation [8], animal models suggest that peripheral inflammation associated with OA may trigger neural inflammation and induce Alzheimer's disease pathology—the most common form of dementia [9]. Given that the number of cases of OA and dementia are each increasing as the population of older adults continues to grow [10, 11], there is an urgent need for effective treatment strategies for OA symptoms since this may also help reduce dementia prevalence.

Two frontline strategies for improving OA symptoms are increasing moderate-to-vigorous physical activity and reducing sedentary behaviour [12–16]. Briefly, moderate-to-vigorous physical activity (MVPA) refers to any behaviour which incurs ≥3.0 metabolic equivalents (METs), while sedentary behaviour (SB) refers to any behaviour which incurs ≤1.5 METs and occurs while sitting or lying down. While OA is linked to declines in joint protective biomarkers such as lubricin and pituitary adenylate cyclase-activating polypeptide (PACAP), and increases in inflammatory markers and apoptotic signaling [17, 18], animal models of OA indicate that MVPA can 1) promote lubricin synthesis [19–21]; 2) down-regulate apoptotic signalling [19]; 3) down-regulate inflammatory markers of OA including interleukin-1 [21]; and 4) may stimulate the production of PACAP [22]. Increased MVPA can also improve strength and balance in adults with arthritis [23], reduce the risk of falls [24], and reduce OA symptoms such as pain, fatigue, and joint stiffness [25]. While less is known about how SB may impact the symptoms of OA, epidemiological evidence suggests that reduced SB is associated with better physical function in adults with OA—independent of MVPA time [12, 13].

There is also strong evidence that both high MVPA and low SB are neuroprotective [26, 27]. Animal models suggest that MVPA reduces pro-inflammatory markers and amyloid β protein levels in transgenic mice predisposed to Alzheimer's disease [28], and human epidemiological data consistently indicates that MVPA is associated with better cognitive function and a lower risk of cognitive decline [27]. Greater amounts of SB

may negatively impact the cellular mechanisms by which MVPA improves cognitive health [29], and may alter the connectivity of the brain such that cognitive function worsens with greater SB [30]. As such, current guidelines suggest that all adults should engage in ≥150 min of MVPA each week and limit discretionary SB as much as possible [26].

Given that 1) increasing MVPA and reducing SB promotes cellular mechanisms which reduce OA associated inflammatory and apoptotic responses [19–22, 28, 29]; and 2) OA associated inflammation and apoptotic signalling increases dementia risk [9], it is plausible that increasing MVPA and reducing SB is an effective frontline dementia prevention strategy for adults with OA. Unfortunately, the uptake of knowledge about the importance of MVPA and SB for controlling OA symptoms and reducing dementia risk has been slow. Among adults living with OA, 87% do not meet current recommendations of ≥150 min/week of MVPA [31], and people with OA spend 61% of all waking hours in SB [32]. Finding strategies to address this knowledge-to-action gap are thus greatly needed since increasing MVPA and reducing SB among adults with OA may provide benefits for both physical and cognitive health.

One promising strategy for increasing MVPA and/or reducing SB is consumer-available, wearable activity-monitoring technology. These devices present several distinct advantages as a MVPA promotion and SB reduction tool including: 1) adults typically perceive activity-monitors as useful [33]; 2) these devices incorporate multiple behavioural change strategies [34]; and 3) clinicians can readily use these devices to help promote behaviour change among their underactive patients [35]. Importantly, we recently determined that a wearable technology enabled counselling program for adults with knee OA increased MVPA by 25 min/day and improved OA symptoms [36]. Within this study, we included secondary measures to determine if increasing MVPA and/or reducing SB among adults with knee OA could also benefit cognitive function. Thus, the aim of the present paper is to determine whether this intervention to increase MVPA and reduce SB among adults with OA also improved cognitive function.

Methods
Study design

This study was a secondary analysis of *Monitor-OA*, a six month randomized controlled trial (RCT) examining the efficacy of a technology-enabled counselling intervention for increasing MVPA and reducing SB in people with knee OA [36]. The study occurred between November 1st 2015 and June 1st 2017. We used a randomized delayed-control design. In this study design, randomization determined the timing of when the intervention was provided (i.e., immediately vs. a 2-month delay).

Participants

We recruited community-dwelling adults from Vancouver, British Columbia who had a physician confirmed diagnosis of knee OA, or passed two criteria for early OA: 1) aged 50+ years; and 2) experienced knee pain during the previous year lasting > 28 separate or consecutive days [37]. Participants were excluded if they 1) had been diagnosed with inflammatory arthritis, connective tissue diseases, fibromyalgia, or gout; 2) used anti-rheumatic drugs or gout medications; 3) had previously underwent knee arthroplasty, or were on the waitlist to receive total knee arthroplasty; 4) had suffered an acute knee injury in the past six months; 5) had a body mass index (BMI) of > 40 kg/m^2; 6) had received a steroid injection or a hyaluronate injection in the last 6 months; 7) were using medications which impaired physical activity tolerance (e.g., beta blockers), or had an inappropriate level of risk for increasing their physical activity. Participants were also excluded if they did not have access to a computer in their home, or did not have a personal email address. Potential participants completed the Physical Activity Readiness Questionnaire (PAR-Q) [38]. If a potential risk was identified by the PAR-Q, physician confirmation was required to ensure the participant was able to be physically active without supervision of a health professional.

The CONSORT (Consolidated Standards of Reporting Trials) flowchart in Fig. 1 shows the number of participants in the treatment arms at each stage of the study [39]. The research protocol was approved by the University of British Columbia Behavioural Research Ethics Board (Application number: H14–01762), and was published in ClinicalTrials.gov (NCT02315664).

Measures

Trained staff members administered all testing procedures. We assessed participants at baseline, 2 months, 4 months, and 6 months follow-up. In this paper we report data from baseline, 2 months, and 4 months.

Demographics

At baseline, we obtained general health history and demographics information by questionnaire. Height and weight

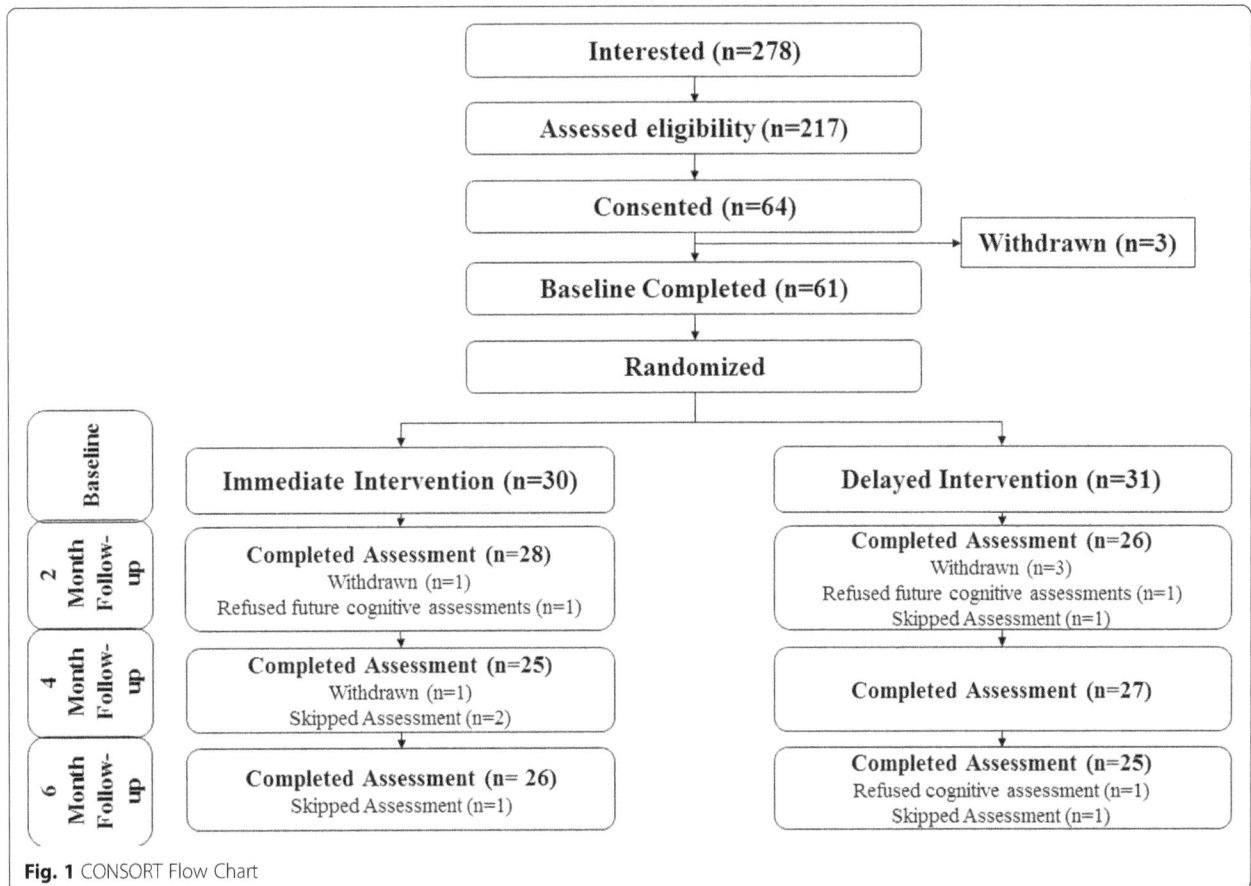

Fig. 1 CONSORT Flow Chart

were ascertained using a calibrated stadiometer and an electronic scale, respectively. This information was used to determine BMI. In addition, we assessed global cognitive function at baseline using the Mini-Mental State Exam and the Montreal Cognitive Assessment [40, 41].

MVPA and SB

We measured MVPA and SB using the SenseWear Mini (Body Media, Pittsburgh, PA, USA), a multi-sensor monitor worn on the upper arm over the triceps [42]. Briefly, the device integrates tri-axial accelerometer data, physiological sensor data and personal demographic information to provide valid and reliable estimates of MVPA and SB [42–44]. Participants wore the device on the non-dominant arm for 7 days at each assessment. For our analyses, we examined time spent in MVPA in periods of 10 or more minutes, and time spent in SB in periods of 20 or more minutes.

Cognitive function

We measured cognitive function using the National Institutes of Health Toolbox Cognition Battery (NIHTB-CB) [45]. Briefly, the NIHTB-CB provides a brief, convenient set of computerized and standardized measures of cognitive function. We examined two specific cognitive subdomains: 1) *episodic memory* using the picture sequence memory task [46]; and 2) *working memory* using the list-sorting task [47]. Empirical evidence suggests increasing MVPA or reducing SB can influence each of these domains of cognitive function [26, 48]. Briefly, the picture sequence memory task assesses episodic memory by having participants remember a sequence of actions embedded within a story. Participants re-arrange several pictures on the computer to match the sequence of events in the story. The list-sorting task assesses working memory by asking participants to repeat the names of orally—and visually—presented stimuli in order of size, from smallest largest. The number of items per set increases from one trial to the next and is discontinued once 2 trials of the same length are failed. Three trials of increasing length are completed. We recorded age-corrected scores for each measure.

Randomization

After completing the baseline assessment, eligible participants were randomly assigned to the *Immediate Intervention* (I-INT) or the *Delayed Intervention* (i.e. control; D-INT) in a 1:1 allocation ratio. Randomization was performed using computer-generated random numbers in variable block sizes. The D-INT received the same intervention as the I-INT after a 2-month wait.

Intervention

Details of the intervention have been described previously [36]. Briefly, the intervention consisted of participants attending a 1.5-h session, where they received: 1) a standardized group education session about the benefits of increasing MVPA and reducing SB; 2) a Fitbit® Flex™; and 3) individual activity counselling with a physiotherapist. The education session was delivered in groups of 2–3 participants. The individual activity counselling session followed the Brief Action Planning approach [49]. The physiotherapist guided participants to identify their MVPA goals (e.g., begin resistance training, start cycling, join a walking group, etc.), develop an action plan (i.e., where they plan to perform their MVPA goal, how often, and for how long), identify barriers and solutions, and then rate their confidence in executing the plan. For SB, the physiotherapists began by asking participants to estimate their sitting time in a normal day. Participants were then asked to identify ways to break up their sitting time into shorter bouts.

Following the education session, participants were provided with a Fitbit Flex™ which they were instructed to wear 24 h/day except during water-based activity (i.e., swimming or bathing) or when charging the device. The Fitbit data were wirelessly synchronized with Fitbit's online Dashboard which could be viewed only by the participants and the study physiotherapist. During the intervention period, the physiotherapist reviewed the individual's MVPA on the Dashboard and progressively modified the activity goals during 4 biweekly phone calls. During these phone calls, we also monitored participant adherence to SB goals using self-report. Specifically, participants were asked at each biweekly phone call whether they fully met, partially met, or did not meet their SB goal. These goals were then modified as needed.

Statistical analyses

We conducted all statistical analyses using R version 3.3.1 in the *lsmeans 2.26–3, lmerTest 2.0–33*, and *mice 2.46.0* packages. Descriptive statistics were used to summarize participant demographics. In order to account for missing data at each follow-up time point, we performed multiple imputation in the *mice 2.46.0* package using predicted mean matching (5 imputations; 20 iterations each), and visually checked for convergence. All statistical models used pooled estimates from all 5 imputed data sets. Plots and graphs were created using *ggplot2 2.2.1*. Our statistical code can be found in Additional file 1.

Main analyses

We evaluated between-group differences (I-INT vs. D-INT) on the outcomes of interest following the primary intervention (i.e., Baseline – 2 Months) using the intention-to-treat principle, as per our primary outcomes paper [36]. Two separate analyses of covariance (ANCOVA) models were conducted, wherein cognitive performance at 2 months was the dependent variable and treatment group was the independent variable of interest; both models controlled for baseline cognitive performance. We estimated group mean changes in cognitive function and corresponding 95% confidence intervals pooled across the 5 imputed datasets, as well as estimated group mean difference (with 95% CI) and estimated Cohen's d effect size.

Secondary analyses

We also examined whether changes in MVPA or SB during the intervention were associated with changes in cognitive function. We created change scores (i.e., I-INT = Baseline − 2 Months; D-INT = Baseline − 4 Months) for MVPA, SB, the list-sorting task, and the picture sequence memory task. We performed four separate multiple linear regression models wherein changes in cognitive performance (i.e., list-sorting memory or picture sequence memory) during the intervention were specified as the dependent variable, and changes in MVPA (or SB) was specified as the independent variable of interest. Each model included 1) baseline score for the cognitive performance variable of interest; 2) baseline MVPA (or SB); and 3) treatment group as covariates of no interest. We report unstandardized beta values and standard errors. Given our sample size, and a two-tailed α = 0.05, we had 80% power to detect a two-sided correlation with a medium effect size of $|\rho| = 0.34$ [50].

Results

Participant characteristics

From 2015 to 2016, 278 people indicated an interest to participate, and 64 met the eligibility criteria (Fig. 1). Of those, we recruited 61 participants (I-INT: $n = 30$; D-INT: $n = 31$). As described in Table 1, there were no group differences in age (I-INT: 61.73 [SD 9.40] years;

D-INT: 62.61 [8.54]), sex (I-INT: 73.33% female; D-INT: 90.32%), BMI (I-INT: 29.16 [5.46] kg/m^2; D-INT: 29.24 [4.82], or time spent in MVPA (I-INT: 83.44 [60.80] minutes/day; D-INT: 86.19 [86.19] minutes/day) and SB (I-INT: 681.96 [111.51] minutes/day; D-INT: 703.05 [161.17] minutes/day) at baseline. Participants in I-INT had a lower picture sequence memory score (I-INT: 102.04 [17.22]; D-INT: 112.53 [14.67]; $p = 0.02$), but there were no differences between groups for list-sorting score (I-INT: 102.05 [17.22]; D-INT: 102.42 [14.64]).

Changes in cognitive function

Group differences in cognitive performance—accounting for baseline cognitive performance—are illustrated in Fig. 2. Briefly, there were no statistically significant differences between groups following the intervention. As described in Table 2, we calculated a small improvement of the I-INT compared to D-INT for picture sequence memory (estimated mean difference: 1.27; 95% CI [− 9.27, 11.81]; $d = 0.10$), and a small improvement of the D-INT compared to the I-INT for list-sorting memory (estimated mean difference: -1.64; 95% CI [− 8.72, 5.44]; $d = − 0.19$).

Correlation between MVPA and SB changes with changes in cognitive function

The relationship between changes in MVPA and changes in cognitive function are illustrated in Fig. 3. There were no statistically significant relationships between changes in MVPA and changes in cognitive function. Increases in MVPA were correlated with changes in list-sorting memory in the expected direction (B = 0.04; 95% CI [− 0.07, 0.14]), however changes in picture sequence memory appeared to be negatively correlated with increases in MVPA (B = − 0.02; 95% CI [− 0.15, 0.12]).

Table 1 Baseline Characteristics

Participant Characteristic	Immediate Intervention (N = 30)	Delayed Intervention (N = 31)	p
Age	61.73 (9.40)	62.61 (8.54)	0.70
%Female	73.33%	90.32%	0.16
Education			
High school or less	16.67%	19.35%	0.92
Some university	33.33%	29.03%	
University degree or higher	50.00%	51.61%	
Body Mass Index (kg/m)	29.16 (5.46)	29.24 (4.82)	0.95
Moderate-to-Vigorous Physical Activity (min/day)	83.44 (60.80)	86.19 (86.19)	0.89
Sedentary Behaviour (min/day)	681.96 (111.51)	703.05 (161.17)	0.55
Mini-Mental State Exam	28.03 (2.62)	28.62 (1.35)	0.28
Montreal Cognitive Assessment	27.27 (2.53)	26.24 (2.86)	0.15
List-Sorting Task	102.05 (13.03)	102.42 (14.64)	0.92
Picture Sequence Memory Task	102.04 (17.22)	112.53 (14.67)	0.02

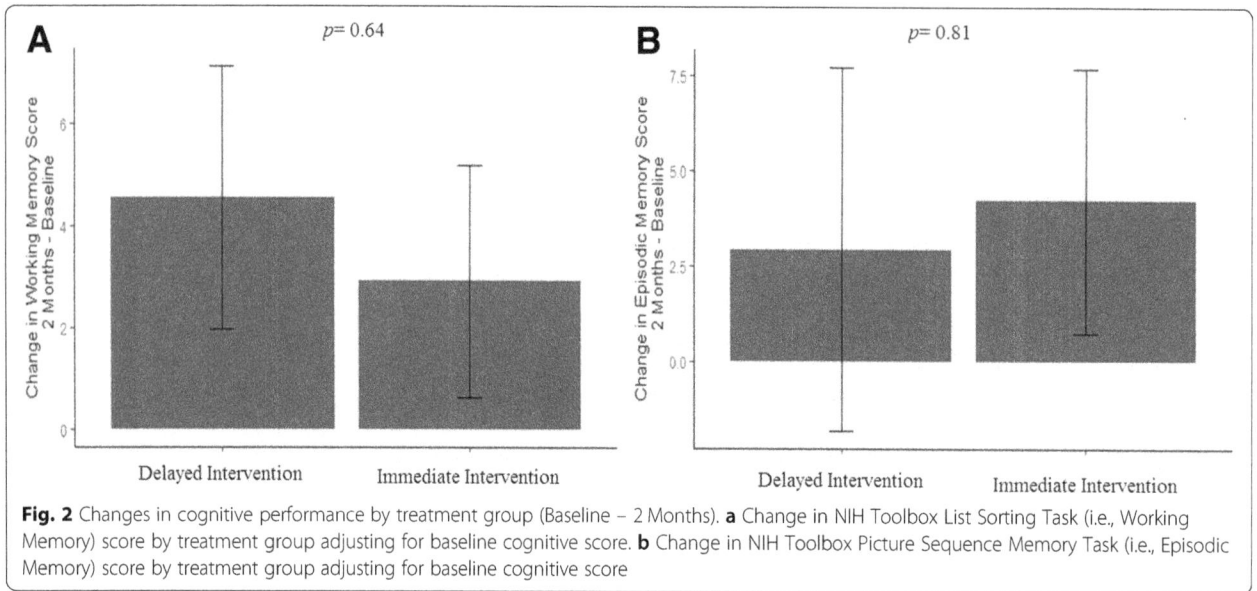

Fig. 2 Changes in cognitive performance by treatment group (Baseline – 2 Months). **a** Change in NIH Toolbox List Sorting Task (i.e., Working Memory) score by treatment group adjusting for baseline cognitive score. **b** Change in NIH Toolbox Picture Sequence Memory Task (i.e., Episodic Memory) score by treatment group adjusting for baseline cognitive score

The relationship between changes in SB and changes in cognitive function are illustrated in Fig. 4. There were no statistically significant relationships between changes in SB and changes in either picture sequence memory (B = – 0.01; 95% CI [– 0.09, 0.07]) or list-sorting memory (B = 0.00; 95% CI [– 0.09, 0.10]).

Discussion

Although we previously determined this intervention can increase MVPA and improve quality of life among adults with knee OA [36], there does not appear to be sufficient evidence that our intervention can also improve cognitive function within this population. However, our results suggest that future research on the role of MVPA and SB for maintaining cognitive health among adults with OA is warranted. Given that most adults with OA are inactive [32], and thus more at risk to future cognitive decline [26, 27], we believe that such research would be valuable. We now discuss potential explanations for our findings.

While there is strong evidence that MVPA in the form of exercise training can improve cognitive function [51], the results of community-based MVPA interventions to promote cognitive health have been far less conclusive [52]. Importantly, the effects of MVPA on cognitive function seem to be largest for individuals who are underactive, while regular MVPA may be mainly

neuroprotective for individuals who are meeting current guidelines [53]. Our participants were already highly active at baseline, and thus changes in MVPA may have had limited impact on cognitive function due to high basal levels. Moreover, the high activity level of our sample at baseline suggests that the results may not be generalizable to most adults with OA—who are sedentary. In order to first determine the efficacy of MVPA as a treatment for maintaining cognitive health for adults with OA, future trials should therefore recruit less active individuals since they 1) are more generalizable to the OA population; and 2) will more likely reap the most benefits from increasing their MVPA.

To date, most of the evidence examining how SB impacts cognitive health comes from epidemiological data [26, 29, 30]. Our study is the first to examine if an intervention to reduce SB can improve cognitive health among adults with OA. The results do not appear to suggest reductions in SB are associated with improvements in cognitive function; however, our intervention did not significantly reduce time spent in SB [36]. Preliminary evidence does suggest reductions in sedentary time may reverse the deleterious physiological effects of SB—such as impaired glucose and lipid metabolism [54]. Healthy glucose and lipid metabolism are strongly linked to better cognitive health [55]. Thus, while our results cannot determine

Table 2 Changes in cognitive function (Baseline – 2 Months) by treatment group

Variable	Immediate Intervention Group Mean [95% CI]	Delayed Intervention Group Mean [95% CI]	Estimated Mean Group Difference [95% CI]	d
List Sorting Task	2.90 [−1.55, 7.35]	4.53 [−0.53, 9.59]	-1.64 [−8.72, 5.44]	−0.19
Picture Sequence Memory Task	4.21 [−2.55, 10.97]	2.95 [−6.36, 12.26]	1.27 [−9.27, 11.81]	0.10

Note: All estimates adjusted for cognitive score at baseline

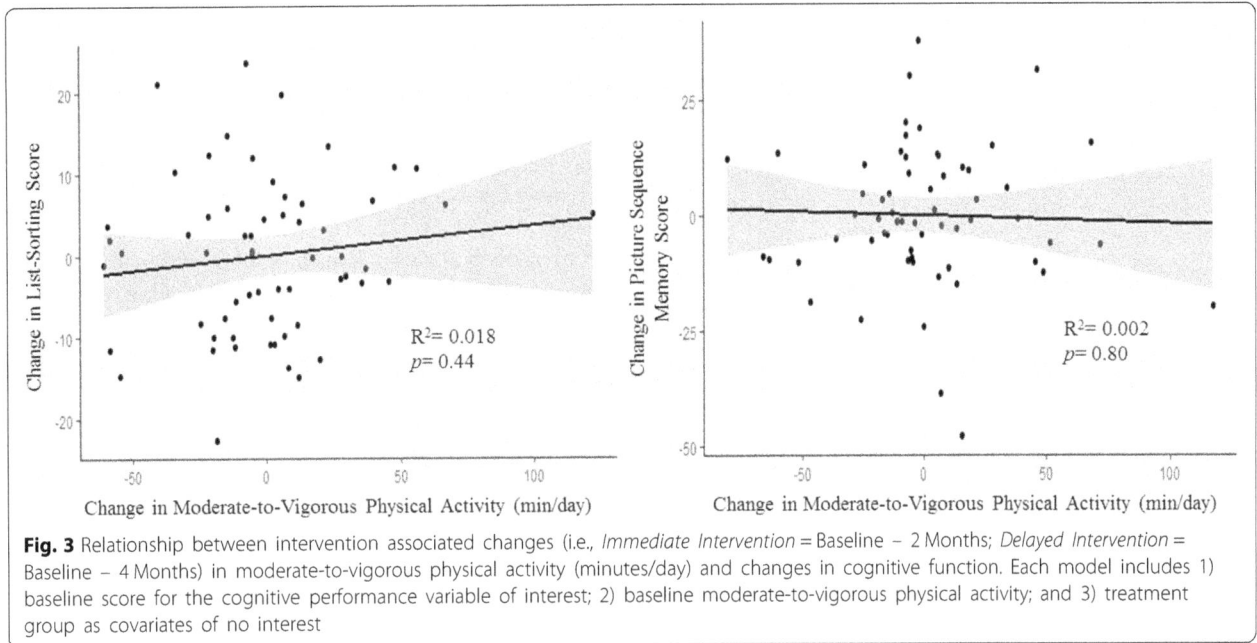

Fig. 3 Relationship between intervention associated changes (i.e., *Immediate Intervention* = Baseline – 2 Months; *Delayed Intervention* = Baseline – 4 Months) in moderate-to-vigorous physical activity (minutes/day) and changes in cognitive function. Each model includes 1) baseline score for the cognitive performance variable of interest; 2) baseline moderate-to-vigorous physical activity; and 3) treatment group as covariates of no interest

whether reducing SB can improve cognitive function, there does appear to be a plausible mechanism by which reduced SB may benefit cognitive function.

This was a secondary analysis of a proof-of-concept RCT, and thus we think the logical next step is for an adequately powered RCT to determine the efficacy of this intervention to promote cognitive health among adults with OA. A recent meta-analysis suggests that MVPA in the form of exercise training has a modest effect size on cognitive function of $d = 0.29$ [51]. Based on this effect size, we post-hoc investigated the necessary sample size to perform an adequately powered RCT to improve cognitive function using G*Power 3.1 [50]. In

order to detect an effect size of the magnitude suggested by Northey and colleagues [51], we would need at least 376 participants to achieve 80% power (assuming a two-sided $\alpha = 0.05$). The study we report herein was thus under-powered, however we would expect the effect sizes for this intervention to increase through two simple strategies. First, future studies should exclude adults that are already physically active since the largest effects of MVPA on health occur for individuals who are inactive [56]. Second, increasing the length of time between assessment points would help reduce the potential for practice effects to occur on cognitive tests [57], and provide adequate time for eliciting changes in

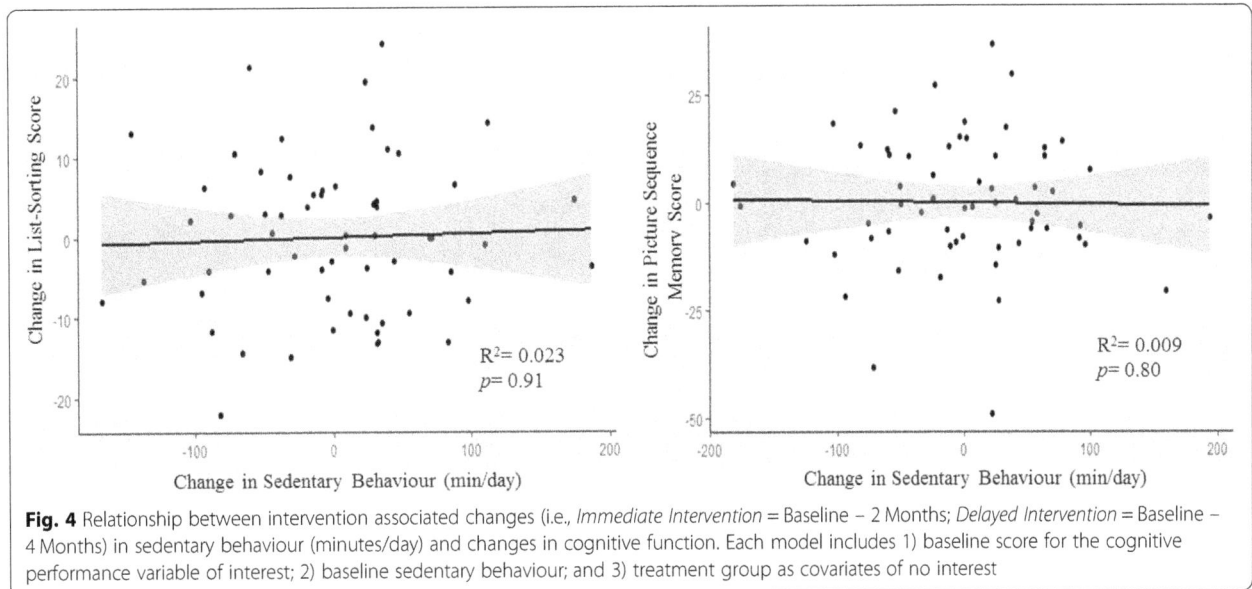

Fig. 4 Relationship between intervention associated changes (i.e., *Immediate Intervention* = Baseline – 2 Months; *Delayed Intervention* = Baseline – 4 Months) in sedentary behaviour (minutes/day) and changes in cognitive function. Each model includes 1) baseline score for the cognitive performance variable of interest; 2) baseline sedentary behaviour; and 3) treatment group as covariates of no interest

cognitive function which evidence suggests are larger after at least 6 months of increased MVPA [48].

Clinical applications

Although we did not find that our intervention significantly improved cognitive function, there are several potential clinical applications to our study. First, we previously demonstrated that clinicians (i.e., physical therapists) can use consumer-available wearable activity-monitors such as a Fitbit to promote MVPA and reduce SB among their patients with OA [36]. Given the health care system has an untapped capacity for promoting changes in MVPA and SB, which to date has not been fully developed [58], a first step towards harnessing this potential to promote behaviour change is for clinicians to track their patients' MVPA and SB using wearable activity-monitors. At minimum, clinicians should query about activity during their consultations with OA patients [59].

Secondly, both OA and SB may increase the risk of cognitive impairment and dementia [7–9, 26, 29, 30]. In contrast, engagement in MVPA reduces dementia risk and promotes overall cognitive and physical health [14–16, 27, 28]. Adults with OA should therefore be encouraged to adhere to the current public health recommendations of engaging in ≥150 min/week of MVPA and limiting their SB as much as possible [26]. Importantly, 87% of adults with OA are underactive [31] and adults with OA spend an average of 61% of the day in SB [32]. MVPA promotion and SB reduction may thus be particularly important for physical and cognitive health in adults with OA.

Limitations and future research

This was a secondary outcomes analysis, and thus our findings are a preliminary investigation of whether increasing MVPA and reducing SB can improve cognitive function in adults with OA. While the SenseWear Mini provides valid and reliable estimates of energy expenditure for both younger and older adults [42, 60], which can be used to derive time spent in MVPA and time spent in SB, we cannot determine whether time estimated as SB was actually spent sitting or lying down. Hence, future studies to examine changes in SB should use measures of body posture such as the activPAL [61], which can accurately determine whether a person is sitting, standing, or walking.

We did not collect information on medication use, however our participants were community-dwelling adults who were healthy enough to start a physical activity program at study entry. We also did not exclude participants based on current activity level and hence the results may not be generalizable to most people with OA—who are often sedentary. Given the high activity level of our participants, the effects of increased MVPA and reduced SB on cognitive function may have been attenuated. We

therefore suggest future studies should recruit underactive adults with OA, since these individuals are likely to benefit from increased MVPA and reduced SB.

There is growing evidence that the effects of MVPA (and potentially SB) are moderated by age and sex [62, 63], however due to our small sample size, it was not feasible for us to control for age and sex within our analyses. As detailed previously [36], our intervention did not reduce SB which is perhaps due to several shortcomings of the counselling program, which we have rectified. Specifically, the intervention now includes a new SB counselling strategy, and a Fitbit-compatible web app with enhances functionality for setting goals and rewarding behaviours that break up prolonged sitting [64]. This paradigm is currently being tested in a RCT (ClinicalTrial.gov identifier: NCT02554474) involving people with rheumatoid arthritis and systematic lupus erythematosus [65].

Conclusion

While strong evidence indicates that increasing MVPA and reducing SB can positively impact OA symptoms, it is not yet clear whether increasing MVPA and reducing SB can also promote cognitive health among this population. However, increasing MVPA and reducing SB among adults with OA should be a public health priority since it can help maintain physical health and reduce the risk of cognitive impairment and dementia. Clinicians should therefore take the time to counsel their patients with OA to engage in ≥150 min/week of MVPA and limit their SB in order to promote physical and cognitive health.

Abbreviations

BMI: Body Mass Index; D-INT: Delayed Intervention; I-INT: Immediate Intervention; METS: Metabolic Equivalents; MVPA: Moderate-to-Vigorous Physical Activity; NIHTB-CB: National Institutes of Health Toolbox Cognition Battery; OA: Osteoarthritis; PACAP: Pituitary Adenylate Cyclase-Activating Peptide; PAR-Q: Physical Activity Readiness Questionnaire; RCT: Randomized Controlled Trial; SB: Sedentary Behaviour

Acknowledgements

We would like to thank the Track-OA research staff for their assistance with the intervention and data collection.

Author contributions

RSF wrote the first draft of the manuscript. LL and TLA conceived the study concept and design. RSF and JRB performed the data analysis and interpreted the results. JRB, LL, PCYC, LMF and TLA wrote portions of the manuscript and provided critical review. All authors have read and approve of the final manuscript.

Funding

Funding for this project was provided by a Canadian Institutes of Health Research Operational Grant (F14–03974), and by the Jack Brown & Family Alzheimer's Research Foundation. The funding bodies did not play a role in the study design. RSF is funded by the University of British Columbia Rehabilitation Sciences Scholarship, the Omer H. Patrick II Memorial Prize, and the Louise McGregor Memorial Award in Neurorehabilitation. TLA is a Canada Research Chair in Physical Activity, Mobility, and Cognitive Heatlth. LCL is a Canada Research Chair in Patient-Oriented Knowledge Translation and holds the Harold Robinson / Arthritis Society Chair in Arthritic Diseases.

Consent for publication
Not applicable.

Competing interests
The authors declare that they have no competing interests.

Author details
[1]Faculty of Medicine, Aging, Mobility and Cognitive Neuroscience Laboratory, Djavad Mowafaghian Centre for Brain Health, Department of Physical Therapy, University of British Columbia, 212-2177 Wesbrook Mall, Vancouver, BC V6T 1Z3, Canada. [2]Faculty of Medicine, Arthritis Research Canada, University of British Columbia, Vancouver, Canada.

References
1. Bombardier C, Hawker G, Mosher D. The impact of arthritis in Canada: today and over the next 30 years. Toronto: Arthritis Alliance of Canada. 2011;2011. http://www.arthritisalliance.ca/images/PDF/eng/Initiatives/20111022_2200_impact_of_arthritis.pdf.
2. Laupattarakasem W, Laopaiboon M, Laupattarakasem P, Sumananont C. Arthroscopic debridement for knee osteoarthritis. Cochrane Database Syst Rev. 2008;1:Cd005118. https://doi.org/10.1002/14651858.CD005118.pub2.
3. Husted JA, Tom BD, Farewell VT, Schentag CT, Gladman DDA. Longitudinal study of the effect of disease activity and clinical damage on physical function over the course of psoriatic arthritis: does the effect change over time? Arthritis Rheum. 2007;56(3):840–9.
4. Sturnieks DL, Tiedemann A, Chapman K, Munro B, Murray SM, Lord SR. Physiological risk factors for falls in older Peoplen with lower limb arthritis. J Rheumatol. 2004;31(11):2272–9.
5. Hatfield GL, Hubley-Kozey CL, Wilson JLA, Dunbar MJ. The effect of total knee arthroplasty on knee joint kinematics and kinetics during gait. J Arthroplast. 2011;26(2):309–18.
6. Beswick AD, Wylde V, Gooberman-Hill R, Blom A, Dieppe P. What proportion of patients report long-term pain after total hip or knee replacement for osteoarthritis? A systematic review of prospective studies in unselected patients. BMJ Open. 2012;2(1):e000435.
7. Huang S-W, Wang W-T, Chou L-C, Liao C-D, Liou T-H, Lin H-W. Osteoarthritis increases the risk of dementia: a nationwide cohort study in Taiwan. Sci Rep. 2015;5:10145.
8. Baker NA, Barbour KE, Helmick CG, Zack M, Al Snih S. Arthritis and cognitive impairment in older adults. Rheumatol Int. 2017;37(6):955–61.
9. Kyrkanides S, Tallents RH, Jen-nie HM, Olschowka ME, Johnson R, Yang M, et al. Osteoarthritis accelerates and exacerbates Alzheimer's disease pathology in mice. J Neuroinflammation. 2011;8(1):112.
10. Prevalence of doctor-diagnosed arthritis and arthritis-attributable activity limitation--United States. 2010-2012. Morb Mortal Wkly Rep. 2013;62(44):869–73.
11. World Health Organization, Alzheimer's Disease International. Dementia: A Public Health Authority. 2012.
12. Lee J, Chang RW, Ehrlich-Jones L, Kwoh CK, Nevitt M, Semanik PA, et al. Sedentary behavior and physical function: objective evidence from the osteoarthritis initiative. Arthritis Care & Research. 2015;67(3):366–73.
13. Song J, Lindquist LA, Chang RW, Semanik PA, Ehrlich-Jones LS, Lee J, et al. Sedentary behavior as a risk factor for physical frailty independent of moderate activity: results from the osteoarthritis initiative. Am J Public Health. 2015;105(7):1439–45.
14. Brosseau L, MacLeay L, Robinson V, Wells G, Tugwell P. Intensity of exercise for the treatment of osteoarthritis. Cochrane Database Syst Rev. 2003;2.
15. Zhang W, Moskowitz R, Nuki G, Abramson S, Altman R, Arden N, et al. OARSI recommendations for the management of hip and knee

osteoarthritis, part I: critical appraisal of existing treatment guidelines and systematic review of current research evidence. Osteoarthr Cartil. 2007;15(9):981–1000.
16. Brosseau L, Wells GA, Tugwell P, Egan M, Dubouloz C, Casimiro L, et al. Ottawa panel evidence-based clinical practice guidelines for therapeutic exercises and manual therapy in the management of osteoarthritis. Phys Ther. 2005;85(9):907–71.
17. Giunta S, Castorina A, Marzagalli R, Szychlinska MA, Pichler K, Mobasheri A, Musumeci G. Ameliorative effects of PACAP against cartilage degeneration. Morphological, immunohistochemical and biochemical evidence from in vivo and in vitro models of rat osteoarthritis. Int J Mol Sci. 2015;16(3):5922–44.
18. Szychlinska MA, Leonardi R, Al-Qahtani M, Mobasheri A, Musumeci G. Altered joint tribology in osteoarthritis: reduced lubricin synthesis due to the inflammatory process. New horizons for therapeutic approaches Annals of Physical and Rehabilitation Medicine. 2016;59(3):149–56.
19. Musumeci G, Loreto C, Leonardi R, Castorina S, Giunta S, Carnazza ML, et al. The effects of physical activity on apoptosis and lubricin expression in articular cartilage in rats with glucocorticoid-induced osteoporosis. J Bone Miner Metab. 2013;31(3):274–84.
20. Musumeci G, Castrogiovanni P, Trovato FM, Imbesi R, Giunta S, Szychlinska MA, et al. Physical activity ameliorates cartilage degeneration in a rat model of aging: a study on lubricin expression. Scand J Med Sci Sports. 2015;25(2):e222–30.
21. Musumeci G, Trovato FM, Pichler K, Weinberg AM, Loreto C, Castrogiovanni P. Extra-virgin olive oil diet and mild physical activity prevent cartilage degeneration in an osteoarthritis model: an in vivo and in vitro study on lubricin expression. J Nutr Biochem. 2013;24(12):2064–75.
22. Juhász T, Szentléleky E, Somogyi CS, Takács R, Dobrosi N, Engler M, et al. Pituitary adenylate cyclase activating polypeptide (PACAP) pathway is induced by mechanical load and reduces the activity of hedgehog signaling in chondrogenic micromass cell cultures. Int J Mol Sci. 2015;16(8):17344–67.
23. Suomi R, Collier D. Effects of arthritis exercise programs on functional fitness and perceived activities of daily living measures in older adults with arthritis. Archives of Physical Medicine Rehabilitation. 2003;84(11):1589–94.
24. Barnett A, Smith B, Lord SR, Williams M, Baumand A. Community-based group exercise improves balance and reduces falls in at-risk older people: a randomised controlled trial. Age Ageing. 2003;32(4):407–14.
25. Semble EL, Loeser RF, Wise CM. Therapeutic exercise for rheumatoid arthritis and osteoarthritis. Semin Arthritis Rheum. 1990;20(1):32–40.
26. Falck RS, Davis JC, Liu-Ambrose T. What is the association between sedentary behaviour and cognitive function? A systematic review British Journal of Sports Medicine. 2017;51:800–11.
27. Hamer M, Chida Y. Physical activity and risk of neurodegenerative disease: a systematic review of prospective evidence. Psychol Med. 2009;39(1):3–11.
28. Adlard PA, Perreau VM, Pop V, Cotman CW. Voluntary exercise decreases amyloid load in a transgenic model of Alzheimer's disease. J Neurosci. 2005;25(17):4217–21.
29. Vaynman S, Gomez-Pinilla F. Revenge of the "sit": how lifestyle impacts neuronal and cognitive health through molecular systems that interface energy metabolism with neuronal plasticity. J of Neurosci Res. 2006;84(4):699–715.
30. Voss MW, Carr LJ, Clark R, Weng T. Revenge of the "sit" II: does lifestyle impact neuronal and cognitive health through distinct mechanisms associated with sedentary behavior and physical activity? Ment Health and Phys Act. 2014;7(1):9–24.
31. Wallis JA, Webster KE, Levinger P, Taylor NF. What proportion of people with hip and knee osteoarthritis meet physical activity guidelines? A systematic review and meta-analysis. Osteoarthr Cartil. 2013;21(11):1648–59.
32. Sliepen M, Mauricio E, Lipperts M, Grimm B, Rosenbaum D. Objective assessment of physical activity and sedentary behaviour in knee osteoarthritis patients–beyond daily steps and total sedentary time. BMC Musculoskelet Disord. 2018;19(1):64.
33. Mercer K, Giangregorio L, Schneider E, Chilana P, Li M, Grindrod K. Acceptance of commercially available wearable activity trackers among adults aged over 50 and with chronic illness: a mixed-methods evaluation. J Med Internet Res. 2016;4(1).
34. Mercer K, Li M, Giangregorio L, Burns C, Grindrod K. Behavior change

techniques present in wearable activity trackers: a critical analysis. J Med Internet Res. 2016;4(2).

35. Falck RS, Landry GJ, Best JR, Davis JC, Chiu BK, Liu-Ambrose T. cross-sectional relationships of physical activity and sedentary behavior with cognitive function in older adults with probable mild cognitive impairment. Phys Ther. 2017.

36. Li LC, Sayre EC, Xie H, Falck RS, Best JR, Liu-Ambrose T, et al. efficacy of a community-based technology-enabled physical activity counselling program for people with knee osteoarthritis: a proof-of-concept study. J Med Internet Res. 2018;20(4):e159.

37. Marra CA, Cibere J, Tsuyuki RT, Soon JA, Esdaile JM, Gastonguay L, et al. improving osteoarthritis detection in the community: pharmacist identification of new, diagnostically confirmed osteoarthritis. Arthritis Care & Research. 2007;57(7):1238–44.

38. Cardinal BJ, Cardinal MK. Preparticipation physical activity screening within a racially diverse, older adult sample: comparison of the original and revised physical activity readiness questionnaires. Res Q Exerc Sport. 2000;71(3):302–7.

39. Begg C, Cho M, Eastwood S, Horton R, Moher D, Olkin I, et al. Improving the quality of reporting of randomized controlled trials: the CONSORT statement. J Am Med Assoc. 1996;276(8):637–9.

40. Folstein MF, Folstein SE, McHugh PR. "Mini-mental state". A practical method for grading the cognitive state of patients for the clinician. J Psychiatr Res. 1975;12(3):189–98.

41. Nasreddine ZS, Phillips NA, Bédirian V, Charbonneau S, Whitehead V, Collin I, et al. The Montreal cognitive assessment, MoCA: a brief screening tool for mild cognitive impairment. Journal of the American Geriatric Society. 2005; 53(4):695–9.

42. Johannsen DL, Calabro MA, Stewart J, Franke W, Rood JC, Welk GJ. Accuracy of armband monitors for measuring daily energy expenditure in health adults. Medicine & Science in Sport & Exercise. 2011;42(11):2134–40.

43. Reece JD, Barry V, Fuller DK, Caputo J. Validation of the SenseWear armband as a measure of sedentary behavior and light activity. J Phys Act Health. 2015;12(9):1229–37.

44. Tierney M, Fraser A, Purtill H, Kennedy N. Study to determine the criterion validity of the SenseWear armband as a measure of physical activity in people with rheumatoid arthritis. Arthritis Care & Research. 2013;65(6):888–95.

45. Weintraub S. Cognition assessment using the NIH toolbox. Neurology. 2013; 80(S3):S54–64.

46. Dikmen SS, Bauer PJ, Weintraub S, Mungas D, Slotkin J, Beaumont JL, et al. Measuring episodic memory across the lifespan: NIH toolbox picture sequence memory test. J Int Neuropsychol Soc. 2014;20(6):611–9.

47. Tulsky DS, Carlozzi N, Chiaravalloti ND, Beaumont JL, Kisala PA, Mungas D, et al. NIH toolbox cognition battery (NIHTB-CB): list sorting test to measure working memory. J Int Neuropsychol Soc. 2014;20(6):599–610.

48. Colcombe S, Kramer AF. Fitness effects on the cognitive function of older adults: a meta-analytic study. Psychol Sci. 2003;14(2):125–30.

49. Gutnick D, Reims K, Davis C, Gainforth H, Jay M, Cole S. Brief action planning to facilitate behavior change and support patient self-management. J Clin Outcomes Manag. 2014;21(1):18–29.

50. Faul F, Erdfelder E, Lang A-G, Buchner A. G* power 3: a flexible statistical power analysis program for the social, behavioral, and biomedical sciences. Behavioral Research Methods. 2007;39(2):175–91.

51. Northey JM, Cherbuin N, Pumpa KL, Smee DJ, Rattray B. Exercise interventions for cognitive function in adults older than 50: a systematic review with meta-analysis. Br J Sports Med. 2018;52:154–60.

52. Sink KM, Espeland MA, Castro CM, Church T, Cohen R, Dodson JA, et al. Effect of a 24-month physical activity intervention vs health education on cognitive outcomes in sedentary older adults: the LIFE randomized trial. J Am Med Assoc. 2015;314(8):781–90.

53. Bherer L, Erickson KI, Liu-Ambrose T. a review of the effects of physical activity and exercise on cognitive and brain functions in older adults. Journal of Aging Research. 2013;2013:657508.

54. Tremblay MS, Colley RC, Saunders TJ, Healy GN, Owen N. Physiological and health implications of a sedentary lifestyle. Appl Physiol Nutr Metab. 2010; 35(6):725–40.

55. Craft S. The role of metabolic disorders in Alzheimer disease and vascular dementia: two roads converged. Arch Neurol. 2009;66(3):300–5.

56. Physical Activity Guidelines Advisory Committee (2008). Physical activity guidelines advisory committee report, 2008. Washington: DC: US Department of Health and Human Services; 2008. p. A1–H14.

57. Falleti MG, Maruff P, Collie A, Darby DG. Practice effects associated with the repeated assessment of cognitive function using the CogState battery at 10-minute, one week and one month test-retest intervals. J Clin Exp Neuropsychol. 2006;28(7):1095–112.

58. Berra K, Rippe J, Manson JE. Making physical activity counseling a priority in clinical practice: the time for action is now. J Am Med Assoc. 2015;314(24):2617–8.

59. Sallis R. Developing healthcare systems to support exercise: exercise as the fifth vital sign. Br J Sports Med. 2011;45(6):473–4.

60. Mackey DC, Manini TM, Schoeller DA, Koster A, Glynn NW, Goodpaster BH, Satterfield S, Newman AB, Harris TB, Cummings SR, Health, Aging, and body composition study. Validation of an armband to measure daily energy expenditure in older adults. Journals of gerontology series a: biomedical sciences and medical Sciences. 2011;66(10):1108–13.

61. Koster A, Shiroma EJ, Caserotti P, Matthews CE, Chen KY, Glynn NW, Harris TB. Comparison of sedentary estimates between activPAL and hip-and wrist-worn ActiGraph. Med Sci Sports Exerc. 2016;48(8):1514.

62. Physical Activity Guidelines Advisory Committee. Physical activity guidelines advisory committee scientific report. Washington, DC: US Department of Health and Human Services; 2018.

63. Barha CK, Davis JC, Falck RS, Nagamatsu LS, Liu-Ambrose T. Sex differences in exercise efficacy to improve cognition: a systematic review and meta-analysis of randomized controlled trials in older humans. Front Neuroendocrinol. 2017;46:71–85.

64. Gupta A, Tong X, Shaw C, Li L, Feehan L, editors. FitViz: A Personal Informatics Tool for Self-management of Rheumatoid Arthritis. International Conference on Human-Computer Interaction; 2017: Springer.

65. Li LC, Feehan LM, Shaw C, Xie H, Sayre EC, Aviña-Zubeita A, et al. A technology-enabled counselling program versus a delayed treatment control to support physical activity participation in people with inflammatory arthritis: study protocol for the OPAM-IA randomized controlled trial. BMC Rheumatology. 2017;1(1):6.

15

Inter- and *intra*-rater reliability for measurement of range of motion in joints included in three hypermobility assessment methods

Angela Schlager[1]*[iD], Kerstin Ahlqvist[1], Eva Rasmussen-Barr[2], Elisabeth Krefting Bjelland[1,3], Ronnie Pingel[1], Christina Olsson[2,4], Lena Nilsson-Wikmar[2,4] and Per Kristiansson[1]

Abstract

Background: Comparisons across studies of generalized joint hypermobility are often difficult since there are several classification methods and methodological differences in the performance exist. The Beighton score is most commonly used and has been tested for *inter-* and *intra*-rater reliability. The Contompasis score and the Hospital del Mar criteria have not yet been evaluated for reliability. The aim of this study was to investigate the *inter-* and *intra*-rater reliability for measurements of range of motion in joints included in these three hypermobility assessment methods using a structured protocol.

Methods: The study was planned in accordance with guidelines for reporting reliability studies. Healthy adults were consecutively recruited (49 for *inter-* and 29 for *intra*-rater assessments). Intra-class correlations, two-way random effects model, (ICC 2.1) with 95% confidence intervals, standard error of measurement, percentage of agreement, Cohen's Kappa (κ) and prevalence-adjusted bias-adjusted kappa were calculated for single-joint measured in degrees and for total scores.

Results: The *inter-* and *intra*-rater reliability in total scores were ICC 2.1: 0.72–0.82 and 0.76–0.86 and for single-joint measurements in degrees 0.44–0.91 and 0.44–0.90, respectively. The difference between ratings was within 5 degrees in all but one joint. Standard error of measurement ranged from 1.0 to 6.9 degrees. The *inter-* and *intra*-rater reliability for prevalence of positive hypermobility findings the Cohen's κ for total scores were 0.54–0.78 and 0.27–0.78 and in single joints 0.21–1.00 and 0.19–1.00, respectively. The prevalence- and bias adjusted Cohen's κ, increased all but two values.

Conclusions: Following a structured protocol, the *inter-* and *intra*-rater reliability was good-to-excellent for total scores and in all but two single joints, measured in degrees. The *inter-* and *intra* rater reliability for prevalence of positive hypermobility findings was fair-to-almost perfect for total scores and slight-to-almost-perfect in single joints.
By using a structured protocol, we attempted to standardize the assessment of range of motion in clinical and in research settings. This standardization could be helpful in the first part of the process of standardizing the tests thus avoiding that assessment of GJH is based on chance.

Keywords: Generalized joint hypermobility, *Inter-* and *intra-* reliability, Beighton score, Contompasis score, Hospital del mar criteria, Joint mobility assessment, Standardized protocol, Goniometer, Range of motion

* Correspondence: angela.schlager@pubcare.uu.se
A Schlager and K Ahlqvist equally contributed to the study as first authors
[1]Department of Public Health and Caring Sciences, Uppsala University, Husargatan 3, Box 564, 752 37 Uppsala, Sweden
Full list of author information is available at the end of the article

Background

Generalized joint hypermobility (GJH), defined as an increased range of motion (ROM) in several joints [1], is associated with longstanding musculoskeletal problems [2]. Many people with GJH seek primary care for pain and activity limitations [3, 4].

Joint ROM varies greatly in the general population [5, 6] and a joint ROM above two standard deviations from the average is suggested to be hypermobile [7]. The prevalence of GJH varies across gender, age, ethnicity and according to assessment methods and their cut-off points [8]. In Sweden, GJH is estimated to be present in approximately 10% of the general population [9].

Although GJH is an important criterion in the diagnosis of many heritable connective tissue disorders [3, 5] no agreed criteria exist [5, 10, 11]. Furthermore, which joints to include in diagnosing GJH has been debated [12]. The Beighton score (BeS) [13], which is a development of the Carter and Wilkinson score [14], is the most common diagnostic test for GJH worldwide [8, 15]. The BeS demonstrates good *inter*- and *intra*-rater reliability [15–17] but with conflicting evidence and methodological flaws [18]. Advantageously, the BeS is quick and easy to perform. However, the BeS only covers five joints particularly hinge joints and is an "all-or-none-test" with no indication regarding the degree of hypermobility [13]. Commonly used cut-off levels in the BeS vary between ≥4 and ≥ 5 for diagnosing GJH in adults [18].

Another assessment method is the Contompasis score (CS), a modification of the BeS which includes one additional joint. The CS is measured by grading the ROM and might be considered more time-consuming [19]. Furthermore, the Hospital del Mar criteria (HdM), which is a development of the Rotés-Querol, offer a wider view of joint mobility by assessing nine joints, including ball-and-socket-joints [12]. To our best knowledge, the *inter*- and *intra*-rater reliability of the CS and the HdM scores have not yet been evaluated.

Comparisons across studies of GJH assessments are hampered because a structured protocol is often lacking [20–23]. Neither the literature nor the criteria for diagnosis of GJH [3] and heritable connective tissue disorders [24] describes the test performances in detail [10, 18]. Although ROM measured in degrees using a goniometer has shown better *inter*-rater reliability, assessment of GJH is often based on visual assessment [15, 17, 25] with a dichotomous principle of judgement. The reliability is also affected by the joint structure, the level of pre-training and experience among the raters [26].

To identify people with GJH and subsequently tailor suitable interventions, reliable clinical assessment methods are important. Thus, there is a need for international consensus regarding performance, cut-off levels and interpretation of clinical assessments based on reliability studies of high quality [11, 18] to reduce the likelihood that the assessment of GJH is based on chance. Before deciding on the validity of these tests the reliability needs to be investigated in a standardized manner [18].

The aim of this study was to investigate the *inter*- and *intra*-rater reliability for measurements of ROM in joints included in three hypermobility assessment methods using a structured protocol.

Methods

Design

An *inter*- and *intra*-reliability study.

This study was planned and developed in accordance with "Guidelines for Reporting Reliability and Agreement Studies" (GRRAS) and "Quality Appraisal of Reliability Studies" (QAREL) [27, 28].

Structured protocol and instruments

This study assessed *inter*- and *intra*-rater reliability of three hypermobility assessment methods, the BeS, the CS and the HdM for measuring joint ROM using a test-retest design which comprised in total 12 single joints. A protocol was developed to standardize the measurement of joint ROM (Additional file 1), which was further expanded from the original versions of the BeS, the CS and the HdM (Additional file 2). Starting position, positioning of the goniometer, anatomical landmarks, stabilization of adjacent structures and performances, using active or passive movement, were described and illustrated using photographs in the new protocol.

The BeS [13] comprises assessments of five joints, passive dorsiflexion of the fifth finger metacarpophalangeal joint, passive apposition of the thumb, passive hyperextension of the elbow and knee as well as forward flexion of the trunk. The first four joints are assessed bilaterally yielding a total score ranging from 0 to 9 [13]. The BeS scores of ≥4 and ≥ 5 points were used as cut-off levels for GJH.

The CS [19] comprises the assessment of six joints, which is similar to the BeS but with one additional joint, the foot flexibility test. Five joints are assessed bilaterally with each joint graded from two to six/or eight points with a total score range from 22 to 72 [19]. A cut-off level of ≥30 points for the CS was used to define GJH. The CS scores was modified because ROM in degrees for the elbow, knee and fifth finger were insufficiently graded and some degrees were represented in two score levels in the original description (Additional file 2).

The HdM [12] comprises the assessment of 10 items, passive apposition of the thumb, passive dorsiflexion of the fifth finger, passive hyperextension of the elbow, external shoulder rotation, hip abduction, patella hypermobility, ankle and foot hypermobility, first metatarsophalangeal joint, knee hyperflexion and easy bruising. Nine joints are assessed unilaterally on the non-dominant side. The last item deals with bruising; "Do you get bruises easily after minimal trauma?" Each hypermobile item scores one point, yielding a total score ranging from 0 to 10. The HdM ≥ 4 and ≥ 5 were set as cut-off levels for GJH [12]. The HdM measurement was modified by measuring passive opposition of the thumb with a goniometer instead of a ruler where < 15 degrees on the goniometer corresponds to < 21 mm on the ruler as used in the original description. Due to the lack of a reference value regarding a positive hypermobility finding for the ankle and the patella, ≥ 45 degrees was considered as hypermobile for the ankle [29, 30]. In addition, the measurement of the patella was standardized to make objective assessment possible (Additional file 1).

A goniometer (Medema Brodin, Kista Sweden, 31 cm or 21 cm with a 180° protractor and movable arms) was used. The small goniometer was used for measurements of the fifth finger and the big toe. Each joint was registered to the nearest 1-degree.

Raters

Two physiotherapists, rater A (KA) and rater B (AS) assessed all of the participants. Both raters had clinical experience in the physical examination of patients with joint hypermobility attending primary care (27 and 24 years of experience respectively). To standardize the performance and to assure similar interpretations of the assessments, the two raters trained un-blinded on three occasions until consensus was reached, for a total of 24 h, before data collection. The training cohort included 21 persons.

Participants

Information regarding the study was sent by e-mail to all 250 employees in a rehabilitation company within primary care in Stockholm, Sweden. The inclusion criteria were men and women aged between 18 and 65 years. For the *inter*-reliability study, we recruited the first consecutive 50 individuals who agreed to participate and who met the inclusion criteria. Of these, the first 30 participants were included in the *intra*-rater reliability study. Individuals with joint inflammatory signs, spasticity, joint-replacement, musculoskeletal injuries during the past 3 months and those who were not fluent in the Swedish language were excluded.

Procedures

Self-reported sociodemographic data concerning gender, age and country of birth were obtained using a questionnaire. The raters examined the participants in separate examination rooms without the presence of other employees. The participants wore shorts and tank tops. No

warming-up sessions were done before assessments. Reference dots were marked by the assessing rater on anatomical landmarks (Additional file 1), and were removed after each assessment session. The rater started each assessment with both oral and visual instructions about how the test would be performed.

The rater instructed the participant to stop the passive movement when they experienced that their joints were at an end-range position. The rater examined if it was possible to move the joint further without causing pain. In measurement of active ROM, the participant was asked: "Is this your maximum ROM?" For *inter*-rater-reliability, the raters assessed the same participant with a minimum of 30 min and a maximum of 7 h between assessments. The raters were blinded with respect to each other's results. To avoid recall bias in the *intra*-rater-reliability study, rater B conducted the repeated assessments 7 to 14 days after the first assessment. The second assessment was performed at the same time of the day as the first.

A timetable assured that the time intervals between assessments were achieved and that the order in which raters assessed the participants varied. The order of the joint assessments changed every third assessment day for both *inter*- and *intra*-rater reliability examinations by starting from the end of the protocol (Additional file 1).

Statistical analysis

Statistical analysis was conducted with R.3.3.1 (The R Project for Statistical Computing, Vienna, Austria). Intra-class correlations, two-way random effects model, ICC (2.1) with 95% confidence intervals (CI), were used to measure the *inter*- and *intra*-rater reliability for the quantitative measurements joint ROM (degrees) and total scores of the three hypermobility assessment methods [31]. The two-way models allow the error to be partitioned between systematic and random error [31, 32]. The ICC specific to the total score of the hypermobility assessment methods was used as the majority of these values were based on measured degrees. An ICC-score of < 0.40 was considered poor, 0.40–0.59 = fair/moderate, 0.60–0.74 = good and ≥ 0.75 = excellent [32]. The standard error of measurement (SEM) quantifies absolute reliability [33] and is referred to as the "typical" error [34]. The SEM was calculated using the residual mean square error from two-way repeated measures ANOVA. The SEM is important since a smaller SEM indicates more reliable results [33]. The value of an accepted SEM is a clinical decision.

For binary variables, the total percentage of agreement (P_a) for prevalence of positive findings was calculated. To assess the proportion of agreement beyond that expected by chance Cohen's Kappa (κ) was used [35]. A kappa value of $\kappa = < 0.00$ is considered as poor, 0.00–0.20 = slight, 0.21–0.40 = fair, 0.41–0.60 = moderate, 0.61–0.80 = substantial and ≥ 0.81almost perfect [36]. Since prevalence and bias affect the magnitude of the kappa coefficient, the prevalence-adjusted bias-adjusted kappa (PABAK) was calculated in addition to the obtained value of kappa [35].

With a significance level at 0.05 and a power of 80%, the sample size in this study was based upon an ICC score of at least 0.82 where a score of 0.6 or higher would be acceptable [37].

Results

Forty-nine adults, 38 women and 11 men, mean (SD) age 39.8 (13.5) years participated in the *inter*-raterreliability study. Twenty-nine adults, 23 women and 6 men, mean (SD) age 39.9 (12.5) years participated in the *intra*-raterreliability study. The majority were Europeans, 96% and 97% respectively. One participant was excluded because of injury. The time interval from assessments in the *inter*-raterreliability study varied from 30 min to 7 h and between eight to 8 days in the *intra*-rater reliability study.

The *inter*- and *intra*rater-reliability for the total score of all assessment methods, using ICC 2.1, was good-to-excellent 0.72–0.82 and 0.76–0.86, respectively (Table 1).

The *inter*-rater reliability for measurements of joint ROM in degrees was good-to-excellent in all but three of the assessed joints (ICC 2.1: 0.67–0.91). For the hips and right calcaneus the reliability was moderate (ICC 2.1: 0.44–0.59). The differences between raters were within 5 degrees (0.1–4.3) in all but one measurement. The SEM ranged from 1.1 to 6.2 degrees (Table 2).

The *intra*-rater reliability for measurements of joint ROM in degrees was good-to-excellent in all but three of the assessed joints (ICC 2.1: 0.60–0.90). For left hip and the calcaneus bilaterally the reliability was moderate (ICC 2.1: 0.44–0.51). The differences between test-retest assessments were within 3 degrees (0.0–2.7) in all but one of the measurements. SEM ranged from 1.0 to 5.7 degrees (Table 3).

For *inter*-rater reliability, the agreement (P_a) for the prevalence of positive hypermobility findings ranged from 80 to 98% for all total scores and Cohen's (κ) was moderate-to-substantial ($\kappa = ≥0.54–0.78$). The PABAK increased the results ($\kappa = ≥0.59–0.96$), (Table 4).

Regarding prevalence of positive hypermobility findings for separate joint assessments, the P_a ranged from 80 to 100%, except for the calcaneus. Cohen's (κ) was substantial-to-almost perfect for 13 of the 21 joint assessments ($\kappa = 0.63–1.00$) while the PABAK was substantial-to-almost perfect in all but three joint assessment ($\kappa = 0.63–1.00$), (Table 4).

For *intra*-rater reliability, the P_a for prevalence of positive hypermobility findings ranged from 72 to 97% for all total assessment scores. Cohen's (κ) was fair-to-substantial ($\kappa = 0.27–0.78$) and the PABAK was moderate-to-almost perfect ($\kappa = 0.45–0.93$), (Table 5). For prevalence of positive hypermobility findings regarding single joint assessments, the P_a ranged from 79 to 100% excpept for the calcaneus. Cohen's (κ) was substantial-to-almost perfect in 13 of the 21 joint assessments ($\kappa = 0.61–1.00$). The PABAK was substantial-to-almost perfect in all but three joint assessment ($\kappa = 0.66–1.00$), (Table 5).

The inter- and *intra*-rater reliability for the prevalence of positive hypermobility findings for the hip- abduction are not reported since none of the participants reached the cut off limit of > 85 degrees (Tables 4 and 5).

Discussion

To the best of our knowledge, this is the first study to investigate the *inter*- and *intra*-rater reliability of the Beighton score, the Contompasis score and the Hospital del Mar criteria. We used a structured protocol including descriptions of testing positions, starting positions, goniometer positions, anatomical landmarks, stabilization of adjacent structures and performance illustrated by photos.

Following this structured protocol with use of a goniometer, all of the three hypermobility assessment methods, the BeS, the CS and the HdM, showed good-to-excellent *inter*- and *intra*-rater reliability for the total scores and for the majority of the single-joint measurements in degrees. The SEM for *inter*- and *intra*-rater reliability ranged from 1.0 to 6.2 degrees.

Previous reliability studies of the BeS using a protocol have presented similar results to those in this study [12, 15–17, 25, 38, 39]. However, comparisons with these studies are complicated as the testing

Table 1 *Inter*-and *intra*-rater reliability of the total score of three hypermobility instruments

Variable	Inter-rater reliability					Intra-rater reliability				
Hypermobility instrument	Rater A mean (SD)	Rater B mean (SD)	P-value	Intra class correlation [1, 2] (95%CI)	Standard error of measurement	Rating 1 mean (SD)	Rating 2 mean (SD)	P-value	Intra class correlation [1, 2] (95%CI)	Standard error of measurement
BeS	1.4 (1.4)	1.3 (1.4)	0.59	0.72 (0.55–0.83)	0.7	1.4 (1.6)	1.1 (1.4)	0.11	0.76 (0.54–0.88)	0.7
HdM	2.7 (1.4)	2.6 (1.5)	0.42	0.81 (0.69–0.89)	0.6	2.5 (1.2)	2.3 (1.2)	0.08	0.86 (0.73–0.93)	0.4
CS	28.9 (4.3)	28.1 (4.1)	0.03	0.82 (0.69–0.89)	1.8	28.4 (3.5)	27.4 (3.8)	0.02	0.79 (0.57–0.90)	1.6

The hypermobility instruments used in this study were: *BeS* Beighton score, *CS* Contompasis score, *HdM* Hospital del Mar

Table 2 *Inter*-rater reliability for measurement of joint mobility measured in degrees in three hypermobility instruments

Joint	Hypermobility instrument	Rater A mean (SD)	Rater B mean (SD)	Difference A-B	P-value	Intra class correlation [1, 2] (95%CI)	Standard error of measurement
5th Finger, left	BeS, CS, HdM	76.9 (13.0)	73.4 (13.8)	3.5	< 0.001	0.85 (0.69–0.92)	4.7
5th Finger, right	BeS, CS, HdM	72.9 (14.6)	70.2 (14.0)	2.7	0.014	0.85 (0.74–0.92)	5.2
Thumb, left	BeS, CS, HdM	24.8 (11.0)	26.4 (10.9)	−1.6	0.017	0.91 (0.83–0.95)	3.2
Thumb, right	BeS, CS, HdM	27.4 (11.1)	27.3 (9.3)	0.1	0.859	0.89 (0.82–0.94)	3.4
Elbow, left	BeS, CS, HdM	5.6 (3.3)	4.4 (3.4)	1.2	0.002	0.69 (0.46–0.82)	1.8
Elbow, right	BeS, CS, HdM	5.4 (3.8)	4.2 (3.9)	1.2	0.005	0.67 (0.46–0.81)	2.1
Shoulder, left	HdM	62.1 (15.5)	60.3 (16.6)	1.8	0.081	0.90 (0.82–0.94)	5.0
Shoulder, right	HdM	63.4 (15.0)	61.4 (15.9)	2.0	0.054	0.89 (0.81–0.94)	5.1
Calcaneus, left	CS	3.2 (2.2)	2.3 (1.8)	0.8	< 0.001	0.68 (0.41–0.83)	1.0
Calcaneus, right	CS	2.9 (1.8)	2.3 (1.5)	0.6	0.011	0.59 (0.36–0.75)	1.0
Ankle, left	HdM	38.1 (5.5)	39.9 (6.2)	−1.8	0.001	0.77 (0.57–0.88)	2.6
Ankle, right	HdM	36.8 (6.2)	39.2 (6.2)	−2.4	< 0.001	0.82 (0.45–0.92)	2.2
Big toe, left	HdM	91.5 (10.9)	97.4 (14.3)	−5.9	< 0.001	0.73 (0.34–0.88)	5.5
Big toe, right	HdM	90.5 (12.2)	94.4(15.3)	−3.9	0.003	0.77 (0.59–0.87)	6.2
Knee extension, left	BeS, CS	3.4 (3.4)	4.0 (3.6)	−0.7	0.023	0.81 (0.68–0.89)	1.5
Knee extension, right	BeS, CS	3.5 (3.1)	4.3 (3.7)	−0.8	0.019	0.76 (0.60–0.86)	1.6
Hip abduction, left	HdM	35.8 (5.0)	32.4 (6.1)	3.4	< 0.001	0.44 (0.13–0.66)	3.8
Hip abduction, right	HdM	34.6 (6.6)	30.2 (5.8)	4.3	< 0.001	0.54 (0.08–0.77)	3.6

The hypermobility instruments used in this study were: *BeS* Beighton score, *CS* Contompasis score, *HdM* Hospital del Mar

procedures vary. This will affect the measurement of joint ROM [40] and thus influence the results [10]. In addition, many studies reported the use of no [21, 22] or an insufficient protocol [23, 25, 41, 42]. Comparisons are further hampered due to differences regarding the use or lack of use of a goniometer, reference lines for the goniometer and for anatomical landmarks, insufficient stabilization of adjacent structures, active or passive testing, testing positions, cut-off levels and statistical methods [15–17, 21, 22, 25, 38, 39, 41, 42].

To the best of our knowledge, this was the first *inter*- and *intra*-rater reliability study of the CS and the HdM and the first reliability study using measurement in degrees for joints included in the three hypermobility assessment methods. The *inter*- and *intra*-rater reliability was good-to-excellent for the majority of the single-joint assessments. Since prevalence and bias affect the magnitude of Cohen's (κ), it is recommended to also calculate the PABAK [35]. Due to adjusting for prevalece and bias, higher PABAK than Cohen's (κ) was found across all the results (Tables 4 and 5).

The difference between and within the raters in the present study was less than five degrees in all but one measurement which is in accordance with other studies [38, 43]. This is within an acceptable measure, as a variation of ±5 degrees in goniometric measurements is generally accepted in the clinic [44, 45].

The *inter-*and *intra*-rater reliability was moderate for some joints, indicating difficulties in the performance of these assessments. Joints without ROM end points, such as the elbow, the fifth finger and the knee might be considered more challenging to measure. This could be the reason why these joints in the BeS showed the lowest kappa values and the lowest P_a for the prevalence of positive hypermobility findings in this study and as well as in other studies [15, 17, 25, 42]. We stabilized the wrist and the fourth finger when measuring the fifth finger ROM since the test phase showed an increased ROM when the adjacent structures were not stabilized. This may affect the prevalence. Therefore, there is a need for consensus in the performance.

We have not found any documentation regarding the selection of joints for the criteria of the GJH.

In addition to study reliability of the BeS with a structured protocol, this study also aimed to establish the *inter*- and *intra*-rater reliability for the measurement of ROM in joints other than those included in the BeS. Children with joint hypermobility assessed with the BeS were equally hypermobile in their ball-and-socket-joints [43]. Thus, the importance of ball-and-socket-joints in adults with GJH requires further study.

Following this structured protocol with standardized assessments provided an excellent *inter*- and *intra*-rater reliability for the measurement of external rotation of the shoulder ICC 2.1: 0.89–0.90 and 0.86–0.87, respectively.

Table 3 *Intra*-rater reliability for measurement of joint mobility measured in degrees in three hypermobility instruments

Joint	Hypermobility instrument	Rating 1 mean (SD)	Rating 2 mean (SD)	Difference 1–2	P-value	Intra class correlation [1, 2] (95%CI)	Standard error of measurement
5th Finger, left	BeS, CS, HdM	71.5 (12.8)	71.6 (13.2)	−0.1	0.908	0.88 (0.77–0.94)	4.5
5th Finger, right	BeS, CS, HdM	71.6 (13.1)	70.4 (12.9)	1.2	0.312	0.88 (0.75–0.94)	4.6
Thumb, left	BeS, CS, HdM	26.3 (8.7)	27.3 (8.9)	−1.0	0.207	0.89 (0.78–0.94)	3.0
Thumb, right	BeS, CS, HdM	28.6 (9.4)	28.6 (8.3)	0.0	1.000	0.90 (0.79–0.95)	2.8
Elbow, left	BeS, CS, HdM	4.8 (4.0)	5.2 (3.5)	−0.4	0.551	0.60 (0.30–0.79)	2.4
Elbow, right	BeS, CS, HdM	5.4 (4.1)	4.2 (4.2)	1.2	0.040	0.71 (0.47–0.86)	2.1
Shoulder, left	HdM	60.4 (15.5)	62.5 (15.6)	−2.1	0.175	0.86 (0.73–0.93)	5.7
Shoulder, right	HdM	61.5 (13.9)	63.0 (15.7)	−1.5	0.288	0.87 (0.74–0.94)	5.3
Calcaneus, left	CS	2.4 (1.5)	1.9 (1.5)	0.5	0.105	0.44 (0.11–0.69)	1.1
Calcaneus, right	CS	2.6 (1.3)	2.4 (1.5)	0.2	0.432	0.51 (0.19–0.74)	1.0
Ankle, left	HdM	40.2 (5.1)	40.0 (6.2)	0.3	0.676	0.81 (0.64–0.91)	2.5
Ankle, right	HdM	39.6 (6.8)	39.6 (6.0)	0.0	0.959	0.85 (0.70–0.93)	2.5
Big toe, left	HdM	99.9 (13.4)	93.5 (14.6)	6.3	< 0.001	0.79 (0.31–0.92)	5.2
Big toe, right	HdM	93.1 (14.8)	90.4 (16.5)	2.7	0.079	0.86 (0.72–0.93)	5.6
Knee extension, left	BeS, CS	4.4 (3.5)	3.9 (3.6)	0.5	0.285	0.77 (0.58–0.89)	1.7
Knee extension, right	BeS, CS	4.8 (3.4)	4.4 (4.1)	0.4	0.515	0.66 (0.40–0.83)	2.2
Hip abduction, left	HdM	30.9 (5.0)	33.4 (5.0)	−2.5	0.010	0.45 (0.11–0.70)	3.6
Hip abduction, right	HdM	28.8 (5.9)	30.5 (6.2)	−1.7	0.062	0.67 (0.40–0.83)	3.4

The hypermobility instruments used in this study were: *BeS* Beighton score, *CS* Contompasis score, *HdM* Hospital del Mar

In accordance with another study [15], we reported low *inter*- and *intra*-rater reliability in measurements of hip-abduction, which may be due to insufficient stabilization of the pelvis. Furthermore, as in the hip-abduction measurement of elbow and calcaneus showed wide confidence intervals. The lack of precision in these measurements, as displayed by the wide CIs, suggests that the reliability should be interpreted with care. For the elbow, this could depend on a large valgus angle that falsely might give an impression of hypermobility [17]. Moreover, it is difficult to evaluate the reliability of the calcaneus tilt since the ROM is within the measurement error of the goniometer. This finding suggests that the calcaneus tilt should be excluded in the assessment of GJH. Other disputable tests included in the HdM are the knee-hyperflexion and the big toe-extension test. Most participants scored positive on these tests even though they were not hypermobile in other joints, suggesting that the risk of a false positive finding in the general population is high. Despite good-to-excellent *inter*- and *intra*-rater reliability, these tests are not adequate to identify joint hypermobility, as also confirmed in another study [23]. We therefore propose that these tests should be removed from the HdM. The remarkably high prevalence of positive hypermobility findings for knee-flexion and big toe-extension

may have resulted in a higher prevalence of hypermobility in the HdM compared to the BeS in this study.

There was a difference in big toe-extension between right and left side for both *inter*- and *intra*-rater reliability, indicating a systematic error. This may be explained by the fact that both raters were right-handed.

None of the participants had hypermobile hip-abduction and few had hypermobile external rotation of the shoulder even though measurements showed hypermobility in other joints. This may indicate that the cut-off value for hypermobility in these joints is too high in the HdM. A too high cut-off value increases the risk of underdiagnosing a possible hypermobility. In accordance with another study [15] cut-off levels for hypermobility above 55 degrees for hip-abduction [30, 46] and above 68 degrees for the shoulder external rotation [46] are supported.

We defined cut-off levels for the three hypermobility assessment methods. A cut-off level of the CS ≥ 30 for GJH was used in this study which corresponds to the BeS cut-off level of ≥4 points [47]. Previous reliability studies concerning the CS also used other cut-off levels [47, 48] than in the original description [19]. A cut-off level of ≥30 for the CS had a lower kappa value compared to a cut-off level of ≥4 or ≥ 5 when using the BeS and the HdM in this study. This may be due to the

Table 4 *Inter*-rater reliability for prevalence of positive hypermobility findings for total score and for single-joints

Total score/single joint	Prevalence of positive findings		Agreement	Reliability		Prevalence Index	Bias Index
	Rater A	Rater B	Prevalence of positive findings (%)				
	n (%)	n (%)		Kappa (95% CI)	Prevalence-adjusted bias-adjusted kappa-value (95% CI)		
BS ≥ 4	3 (6)	4 (8)	94	0.54 (0.26–0.82)	0.88 (0.66–0.97)	0.86	0.02
BS ≥ 5	2 (4)	1 (2)	98	0.66 (0.39–0.92)	0.96 (0.78–1.00)	0.94	−0.02
HdM ≥ 4	13 (27)	11 (22)	92	0.78 (0.50–1.06)	0.84 (0.61–0.95)	0.51	0.04
HdM ≥ 5	7 (14)	8 (16)	94	0.76 (0.48–1.04)	0.88 (0.66–0.97)	0.69	0.02
CS ≥ 30	18 (37)	14 (29)	80	0.54 (0.26–0.81)	0.59 (0.31–0.80)	0.35	−0.08
5th Finger, left	11 (22)	7 (14)	92	0.73 (0.46–1.00)	0.84 (0.61–0.95)	0.63	0.08
5th Finger, right	7 (14)	4 (8)	94	0.70 (0.43–0.96)	0.88 (0.66–0.97)	0.78	−0.06
Thumb, left	11 (22)	11 (22)	100	1.00 (0.72–1.28)	1.00 (0.79–1.00)	0.55	0.00
Thumb, right	7 (14)	6 (12)	98	0.91 (0.63–1.19)	0.96 (0.78–1.00)	0.73	−0.02
Elbow, left	8 (16)	5 (10)	82	0.21 (−0.06–0.48)	0.63 (0.36–0.82)	0.73	−0.06
Elbow, right	7 (14)	7 (14)	88	0.50 (0.22–0.78)	0.76 (0.50–0.91)	0.71	0.00
Shoulder, left	1 (2)	2 (4)	98	0.66 (0.39–0.92)	0.96 (0.78–1.00)	0.94	0.02
Shoulder, right	5 (10)	4 (8)	94	0.63 (0.36–0.91)	0.88 (0.66–0.97)	0.82	−0.02
Calcaneus, left	30 (61)	22 (45)	76	0.52 (0.26–0.79)	0.51 (0.22–0.73)	− 0.06	0.16
Calcaneus, right	28 (57)	19 (39)	73	0.49 (0.22–0.75)	0.47 (0.18–0.70)	0.04	−0.18
Ankle, left	7 (14)	11 (22)	80	0.33 (0.06–0.60)	0.59 (0.31–0.80)	0.63	0.08
Ankle, right	6 (12)	11 (22)	86	0.51 (0.25–0.77)	0.71 (0.46–0.88)	0.65	0.10
Big toe, left	31 (63)	35 (71)	84	0.63 (0.36–0.91)	0.67 (0.41–0.85)	−0.35	0.08
Big toe, right	28 (57)	32 (65)	84	0.66 (0.38–0.93)	0.67 (0.41–0.85)	−0.22	0.08
Knee extension, left	3 (6)	6 (12)	90	0.40 (0.13–0.66)	0.80 (0.56–0.93)	0.82	0.06
Knee extension, right	1 (2)	5 (10)	92	0.31 (0.11–0.51)	0.84 (0.61–0.95)	0.88	0.08
Knee flexion, left	39 (80)	37 (76)	92	0.77 (0.49–1.04)	0.84 (0.61–0.95)	−0.55	− 0.04
Knee flexion, right	38 (78)	36 (73)	92	0.78 (0.50–1.06)	0.84 (0.61–0.95)	− 0.51	− 0.04
Trunk flexion	12 (24)	11 (22)	98	0.94 (0.66–1.22)	0.96 (0.78–1.00)	0.53	−0.02
Patella, left	4 (8)	4 (8)	100	1.00 (0.72–1.28)	1.00 (0.79–1.00)	0.84	0.00
Patella, right	4 (8)	5 (10)	98	0.88 (0.60–1.16)	0.96 (0.78–1.00)	0.82	0.02
Hip abduction, left	0 (0)	0 (0)	NA	NA	NA		
Hip abduction, right	0 (0)	0 (0)	NA	NA	NA		

The hypermobility instruments used in this study were: *BS* Beighton score, *CS* Contompasis score, *HdM* Hospital del Mar, *NA* Not applicable, none of the participants reached the cut off limit

fine-scale grading of the CS, suggesting that the CS is more sensitive to measurement differences. Another possible explanation could be the small ROM of the calcaneus tilt and the cut-off levels for hypermobility making the judgement less reliable as mentioned above.

The strength of this study is that it was planned and developed in accordance with GRRAS [27] and QAREL [28]. It included a structured protocol with use of size-adjusted goniometers and a comprehensive description of the procedures for performing the assessments illustrated by photographs as recommended [18]. Two experienced physiotherapists, who had trained before the study, performed the measurements. The experience of the rater is important [15] as confirmed in another study showing that *inter*-rater variability increased as the level of medical education decreased [42]. Furthermore, the stability of joint ROM was taken into account for time intervals of assessments.

The raters stabilized adjacent structures to reduce the risk of false positive hypermobility findings and mainly used passive tests to assure that the end-range position was reached, since passive ROM is greater than active [30].

This study described testing positions since this impact the ROM and an optimal position should facilitate reaching the end-range position. Testing position

Table 5 *Intra*-rater reliability for prevalence of positive hypermobility findings for total score and for single-joints

Total score/single joint	Prevalence of positive findings		Agreement	Reliability		Prevalence index	Bias index
	Rater A n (%)	Rater B n (%)	Prevalence of positive findings (%)	Kappa (95% CI)	Prevalence-adjusted bias-adjusted kappa-value (95% CI)		
BeS ≥ 4	3 (10)	2 (7)	97	0.78 (0.43–1.14)	0.93 (0.64–1.00)	0.83	−0.03
BeS ≥ 5	3 (10)	1 (3)	93	0.47 (0.16–0.78)	0.86 (0.54–0.98)	0.86	−0.07
HdM ≥ 4	7 (24)	4 (14)	90	0.67 (0.33–1.01)	0.79 (0.45–0.96)	0.62	−0.10
HdM ≥ 5	2 (7)	3 (10)	97	0.78 (0.43–1.14)	0.93 (0.64–1.00)	0.83	0.03
CS ≥ 30	9 (31)	5 (17)	72	0.27 (−0.07–0.60)	0.45 (0.06–0.75)	0.52	−0.14
5th Finger, left	3 (10)	3 (10)	100	1.00 (0.64–1.36)	1.00 (0.66–1.00)	0.79	0.00
5th Finger, right	3 (10)	2 (7)	97	0.78 (0.43–1.14)	0.93 (0.64–1.00)	0.83	−0.03
Thumb, left	8 (28)	5 (17)	90	0.71 (0.36–1.06)	0.79 (0.45–0.96)	0.55	−0.10
Thumb, right	5 (17)	2 (7)	90	0.52 (0.20–0.84)	0.79 (0.45–0.96)	0.76	−0.10
Elbow, left	5 (17)	4 (14)	90	0.61 (0.25–0.97)	0.79 (0.45–0.96)	0.69	−0.03
Elbow, right	6 (21)	4 (14)	93	0.76 (0.41–1.11)	0.86 (0.54–0.98)	0.66	−0.07
Shoulder, left	1 (3)	1 (3)	100	1.00 (0.64–1.36)	1.00 (0.66–1.00)	0.93	0.00
Shoulder, right	2 (7)	3 (10)	90	0.35 (−0.01–0.70)	0.79 (0.45–0.96)	0.83	0.03
Calcaneus, left	14 (48)	10 (34)	66	0.30 (−0.05–0.65)	0.31 (−0.09–0.64)	0.17	− 0.14
Calcaneus, right	13 (45)	10 (34)	76	0.50 (0.15–0.86)	0.52 (0.13–0.79)	0.21	−0.10
Ankle, left	5 (17)	6 (21)	90	0.66 (0.30–1.03)	0.79 (0.45–0.96)	0.62	0.03
Ankle, right	7 (24)	6 (21)	83	0.51 (0.14–0.87)	0.66 (0.28–0.88)	0.55	−0.03
Big toe, left	24 (83)	18 (62)	79	0.51 (0.19–0.83)	0.59 (0.21–0.84)	−0.45	−0.21
Big toe, right	15 (52)	16 (55)	83	0.65 (0.29–1.02)	0.66 (0.28–0.88)	−0.07	0.03
Knee extension, left	4 (14)	3 (10)	97	0.84 (0.48–1.20)	0.93 (0.64–1.00)	0.76	−0.03
Knee extension, right	3 (10)	4 (14)	83	0.19 (−0.17–0.55)	0.66 (0.28–0.88)	0.76	0.03
Knee flexion, left	21 (72)	22 (76)	90	0.73 (0.37–1.09)	0.79 (0.45–0.96)	−0.48	0.03
Knee flexion, right	22 (76)	23 (79)	97	0.90 (0.54–1.26)	0.93 (0.64–1.00)	−0.55	0.03
Trunk flexion	6 (21)	6 (21)	100	1.00 (0.64–1.36)	1.00 (0.66–1.00)	0.59	0.00
Patella, left	2 (7)	3 (10)	97	0.78 (0.43–1.14)	0.93 (0.64–1.00)	0.83	0.03
Patella, right	2 (7)	5 (17)	90	0.52 (0.20–0.84)	0.79 (0.45–0.96)	0.76	0.10
Hip abduction, left	0 (0)	0 (0)	NA	NA	NA		
Hip abduction, right	0 (0)	0 (0)	NA	NA	NA		

The hypermobility instruments used in this study were: *BeS* Beighton score, *CS* Contompasis score, *HdM* Hospital del Mar, *NA* Not applicable, none of the participants reached the cut off limit

of adjacent joints is also important. For example, the position of the wrist and the elbow will impact the ROM of the thumb and the fifth finger [13, 38, 39].

A limitation in the present study is that the degree of agreement set at 80% in the training phase was not specified as recommended by "The International Federation for Manual/Musculoskeletal Medicine" (FIMM) [49]. The rater only measured each subject once to imitate clinical practice. Additionally, another study reported that mobility of joints increased significantly in consecutive measurements [38]. Furthermore, our aim was to measure the participant at the same time point at all testing occasions as it might be important to take this into consideration. However, about half of the participants were not assessed at the same time of the day. This may have influenced the results.

Since both raters were experienced, the use of a third, less experienced rater might have increased the generalizability in a clinical context. However, the generalizability also depends on the raters´ ability to follow the testing procedures in a structured protocol. In our study, the raters were experienced. Still, the reliability was not excellent for all measures. For instance, a ROM measurement close to the cut off level for a positive hypermobility finding could be interpreted as positive by one rater and negative by the other. Future implementation of new tools to measure ROM will hopefully increase the accuracy.

The choice of using a general population instead of a population diagnosed with GJH might be considered a limitation. However, our main focus was to standardize assessment of joint ROM in degrees, regardless whether the participant was hypermobile or not. The decision to measure joint ROM in a general population with an expected variation in joint mobility aimed to generalize our result to a broader context.

If joint hypermobility is suspected after screening in clinical practice, a standardized joint assessment should be performed for diagnosing GJH. Moreover, to be able to compare GJH studies and to reach international consensus regarding diagnosing GJH-related disorders, a description with standardization of procedures for performing assessments of ROM is needed [18].

Conclusions

The *inter-* and *intra-*rater reliability for total scores was good-to-excellent for the BeS, the CS and the HdM following a structured protocol. However, the *inter-* and *intra-*rater reliability was poor-to-moderate in some single joint measurements, indicating difficulties in the performance of these tests. This study includes a structured protocol with a comprehensive description of the performance of joint mobility measurement in several joints. This could be helpful in the first part of the process of standardizing the tests. Standardization for measurement of GJH is needed to provide that the criteria for assessment of GJH is not based on chance and may contribute to minimizing the risk of scoring healthy individuals with GJH. Future studies of reliability and validity should use a standardized protocol to assess persons with GJH. Furthermore, joint measurements other than those included in the BeS are needed, particularly tests assessing ball-and-socket-joints to consider whether these joints are important when diagnosing GJH. In addition, the study indicates that the cut-off value for hypermobility is too high in some joints and needs to be further studied.

Abbreviations
ANOVA: analysis of variance; BeS: Beighton score; CI: Confidence interval; FIMM: International Federation for Manual/Musculoskeletal Medicine; GJH: Generalized joint hypermobility; GRRAS: Guidelines for Reporting Reliability and Agreement Studies; HdM: Hospital del Mar criteria; ICC: Intra class correlation; P_a: Total percentage of agreement; PABAK: Prevalence-adjusted bias-adjusted kappa; QAREL: Quality Appraisal of Reliability Studies; ROM: Range of motion; SD: Standard deviation; SEM: Standard error of measurement; κ: Kappa

Acknowledgements
The authors would like to thank Aleris Rehab Stockholm which made it possible to conduct this study. A special thanks to Aleris Rehab in Liljeholmen and Skärholmen who lent the examination rooms.

Funding
This work was supported by the Aleris Research Fund; Primary Care Research Fund in Region Uppsala and County Council, Uppsala.

Authors' contributions
AS and KA equally contributed to the study as first authors and wrote the manuscript. They made substantial contributions to conception and design, acquisition, analysis and interpretation of data. ERB, EKB, RP, CO, LNW, PK contributed in designing the study. All authors contributed with interpretation of the results and writing the manuscript. RP contributed to the data analysis. All authors critically revised and approved the final version of the manuscript.

Competing interest
The authors declare that they have no competing interests.

Consent for publication
Not applicable.

Author details
[1]Department of Public Health and Caring Sciences, Uppsala University, Husargatan 3, Box 564, 752 37 Uppsala, Sweden. [2]Karolinska Institutet, Department of Neurobiology, Care Sciences and Society, Division of Physiotherapy, Huddinge, Sweden. [3]Department of Obstetrics and Gynecology, Akershus University Hospital, Lørenskog, Norway. [4]Academic Primary Healthcare Centre, Stockholm County Council, Huddinge, Sweden.

References
1. Ross J, Grahame R. Joint hypermobility syndrome. BMJ. 2011;342:c7167.
2. Engelbert RH, Juul-Kristensen B, Pacey V, de Wandele I, Smeenk S, Woinarosky N, et al. The evidence-based rationale for physical therapy treatment of children, adolescents, and adults diagnosed with joint hypermobility syndrome/hypermobile Ehlers Danlos syndrome. Am J Med Genet C Semin Med Genet. 2017;175:158–67.
3. Grahame R, Bird HA, Child A. The revised (Brighton 1998) criteria for the diagnosis of benign joint hypermobility syndrome (BJHS). J Rheumatol. 2000;27:1777–9.
4. Rombaut L, Malfait F, De Wandele I, Thijs Y, Palmans T, De Paepe A, et al. Balance, gait, falls, and fear of falling in women with the hypermobility type of Ehlers-Danlos syndrome. Arthritis Care Res. 2011;63:1432–9.
5. Grahame R. The hypermobility syndrome. Ann Rheum Dis. 1990;49:199–200.
6. Silman AJ, Haskard D, Day S. Distribution of joint mobility in a normal population: results of the use of fixed torque measuring devices. Ann Rheum Dis. 1986;45:27–30.
7. Remvig L, Jensen DV, Ward RC. Are diagnostic criteria for general joint hypermobility and benign joint hypermobility syndrome based on reproducible and valid tests? A review of the literature. J Rheumatol. 2007; 34:798–803.
8. Hakim A, Grahame R. Joint hypermobility. Best Pract Res Clin Rheumatol. 2003;17:989–1004.
9. Larsson LG, Baum J, Mudholkar GS, Srivastava DK. Hypermobility: prevalence and features in a Swedish population. Br J Rheumatol. 1993;32:116–9.
10. Remvig L, Engelbert RH, Berglund B, Bulbena A, Byers PH, Grahame R, et al. Need for a consensus on the methods by which to measure joint mobility and the definition of norms for hypermobility that reflect age, gender and ethnic-dependent variation: is revision of criteria for joint hypermobility syndrome and Ehlers-Danlos syndrome hypermobility type indicated? Rheumatology (Oxford). 2011;50:1169–71.
11. Remvig L, Flycht L, Christensen KB, Juul-Kristensen B. Lack of consensus on tests and criteria for generalized joint hypermobility, Ehlers-Danlos syndrome: hypermobile type and joint hypermobility syndrome. Am J Med Genet A. 2014;164a:591–6.
12. Bulbena A, Duro JC, Porta M, Faus S, Vallescar R, Martin-Santos R. Clinical assessment of hypermobility of joints: assembling criteria. J Rheumatol. 1992;19:115–22.
13. Beighton P, Solomon L, Soskolne CL. Articular mobility in an African population. Ann Rheum Dis. 1973;32:413–8.

14. Carter C, Wilkinson J. Persistent joint laxity and congenital dislocation of the hip. J Bone Joint Surg Br. 1964;46:40–5.

15. Juul-Kristensen B, Rogind H, Jensen DV, Remvig L. Inter-examiner reproducibility of tests and criteria for generalized joint hypermobility and benign joint hypermobility syndrome. Rheumatology (Oxford). 2007;46: 1835–41.

16. Boyle KL, Witt P, Riegger-Krugh C. Intrarater and interrater reliability of the Beighton and Horan joint mobility index. J Athl Train. 2003;38:281–5.

17. Junge T, Jespersen E, Wedderkopp N, Juul-Kristensen B. Inter-tester reproducibility and inter-method agreement of two variations of the Beighton test for determining generalised joint hypermobility in primary school children. BMC Pediatr. 2013;13:214.

18. Juul-Kristensen B, Schmedling K, Rombaut L, Lund H, Engelbert RH. Measurement properties of clinical assessment methods for classifying generalized joint hypermobility-a systematic review. Am J Med Genet C Semin Med Genet. 2017;175:116–47.

19. McNerney JE, Johnston WB. Generalized ligamentous laxity, hallux abducto valgus and the first metatarsocuneiform joint. J Am Podiatr Assoc. 1979;69: 69–82.

20. Mikkelsson M, Salminen JJ, Kautiainen H. Joint hypermobility is not a contributing factor to musculoskeletal pain in pre-adolescents. J Rheumatol. 1996;23:1963–7.

21. Hicks GE, Fritz JM, Delitto A, Mishock J. Interrater reliability of clinical examination measures for identification of lumbar segmental instability. Arch Phys Med Rehabil. 2003;84:1858–64.

22. Evans AM, Rome K, Peet L. The foot posture index, ankle lunge test, Beighton scale and the lower limb assessment score in healthy children: a reliability study. J Foot Ankle Res. 2012;5:1.

23. Ohman A, Westblom C, Henriksson M. Hypermobility among school children aged five to eight years: the hospital del mar criteria gives higher prevalence for hypermobility than the Beighton score. Clin Exp Rheumatol. 2014;32:285–90.

24. Beighton P, De Paepe A, Steinmann B, Tsipouras P, Wenstrup RJ. Ehlers-Danlos syndromes: revised nosology, Villefranche, 1997. Ehlers-Danlos National Foundation (USA) and Ehlers-Danlos support group (UK). Am J Med Genet. 1998;77:31–7.

25. Aartun E, Degerfalk A, Kentsdotter L, Hestbaek L. Screening of the spine in adolescents: inter- and intra-rater reliability and measurement error of commonly used clinical tests. BMC Musculoskelet Disord. 2014;15:37.

26. van de Pol RJ, van Trijffel E, Lucas C. Inter-rater reliability for measurement of passive physiological range of motion of upper extremity joints is better if instruments are used: a systematic review. J Physiother. 2010;56:7–17.

27. Kottner J, Audige L, Brorson S, Donner A, Gajewski BJ, Hrobjartsson A, et al. Guidelines for reporting reliability and agreement studies (GRRAS) were proposed. Int J Nurs Stud. 2011;48:661–71.

28. Lucas NP, Macaskill P, Irwig L, Bogduk N. The development of a quality appraisal tool for studies of diagnostic reliability (QAREL). J Clin Epidemiol. 2010;63:854–61.

29. Wahlstedt C, Rasmussen-Barr E. Anterior cruciate ligament injury and ankle dorsiflexion. Knee Surg Sports Traumatol Arthrosc. 2015;23:3202–7.

30. Clarkson H M, editor. Musculoskeletal assessment: joint motion and muscle testing. 3rd ed. Philadelphia, USA: Lippincott Williams & Wilkins; 2013.

31. Shrout PE, Fleiss JL. Intraclass correlations: uses in assessing rater reliability. Psychol Bull. 1979;86:420–8.

32. Portney L, Watkins M, editors. Foundations of clinical research: applications to practice. 3rd ed. upper Saddle River. USA: Pearson Prentice Hall; 2009. p. 892.

33. Weir JP. Quantifying test-retest reliability using the intraclass correlation coefficient and the SEM. J Strength Cond Res. 2005;19:231–40.

34. Hopkins WG. Measures of reliability in sports medicine and science. Sports Med. 2000;30:1–15.

35. Sim J, Wright CC. The kappa statistic in reliability studies: use, interpretation, and sample size requirements. Phys Ther. 2005;85:257–68.

36. Landis JR, Koch GG. The measurement of observer agreement for categorical data. Biometrics. 1977;33:159–74.

37. Walter SD, Eliasziw M, Donner A. Sample size and optimal designs for reliability studies. Stat Med. 1998;17:101 10.

38. Dijkstra PU, de Bont LG, van der Weele LT, Boering G. Joint mobility measurements: reliability of a standardized method. Cranio. 1994;12:52–7.

39. Hirsch C, Hirsch M, John MT, Bock JJ. Reliability of the Beighton hypermobility index to determinate the general joint laxity performed by dentists. J Orofac Orthop. 2007;68:342–52.

40. Prushansky T, Dvir Z. Cervical motion testing: methodology and clinical implications. J Manip Physiol Ther. 2008;31:503–8.

41. Karim A, Millet V, Massie K, Olson S, Morganthaler A. Inter-rater reliability of a musculoskeletal screen as administered to female professional contemporary dancers. Work. 2011;40:281–8.

42. Hansen ADR, Kristensen JH, Baggerss J, Remvig L. Interexaminer reliability of selected tests for hypermobility. J Orth Med. 2002;25:48–51.

43. Smits-Engelsman B, Klerks M, Kirby A. Beighton score: a valid measure for generalized hypermobility in children. J Pediatr. 2011;158:119–23 23.e1-4.

44. Boone DC, Azen SP, Lin CM, Spence C, Baron C, Lee L. Reliability of goniometric measurements. Phys Ther. 1978;58:1355–60.

45. Smith DS. Measurement of joint range--an overview. Clin Rheum Dis. 1982; 8(3):523–31.

46. Greene W, Heckman J, editors. American Academy of Orthopaedic surgeons. The clinical measurement of joint motion. First ed. Illinois: Rosemont; 1994.

47. Nilsson C, Wykman A, Leanderson J. Spinal sagittal mobility and joint laxity in young ballet dancers. A comparative study between first-year students at the Swedish ballet school and a control group. Knee Surg Sports Traumatol Arthrosc. 1993;1:206–8.

48. McCormack M, Briggs J, Hakim A, Grahame R. Joint laxity and the benign joint hypermobility syndrome in student and professional ballet dancers. J Rheumatol. 2004;31:173–8.

49. Patijn J, editor. FIMM Scientific Committee. Reproducibility and validity studies of Diagnostic Procedures in Manual/Musculoskeletal Medicine. Protocol formats. 3rd ed. Avaliable from: http://www.fimm-online.com/pub/en/data/objects/reproduciblity_validity.pdf.

16

Motion analysis of the wrist joints in Chinese rheumatoid arthritis patients

Lijuan Zhang[1,2†], Haixia Cao[1†], Qiuxiang Zhang[1], Ting Fu[1], Rulan Yin[1], Yunfei Xia[1], Liren Li[1,3*] and Zhifeng Gu[1*]

Abstract

Background: The wrist is often severely affected in rheumatoid arthritis (RA) patients; however, little is known about the potential risk factors of the reduced wrist range of motion. In this study, we explored a broad range of possible risk factors of wrist range of motion in RA patients. We also determined whether measurements of wrist range of motion reflect Sharp score for the wrists.

Methods: Active wrist volar flexion, dorsal flexion, radial deviation and ulnar deviation were assessed using a goniometer. RA patients underwent standardized laboratory and radiographic examinations and completed several questionnaires. A linear regression model was used to study association between the wrist range of motion and independent variables. In addition, Spearman and Pearson correlation analysis were used to compare influence factors and outcome measurements between the measurements of wrist range of motion and Sharp score for the wrists.

Results: In this study, lower socioeconomic status, longer disease duration, severe pain, higher disease activity and drug treatments were associated with reduced wrist range of motion in RA patients ($n = 102$, 86.3% female, mean $\pm$ SD age, 55.0 $\pm$ 11.7 years, and mean $\pm$ SD disease duration, 8.4 $\pm$ 8.7 years). Furthermore, wrist range of motion was highly correlated with Sharp score for the wrists ($P < 0.05$).

Conclusions: Socioeconomic status and disease-specific factors were significantly associated with wrist range of motion in RA patients. The results indicated that rheumatologists and nurses should note the measurements of wrist range of motion in RA patients, especially those with a low socioeconomic status, a long disease duration, severe pain, and high disease activity to develop strategies to improve their quality of life.

Background

Rheumatoid arthritis (RA) is a chronic, inflammatory, progressive autoimmune disease that causes pain, limited range of motion (ROM) of joints, and joints destruction [1], and seriously impacts patients' psychological [2] and physical [3] well-being. The wrist was affected in 50% of patients with RA during the first 2 years after onset of the disease, increasing to more than 90% after 10 years [4]. There was increasing evidence that reduced wrist ROM was associated with RA patients' functional disability [1, 5]. Furthermore, evaluation of wrist ROM was important in the therapeutic

approach to patients with RA [6], and increasing joints motion was a particular goal of the surgical treatments for rheumatic wrist joints [5]. Therefore, it is important to examine which factors have influence on ROM, especially in the wrist.

Several studies have suggested that ROM was associated with age, gender [7], disease duration [8], pain [9, 10], disease activity [10], medical therapy [11, 12], laboratory indexes [13], and disability [1, 14]. It has been reported that RA patients had a higher prevalence of anxiety and depression compared with the general population [2], and the disease exerted an unfavorable impact on the quality of life [3]. Our group has reported that socioeconomic status (SES) was significantly associated with patients' anxiety/depression and quality of life in rheumatic diseases [15, 16], but exact figures about the

---

* Correspondence: larry017@163.com; guzf@ntu.edu.cn
†Lijuan Zhang and Haixia Cao contributed equally to this work.
[1]Department of Rheumatology, Affiliated Hospital of Nantong University, 20th Xisi Road, 226001 Nantong, People's Republic of China
Full list of author information is available at the end of the article

associations among SES, anxiety/depression, quality of life, and wrist ROM in RA patients were scarce. To minimize activity limitations and maintain quality of life, it is important for health professionals to increase RA patients' ROM and provide effective treatments.

To date, Sharp score has assumed a paramount position in the evaluation of RA patients with joint damage in hand-wrist joints. Previous studies have reported that female [17], age [18, 19], body mass index (BMI) [20–22], socioeconomic status (SES) [23], disease duration [20, 24, 25], disease activity [26, 27], comorbid conditions [28, 29], erythrocyte sedimentation rate (ESR) [17], and rheumatoid factor (RF) [24, 30–32] were associated with joint destruction. However, little is known about the associations between Sharp score and the wrist ROM. Only a study from the USA reported that the number of deformed joints, which was rated on each of 48 joints as normal or abnormal in terms of alignment and ROM, was highly correlated with the total Sharp score in RA patients [33]. In the present study, the relationships between influence factors or outcomes values and Sharp score or ROM measurements for the wrists were analyzed.

Therefore, the aims of the present study were the following: (1) to explore a broad range of possible risk factors of wrist ROM in patients with RA; (2) to determine whether RA patients' ROM measurements reflect Sharp score for the wrists.

Methods
Study participants
Patients who fulfilled the American College of Rheumatology (ACR) criteria (1987 or 2012) for RA were recruited from the Affiliated Hospital of Nantong University from January 2015 to April 2016. Of the RA patients who were consecutively invited to participate in a single-centered cross-sectional study, 102 (91.1% of the patients) took part and completed the relevant questionnaires. Patients were excluded based on either of the following: (1) they were less than 18 years old; (2) they did not complete the questionnaire; (3) they did not complete the measurements of ROM and Sharp score for the wrists. This cross-sectional study was approved by the Ethics Committee of the Affiliated Hospital of Nantong University, and a written informed consent was obtained from each RA patient.

Primary outcomes
Active ROM was measured bilaterally in the wrist with a goniometer. The goniometer was applied superficially at the dorsum of each respective joint. The angle of wrist volar flexion, dorsal flexion, radial deviation, and ulnar deviation were measured relative to a position of zero degrees. Participants had to carry out the motion with their muscle strength to increase the angle and keep their joints in position. Measurements were carried out by two trained physiotherapists under the supervision of a rheumatologist. Two physiotherapists were trained with procedures among 30 healthy subjects before the trial. They were kept unaware of the measurement data of their counterpart. Measurement procedures were standardized prior to the study. The values used for analysis were the means of the right and left sides.

Independent variables
At baseline, sociodemographic and disease characteristic [including gender, age (years), BMI (kg/m^2), disease duration (years), education (years), employment status, income/person/month (Yuan), health insurance, and comorbid conditions] were recorded.

One experienced rheumatologist (GZ) and two rheumatologists (XY and GG) scored joint damage at the same time. Radiographs of both wrists were scored using the van der Heijde-modified Sharp Score (HSS). The total score for the wrists ranged from 0 to 87, with the erosion score (E score) ranging from 0 to 35 and the joint space narrowing score (JSN score) ranging from 0 to 32. All were read by the examiners without the knowledge of the patient identity [34].

As described previously [35], hand grip and pinch strength were measured with a hydraulic hand grip and pinch dynamiter [36]. Physical function was evaluated by the Health Assessment Questionnaire (HAQ) [37]. The Hospital Anxiety and Depression Scale (HADS) was used to assess levels of anxiety and depression [38]. Participants' health status was assessed using the Short Form 36 (SF-36) [39, 40]. Disease activity was estimated with the valid and reliable 28-joint Disease Activity Score (DAS28) [41–43]. Several serological markers, ESR, C-reactive protein (CRP), and RF measured at the time of diagnosis were examined [44].

The personal medication information was gained by querying the electronic medical records combined with self-reports of patients, including the use of NSAIDs, DMARDs, corticosteroids, and biologics.

We have described questionnaire and measurement administration in detail previously [35]. Briefly, written questionnaires were provided on paper, and all participants completed the questionnaires under a physician's supervision in a clinical setting.

Statistical analysis
The data were expressed as the mean ± SD for continuous variables and as frequencies (%) for categorical variables. Descriptive analyses were performed to investigate the participants' characteristics. The Spearman and Pearson correlations analysis were used to compare the

influence factors and outcome measurements between Sharp score and the ROM measurements for the wrists.

Furthermore, variables shown to be significantly associated with the primary outcome in the Spearman and Pearson correlations analysis were included in the multivariable regression analysis to identify the independent factors of wrist ROM. Statistical significance was set at $P < 0.05$ (two-sided). Standardized regression coefficients (β) and the R-squared (R^2) were presented to show the relative importance of the independent variables when compared to each other, and the proportion of the variance in the wrist ROM accounted for by the factors in the multivariable regression model, respectively [45]. Analyses were completed using SPSS version 20.0.

Results

Sample characteristics

Ten RA patients did not complete the questionnaires due to lack of interest, resulting in the enrollment of 102 RA patients in the current study. Table 1 presented the baseline participant characteristics included in our analysis. The mean ± SD age of the respondents was 55.0 ± 11.7 years, and 86.3% were female. The mean ± SD disease duration was 8.4 ± 8.7 years, and 93.1 and 35.3% had health insurance and comorbid condition, respectively. The participants tended to have lower income (< 3000 Yuan; 87.2%) and lower than a high school level of education (71.6%). The mean ± SD pain and DAS28 scores of the participants were 43.1 ± 27.2 and 3.7 ± 1.5, respectively. The patients tended to use DMARDs (91.3%), and 78.4% were RF positive. The mean (range) wrist ROM scores, grip/pinch strength, Sharp score, the HAQ score, the HADS anxiety and depression scores, and the scores of SF-36 PCS and MCS were shown in Table 2.

Higher sharp score was significantly associated with reduced ROM for the wrists

As shown in Table 2, the mean (range) ROM scores varied from 13.1 (0 to 35) to 38.7 (0 to 80) degrees in the wrist joint actions, which were much lower than the normal reference. This result was in accordance with previous findings [1, 5, 14]. The correlation between the ROM scores of the wrist joint actions ranged from 0.44 to 0.67. This finding confirms the conclusion of Steultjens, et al... that joint ROM cannot be regarded as a unidimensional physical characteristic of osteoarthritis (OA) patients [46]. Furthermore, Orces CH, et al [33] reported that the number of deformed joints was significantly associated with the total Sharp score. We also found that a higher Sharp score was highly correlated with a lower ROM in the wrist (Table 3). Thus, this raised an interesting question of whether RA patients' ROM measurements might reflect Sharp score for the wrists.

Table 1 Baseline characteristics of 102 patients with rheumatoid arthritis

Characteristic/factor	Value
Gender, female, no. (%)	88 (86.3)
Age, mean ± SD years	55.0 ± 11.7
BMI, mean ± SD kg/m2	22.6 ± 3.3
Disease duration, mean ± SD years	8.4 ± 8.7
Education, years, no. (%)	
≤ 9 years	73 (71.6)
> 9 years	29 (28.4)
Employment status, no. (%)	
Full-time work	63 (61.8)
Part-time work	37 (36.2)
Unemployed	2 (2.0)
Income/person/month, Yuan, no. (%)	54 (52.9)
≤ 1000 Yuan	35 (34.3)
1000–3000 Yuan	12 (11.8)
3000–5000 Yuan	1 (1.0)
≥ 5000 Yuan	95 (93.1)
Health insurance, yes, no. (%)	36 (35.3)
Comorbid condition, yes, no. (%)	43.1 ± 27.2
VAS pain (range 0–100), mean ± SD	4.1 ± 6.0
28-TJC, mean ± SD	54 (52.9)
28-SJC, mean ± SD	2.6 ± 3.8
DAS28, mean ± SD	3.7 ± 1.5
NAIDS usage, yes, no. (%)	42 (41.2)
DMARDs usage, yes, no. (%)	93 (91.2)
Corticosteroids usage, yes, no. (%)	43 (42.2)
Biologics usage, yes, no. (%)	4 (3.9)
ESR, mean ± SD mm/h	25.7 ± 24.9
CRP, mean ± SD mg/L	15.5 ± 24.5
RF positivity, yes, no. (%)	80 (78.4)

BMI Body mass index, *VAS* Visual analog scale, *TJC* Tender joint count, *SJC* Swollen joint count, *DAS28* Disease activity score in 28 joints, *NSAID* Nonsteroidal anti-inflammatory drugs, *DMARD* Disease modifying anti-rheumatic drugs, *ESR* Erythrocyte sedimentation rate, *CRP* C-reactive protein, *RF* Rheumatoid factor

SES, disease activity, laboratory indexes and outcome measures were significantly associated with sharp score and ROM for the wrists

As indicated in Table 4, both Sharp score and the ROM for the wrists were correlated to a similar degree with disease duration, employment status, income, comorbid conditions, grip/pinch strength, the HAQ score, the SF-36 PCS and MCS scores (Table 4).

SES and RA disease-specific factors were the potential risk factors of wrist ROM

We used stepwise linear regression analysis to investigate the potential risk factors of wrist ROM, as shown in Table 5. Only the independent variables that were significantly associated with wrist ROM were entered into

Table 2 Clinical characteristics of 102 patients with rheumatoid arthritis

Characteristic/factor	Value	Range
Wrist volar flexion ‡, mean ± SD degrees	38.7 ± 18.7	0 to 80
Wrist dorsal flexion ‡, mean ± SD degrees	35.2 ± 17.2	0 to 65
Wrist ulnar deviation ‡, mean ± SD degrees	29.7 ± 14.0	0 to 63
Wrist radial deviation ‡, mean ± SD degrees	13.1 ± 7.8	0 to 35
Sharp score for the wrists, mean ± SD	8.6 ± 6.5	0 to 52
Grip strength ‡, mean ± SD kg	13.2 ± 8.6	0 to 40
Pinch strength ‡, mean ± SD kg	3.3 ± 2.2	0 to 11
HAQ score (range 0–3), mean ± SD	0.4 ± 0.6	0 to 2.6
HADS-anxiety score (range 0–21), mean ± SD	9.3 ± 2.7	4 to 17
HADS-depression score (range 0–21), mean ± SD	8.9 ± 2.4	4 to 15
PCS score (range 0–100), mean ± SD	43.9 ± 22.9	2.5 to 92.8
MCS score (range 0–100), mean ± SD	53.0 ± 22.2	1 to 100

‡ Mean of right and left sides. *HAQ* Health assessment questionnaire, *HADS* Hospital anxiety and depression scale, *PCS* Physical components summary, *MCS* Mental components summary

model. We found that SES and RA disease-specific factors were the important predictors of wrist ROM. In addition, we found that there were significant correlations between corticosteroids usage and lower wrist dorsal flexion, which was in contrast with a previous finding [12]. It might be explained that the radiological and functional damage of the wrist is likely to be a direct by-product of the more severe disease features, while steroid usage is likely to be a consequence of the individual clinical profile with more persistent and/or high disease activity.

Discussion

This study provided evidence that Chinese RA patients were characterized with reduced wrist ROM, higher Sharp score for the wrists, decreased grip/pinch strength, lower PCS and MCS scores, higher HAQ score, and HADS anxiety and depression scores, which was similar to previous studies from other countries [1–3, 5, 8, 14]. SES, RA disease-specific factors, and drug treatments were significantly associated with wrist ROM. In addition, the ROM measurements might reflect Sharp score for the wrists with regard to the influence factors

and negative outcomes. To our knowledge, this is the first study exploring the relationships among SES, disease activity, Sharp score, anxiety/depression, quality of life, and wrist ROM in RA patients.

Khadr Z et al. reported that reduced ROM was associated with old age and female gender in a population of elderly people [7]. In contrast, our study reported that there were no relationships between old age, female gender and lower wrist ROM. One possible explanation for the different results is the existence of cultural diversity and the different participants included in the studies with either Chinese or Western cohorts. Previous studies reported that RA could result in a high economic burden on the individual and the society [47]. Our group reported that SES was significantly associated with patients' anxiety/depression and quality of life in rheumatic diseases [15, 16]. It was well known that SES is a multifactor. Occupation [48–50], education, and income [51] were frequently used as measures of SES. Whether SES is associated with ROM remains unknown. In the current study, we found that RA patients with lower education level, lower income, lower employment status, and without health insurance were prone to suffer from

Table 3 Correlation between the wrist ROM and Sharp score for the wrists (N = 102)

Variable	Wrist volar flexion (degrees)		Wrist dorsal flexion (degrees)		Wrist ulnar deviation (degrees)		Wrist radial deviation (degrees)	
	r	P	r	P	r	P	r	P
Wrist volar flexion ‡ (degrees)								
Wrist dorsal flexion ‡ (degrees)	0.67**	0.000						
Wrist ulnar deviation ‡ (degrees)	0.62**	0.000	0.64**	0.000				
Wrist radial deviation ‡ (degrees)	0.47**	0.000	0.44**	0.000	0.48**	0.000		
Sharp score for the wrists	− 0.62**	0.000	− 0.63**	0.000	− 0.67**	0.000	− 0.42**	0.000

‡ Mean of right and left sides. *P < 0.05, **P < 0.01

Table 4 Correlations among the wrist ROM, Sharp score for the wrists, and the variables used in this study (N = 102)

Variable	Sharp score for the wrists		Wrist volar flexion ‡ (degrees)		Wrist dorsal flexion ‡ (degrees)		Wrist ulnar deviation ‡ (degrees)		Wrist radial deviation ‡ (degrees)	
	r	P	r	P	r	P	r	P	r	P
Gender	0.15	0.129	0.02	0.858	0.03	0.746	0.03	0.775	0.18	0.065
Age, years	−0.08	0.451	−0.17	0.096	−0.08	0.434	−0.04	0.659	−0.04	0.713
BMI, kg/m2	−0.06	0.561	−0.03	0.794	−0.12	0.233	−0.08	0.454	−0.08	0.404
Disease duration, years	0.47**	0.000	−0.30**	0.002	−0.46**	0.000	−0.39**	0.000	−0.13	0.200
Education, years	−0.07	0.515	0.26**	0.008	0.20*	0.048	0.21*	0.037	0.16	0.118
Employment status	−0.22*	0.025	0.26*	0.008	0.07	0.458	0.25*	0.012	0.04	0.660
Income/person/month, Yuan	−0.31**	0.002	0.40**	0.000	0.31**	0.002	0.30**	0.002	0.12	0.224
Health insurance	0.05	0.624	0.12	0.248	0.25*	0.012	0.22*	0.027	0.16	0.108
Comorbid condition	0.23*	0.021	−0.18	0.078	−0.27**	0.006	−0.26**	0.007	−0.12	0.215
VAS pain	0.31**	0.002	−0.41**	0.000	−0.40**	0.000	−0.43**	0.000	−0.34**	0.001
28-TJC	0.12	0.229	−0.30**	0.003	−0.30**	0.002	−0.28**	0.005	−0.20*	0.043
28-SJC	0.16	0.102	−0.23*	0.021	−0.25*	0.011	−0.13	0.195	−0.21*	0.038
DAS28	0.27*	0.017	−0.32**	0.001	−0.30**	0.002	−0.31**	0.002	−0.39**	0.000
NAIDS usage	−0.02	0.866	−0.05	0.634	−0.04	0.702	0.00	0.976	0.05	0.627
DMARDs usage	0.00	0.995	0.08	0.438	−0.01	0.958	−0.07	0.477	−0.05	0.604
Corticosteroids usage	0.06	0.529	−0.17	0.080	−0.27**	0.007	−0.11	0.258	−0.06	0.547
Biologics usage	0.04	0.456	0.08	0.438	0.00	0.949	0.05	0.567	0.05	0.447
ESR, mm/h	0.14	0.161	−0.21*	0.039	−0.20*	0.041	−0.24*	0.014	−0.38**	0.000
CPR, mg/L	0.12	0.214	- 0.24*	0.014	−0.29**	0.003	−0.27**	0.006	−0.36**	0.000
RF positivity	0.14	0.155	−0.05	0.619	−0.08	0.448	−0.14	0.163	−0.28**	0.005
Grip strength ‡ (kg)	−0.39**	0.000	0.40**	0.000	0.37**	0.000	0.47**	0.000	0.37**	0.000
Pinch strength ‡ (kg)	−0.30**	0.002	0.29**	0.003	0.25*	0.013	0.32**	0.001	0.24*	0.017
HAQ score	0.35**	0.000	−0.49**	0.000	−0.49**	0.000	−0.47**	0.000	−0.41**	0.000
HADS-anxiety score	0.16	0.109	−0.10	0.322	−0.25*	0.012	−0.06	0.555	−0.24*	0.019
HADS-depression score	0.05	0.610	−0.21*	0.040	−0.20*	0.047	−0.12	0.250	−0.23*	0.020
PCS score	−0.25*	0.011	0.41**	0.000	0.38**	0.000	0.31**	0.002	0.29**	0.003
MCS score	−0.22*	0.023	0.26**	0.008	0.32**	0.001	0.21*	0.030	0.19	0.113

‡ Mean of right and left sides. *BMI* Body mass index, *VAS* Visual analog scale, *TJC* Tender joint count, *SJC* Swollen joint count, *DAS28* Disease activity score in 28 joints, *NSAID* Nonsteroidal antl-Inflammatory drugs, *DMARD* Disease modifying antirheumatic drugs, *ESR* Erythrocyte sedimentation rate, *CRP* C-reactive protein, *RF* Rheumatoid factor, *HAQ* Health assessment, questionnaire, *HADS* Hospital anxiety and depression scale, *PCS* Physical components summary, *MCS* Mental components summary. *P < 0.05, **P < 0.01

lower wrist ROM. Due to work-related income reduction, lower education level, and lack of health insurance, RA patients might have a lower adherence rate to medication, which could lead to higher disease activity, more severe joints damage, and loss of physical function [33].

With regard to clinical factors, we found that longer disease duration was significantly associated with lower wrist ROM. This result was in line with the finding of Goodson A and co-workers [8]. When RA progresses, the wrist is increasingly affected [bone erosions and rigid], which possibly lowers the ROM. Furthermore, the current study also revealed that patients with comorbid conditions tended to suffer from reduced wrist ROM, which showed that comorbidity was an important

predictor of functional status in RA patients [52]. Pain is a major symptom in RA and is the leading reason for patients seeking medical care [53, 54]. Our study demonstrated significant negative correlations among pain, disease activity, and lower wrist ROM, which were similar to previous study [1]. This result may be attributed to the fact that painful movement and the swelling of soft tissues around the joints are additional important factors contributing to decreased joints mobility in RA. Additionally, we found that there were significant correlations between corticosteroids usage and lower wrist dorsal flexion, which was in contrast with a previous finding [12], which might be explained by the likely dependence of the steroid usage on the more aggressive or

Table 5 Results of the multivariable analysis of the association between factors and the ROM scores of the different wrist joint actions (degrees) (N = 102)

Factor	Wrist volar flexion ‡ (degrees)			Wrist dorsal flexion ‡ (degrees)			Wrist ulnar deviation ‡ (degrees)			Wrist radial deviation ‡ (degrees)		
	B(95% CI)	β	P	B(95% CI)	β	P	B(95% CI)	β	P	B(95% CI)	β	P
Education, years							6.11 (1.04, 11.18)	0.20	0.019			
Income/person /month, Yuan	7.00 (2.75, 11.25)	0.28	0.001	4.10 (0.39, 7.82)								
Employment status	5.30 (0.17, 10.42)	0.17	0.043				4.58 (0.83, 8.33)	0.20	0.017			
Disease duration, years	−0.46 (−0.82, −0.10)	−0.21	0.012	−0.76 (−1.08, −0.45)	−0.39	0.000	−0.56 (−0.82, −0.29)	−0.35	0.000			
VAS pain	−0.23 (−0.34, −0.11)	−0.33	0.000	−0.18 (−0.29, −0.08)	−0.29	0.001	−0.17 (−0.26, −0.09)	−0.33	0.000			
DAS28										−2.02 (−2.97, −1.08)	−0.39	0.000
Corticosteroids usage				−7.31(−12.79, −1.84)	−0.21	0.009						
R^2		0.34			0.40			0.37			0.15	

‡ Mean of right and left sides. *VAS* Visual analog scale, *DAS28* Disease activity score in 28 joints, *B* Regression coefficient, *95% CI* 95% confidence interval of B, *β* Standardized regression coefficient, R^2 R-squared

refractory forms of RA where corticosteroids were more frequently used. Furthermore, we also found that ESR, CRP, and RF were associated with wrist ROM, which were in line with a previous study [13]. This finding may be attributed to the fact that the higher levels of ESR and CRP, and positive RF result in higher inflammatory activity, causing pain and swelling of the joints.

Interestingly, we found that there were significant association between ROM and Sharp score for the wrists. This finding indicated that ROM measurements might reflect Sharp score for the wrists. However, no causal conclusion could be inferred because the study was cross-sectional in design. Additional clinical trials are required, and the present study just provided a first step towards more focused studies in the future.

To identify which variables were most significantly correlated with lower wrist ROM, a stepwise linear regression analysis was used. Only independent variables individually associated with the primary outcome with a P-value < 0.05 were entered into a multivariable regression model. We found that SES, RA disease-specific factors, and drug treatments were significantly associated with wrist ROM, which indicated that SES and RA disease-specific factors were independent risk factors of lower wrist ROM. However, steroid usage is likely to be a consequence of the individual clinical profile with more persistent and/or high disease activity.

However, this study has some limitations. First, the sample size was relatively small and all participants were from a single hospital. Second, the intra- and inter-observer reliabilities of the ROM measurements were not tested. Therefore, it might lead to possible biases of the measurements. However, to minimize the bias, all measurements were taken by two trained physiotherapists under the supervision of a rheumatologist.

Third, the inter-rater reliability of Sharp score also could not be tested. However, to ensure the accuracy of Sharp score for the wrists, three rheumatologists evaluated wrist joint damage according to the HSS at the same time, and all readers were blind to the results. In addition, the questionnaires used in this study were all self-reported, which might result in possible biases of the outcomes.

Conclusions

SES, RA disease-specific factors, and drug treatments were significantly associated with the wrist ROM in RA patients. Additionally, our study suggested that ROM measurements might reflect Sharp score for the wrists with regard to influence factors and outcome measurements. The results indicated that rheumatologists and nurses should be aware of the RA patients' wrist ROM measurements, especially those with low SES, long disease duration, severe pain, and high disease activity to develop strategies to improve RA patients' quality of life.

Abbreviations
ACR: American College of Rheumatology; BMI: Body mass index; BP: Body pain; CI: Confidence intervals; CRP: C-reactive protein; DAS28: Disease activity score in 28 joints; DMARDs: Disease-modifying antirheumatic drugs; ESR: Erythrocyte sedimentation rate; GH: General health; HADS: Hospital Anxiety and Depression Scale; HAQ: Health Assessment Questionnaire; JSN: Joint space narrowing; MCS: Mental Component Summary; MH: Mental health; PCS: Physical Component Summary; PF: Physical function; RA: Rheumatoid arthritis; RE: Role emotional; RF: Rheumatoid factor; ROM: Range of motion; RP: Role physical; SD: Standard deviation; SES: Socioeconomic status; SF: Social function; SF-36: The Short Form 36 Health survey; VAS: Visual analog scale; VT: Vitality

Acknowledgments
We would like to thank Biyu Shen and Yan Sang for their assistance with this study.

Funding
This study was supported by Grants from the Chinese National Natural Science Foundation (Grant no. 81671616 and 81471603); Jiangsu Provincial Commission of Health and Family Planning Foundation (Grant no. H201317 and H201623); Science Foundation of Nantong City (Grant no. MS32015021, MS2201564 and MS22016028); Science and Technology Foundation of Nantong City (Grant no. HS2014071 and HS2016003); the College graduate research and innovation of Jiangsu Province (Grant no. KYZZ15_0353 and KYZZ16_0358).

Authors' contributions
LZ and HXC have contributed to study design, data collection, data analysis, interpretation of results, and preparation of the manuscript. QZ, TF, RY, XY, LL and ZG have contributed to study design, preparation of the manuscript. All authors read and approved the final manuscript.

Consent for publication
Not applicable.

Competing interests
The authors declare that they have no competing interests.

Author details
[1]Department of Rheumatology, Affiliated Hospital of Nantong University, 20th Xisi Road, 226001 Nantong, People's Republic of China. [2]Department of Rheumatology, Ruijin Hospital, Shanghai Jiao Tong University School of Medicine, 197 Ruijin 2nd Road, Shanghai 200025, China. [3]School of Nursing, Nantong University, 19th Qixiu Road, 226001 Nantong, People's Republic of China.

References
1. Hakkinen A, Kautiainen H, Hannonen P, Ylinen J, Arkela-Kautiainen M, Sokka T. Pain and joint mobility explain individual subdimensions of the health assessment questionnaire (HAQ) disability index in patients with rheumatoid arthritis. Ann Rheum Dis. 2005;64(1):59–63.
2. Cordingley L, Prajapati R, Plant D, Maskell D, Morgan C, Ali FR, et al. Impact of psychological factors on subjective disease activity assessments in patients with severe rheumatoid arthritis. Arthritis Care Res (Hoboken). 2014; 66(6):861–8.
3. Loza E, Jover JA, Rodriguez L, Carmona L, Group ES. Multimorbidity: prevalence, effect on quality of life and daily functioning, and variation of this effect when one condition is a rheumatic disease. Semin Arthritis Rheum. 2009;38(4):312–9.
4. Trieb K. Treatment of the wrist in rheumatoid arthritis. J Hand Surg Am. 2008;33(1):113–23.
5. Yayama T, Kobayashi S, Kokubo Y, Inukai T, Mizukami Y, Kubota M, et al. Motion analysis of the wrist joints in patients with rheumatoid arthritis. Mod Rheumatol. 2007;17(4):322–6.
6. Vliet Vlieland TP, van den Ende CH, Breedveld FC, Hazes JM. Evaluation of joint mobility in rheumatoid arthritis trials: the value of the EPM-range of motion scale. J Rheumatol. 1993;20(12):2010–4.
7. Khadr Z, Yount K. Differences in self-reported physical limitation among older women and men in Ismailia, Egypt. J Gerontol B Psychol Sci Soc Sci. 2012;67(5):605–17.
8. Goodson A, McGregor AH, Douglas J, Taylor P. Direct, quantitative clinical assessment of hand function: usefulness and reproducibility. Man Ther. 2007;12(2):144–52.
9. Holla JF, Steultjens MP, van der Leeden M, Roorda LD, Bierma-Zeinstra SM, den Broeder AA, et al. Determinants of range of joint motion in patients with early symptomatic osteoarthritis of the hip and/or knee: an exploratory study in the CHECK cohort. Osteoarthr Cartil. 2011;19(4):411–9.
10. Slungaard B, Mengshoel AM. Shoulder function and active motion deficit in patients with rheumatoid arthritis. Disabil Rehabil. 2013;35(16):1357–63.
11. Nishikawa M, Owaki H, Kaneshiro S, Fuji T. Eight-year preservation of knee function with radiographic healing phenomena after anti-tumor necrosis factor-alpha therapy for a severely erosive knee in a young patient with rheumatoid arthritis. Acta Reumatol Port. 2015;40(1):72–6.
12. Wallen M, Gillies D. Intra-articular steroids and splints/rest for children with juvenile idiopathic arthritis and adults with rheumatoid arthritis. Cochrane Database Syst Rev. 2006;1:CD002824.
13. Yoshida A, Higuchi Y, Kondo M, Tabata O, Ohishi M. Range of motion of the temporomandibular joint in rheumatoid arthritis: relationship to the severity of disease. Cranio. 1998;16(3):162–7.
14. Badley EM, Wagstaff S, Wood PH. Measures of functional ability (disability) in arthritis in relation to impairment of range of joint movement. Ann Rheum Dis. 1984;43(4):563–9.
15. Shen B, Tan W, Feng G, He Y, Liu J, Chen W, et al. The correlations of disease activity, socioeconomic status, quality of life, and depression/anxiety in Chinese patients with systemic lupus erythematosus. Clin Dev Immunol. 2013;2013:270878. https://doi.org/10.1155/2013/270878.
16. Shen B, Feng G, Tang W, Huang X, Yan H, He Y, et al. The quality of life in Chinese patients with systemic lupus erythematosus is associated with disease activity and psychiatric disorders: a path analysis. Clin Exp Rheumatol. 2014;32(1):101–7.
17. Syversen SW, Gaarder PI, Goll GL, Odegard S, Haavardsholm EA, Mowinckel P, et al. High anti-cyclic citrullinated peptide levels and an algorithm of four variables predict radiographic progression in patients with rheumatoid arthritis: results from a 10-year longitudinal study. Ann Rheum Dis. 2008; 67(2):212–7.
18. Santiago-Casas Y, Gonzalez-Rivera TC, Castro-Santana LE, Rios G, Martinez D, Rodriguez VE, et al. Impact of age on clinical manifestations and outcome in Puerto Ricans with rheumatoid arthritis. Ethn Dis. 2010;20(1 Suppl 1):S1–191-5.
19. Mangnus L, van Steenbergen HW, Lindqvist E, Brouwer E, Reijnierse M, Huizinga TW, et al. Studies on ageing and the severity of radiographic joint damage in rheumatoid arthritis. Arthritis Res Ther. 2015;17:222.
20. Ickinger C, Musenge E, Tikly M. Patterns and predictors of joint damage as assessed by the rheumatoid arthritis articular damage (RAAD) score in south Africans with established rheumatoid arthritis. Clin Rheumatol. 2013;32(12):1711–7.
21. Baker JF, George M, Baker DG, Toedter G, Von Feldt JM, Leonard MB. Associations between body mass, radiographic joint damage, adipokines and risk factors for bone loss in rheumatoid arthritis. Rheumatology (Oxford). 2011;50(11):2100–7.
22. Vidal C, Barnetche T, Morel J, Combe B, Daien C. Association of Body Mass Index Categories with disease activity and radiographic joint damage in rheumatoid arthritis: a systematic review and Metaanalysis. J Rheumatol. 2015;42(12):2261–9.
23. Molina E, Del Rincon I, Restrepo JF, Battafarano DF, Escalante A. Association of socioeconomic status with treatment delays, disease activity, joint damage, and disability in rheumatoid arthritis. Arthritis Care Res (Hoboken). 2015;67(7):940–6.
24. Terao C, Yamakawa N, Yano K, Markusse IM, Ikari K, Yoshida S, et al. Rheumatoid factor is associated with the distribution of hand joint destruction in rheumatoid arthritis. Arthritis Rheumatol. 2015;67(12):3113–23.
25. Renner N, Kronke G, Rech J, Uder M, Janka R, Lauer L, et al. Anti-citrullinated protein antibody positivity correlates with cartilage damage and proteoglycan levels in patients with rheumatoid arthritis in the hand joints. Arthritis Rheumatol. 2014;66(12):3283–8.
26. Drossaers-Bakker KW, de Buck M, van Zeben D, Zwinderman AH, Breedveld FC, Hazes JM. Long-term course and outcome of functional capacity in rheumatoid arthritis: the effect of disease activity and radiologic damage over time. Arthritis Rheum. 1999;42(9):1854–60.
27. Smolen JS, Van Der Heijde DM, St Clair EW, Emery P, Bathon JM, Keystone E, et al. Predictors of joint damage in patients with early rheumatoid arthritis treated with high-dose methotrexate with or without concomitant infliximab: results from the ASPIRE trial. Arthritis Rheum. 2006;54(3):702–10.
28. Tekaya R, Sahli H, Zribi S, Mahmoud I, Ben Hadj Yahia C, Abdelmoula L, et al. Obesity has a protective effect on radiographic joint damage in rheumatoid arthritis. Tunis Med. 2011;89(5):462–5.
29. Mikuls TR, Payne JB, Yu F, Thiele GM, Reynolds RJ, Cannon GW, et al. Periodontitis and Porphyromonas gingivalis in patients with rheumatoid arthritis. Arthritis Rheumatol. 2014;66(5):1090–100.
30. Aletaha D, Alasti F, Smolen JS. Rheumatoid factor determines structural progression of rheumatoid arthritis dependent and independent of disease activity. Ann Rheum Dis. 2013;72(6):875–80.

31. Lindqvist E, Eberhardt K, Bendtzen K, Heinegard D, Saxne T. Prognostic laboratory markers of joint damage in rheumatoid arthritis. Ann Rheum Dis. 2005;64(2):196–201.

32. van der Heijde DM, van Riel PL, van Leeuwen MA, van 't Hof MA, van Rijswijk MH, van de Putte LB. Prognostic factors for radiographic damage and physical disability in early rheumatoid arthritis. A prospective follow-up study of 147 patients. Br J Rheumatol. 1992;31(8):519–25.

33. Orces CH, Del Rincon I, Abel MP, Escalante A. The number of deformed joints as a surrogate measure of damage in rheumatoid arthritis. Arthritis Rheum. 2002;47(1):67–72.

34. Rossi F, Di Dia F, Galipo O, Pistorio A, Valle M, Magni-Manzoni S, et al. Use of the sharp and Larsen scoring methods in the assessment of radiographic progression in juvenile idiopathic arthritis. Arthritis Rheum. 2006;55(5):717–23.

35. Ji J, Zhang L, Zhang Q, Yin R, Fu T, Li L, et al. Functional disability associated with disease and quality-of-life parameters in Chinese patients with rheumatoid arthritis. Health Qual Life Outcomes. 2017;15:89.

36. Grindulis KA, Calverley M. Grip strength: peak or sustained pressure in rheumatoid arthritis? J Chronic Dis. 1983;36(12):855–8.

37. Welsing PM, van Gestel AM, Swinkels HL, Kiemeney LA, van Riel PL. The relationship between disease activity, joint destruction, and functional capacity over the course of rheumatoid arthritis. Arthritis Rheum. 2001;44(9):2009–17.

38. Wang W, Chair SY, Thompson DR, Twinn SF. A psychometric evaluation of the Chinese version of the hospital anxiety and depression scale in patients with coronary heart disease. J Clin Nurs. 2009;18(17):2436–43.

39. Emery P, Kavanaugh A, Bao Y, Ganguli A, Mulani P. Comprehensive disease control (CDC): what does achieving CDC mean for patients with rheumatoid arthritis? Ann Rheum Dis. 2015;74(12):2165–74.

40. Li L, Wang HM, Shen Y. Chinese SF-36 health survey: translation, cultural adaptation, validation, and normalisation. J Epidemiol Community Health. 2003;57(4):259–63.

41. Prevoo ML, van 't Hof MA, Kuper HH, van Leeuwen MA, van de Putte LB, van Riel PL. Modified disease activity scores that include twenty-eight-joint counts. Development and validation in a prospective longitudinal study of patients with rheumatoid arthritis. Arthritis Rheum. 1995;38(1):44–8.

42. van der Heijde DM, van 't Hof MA, van Riel PL, Theunisse LA, Lubberts EW, van Leeuwen MA, et al. Judging disease activity in clinical practice in rheumatoid arthritis: first step in the development of a disease activity score. Ann Rheum Dis. 1990;49(11):916–20.

43. Sokka T, Kankainen A, Hannonen P. Scores for functional disability in patients with rheumatoid arthritis are correlated at higher levels with pain scores than with radiographic scores. Arthritis Rheum. 2000;43(2):386–9.

44. Kim HH, Kim J, Park SH, Kim SK, Kim OD, Choe JY. Correlation of anti-cyclic citrullinated antibody with hand joint erosion score in rheumatoid arthritis patients. Korean J Intern Med. 2010;25(2):201–6.

45. Fichna J, Janecka A, Costentin J, Do Rego JC. The endomorphin system and its evolving neurophysiological role. Pharmacol Rev. 2007;59(1):88–123.

46. Steultjens MP, Dekker J, van Baar ME, Oostendorp RA, Bijlsma JW. Range of joint motion and disability in patients with osteoarthritis of the knee or hip. Rheumatology (Oxford). 2000;39(9):955–61.

47. Huscher D, Merkesdal S, Thiele K, Zeidler H, Schneider M, Zink A, et al. Cost of illness in rheumatoid arthritis, ankylosing spondylitis, psoriatic arthritis and systemic lupus erythematosus in Germany. Ann Rheum Dis. 2006;65(9):1175–83.

48. Meszaros ZS, Perl A, Faraone SV. Psychiatric symptoms in systemic lupus erythematosus: a systematic review. J Clin Psychiatry. 2012;73(7):993–1001.

49. Stansfeld SA, Head J, Marmot MG. Explaining social class differences in depression and well-being. Soc Psychiatry Psychiatr Epidemiol. 1998;33(1):1–9.

50. Mackenbach JP, Kunst AE, Cavelaars AE, Groenhof F, Geurts JJ. Socioeconomic inequalities in morbidity and mortality in western Europe. The EU Working Group on Socioeconomic Inequalities in Health. Lancet. 1997;349(9066):1655–9.

51. Criswell LA, Katz PP. Relationship of education level to treatment received for rheumatoid arthritis. J Rheumatol. 1994;21(11):2026–33.

52. Michaud K, Wallenstein G, Wolfe F. Treatment and nontreatment predictors of health assessment questionnaire disability progression in rheumatoid arthritis: a longitudinal study of 18,485 patients. Arthritis Care Res (Hoboken). 2011;63(3):366–72.

53. Heiberg T, Kvien TK. Preferences for improved health examined in 1,024 patients with rheumatoid arthritis: pain has highest priority. Arthritis Rheum. 2002;47(4):391–7.

54. Sokka T. Assessment of pain in patients with rheumatic diseases. Best Pract Res Clin Rheumatol. 2003;17(3):427–49.

17

Structural validity of the Dutch version of the disability of arm, shoulder and hand questionnaire (DASH-DLV) in adult patients with hand and wrist injuries

M. E. van Eck(iD), C. M. Lameijer and M. El Moumni[*]

Abstract

Background: Fractures of the hand and wrist are one of the most common injuries seen in adults. The Disabilities of the Arm, Shoulder and Hand (DASH) questionnaire has been developed as a patient-reported assessment of pain and disability to evaluate the outcome after hand and wrist injuries. Patient reported outcomes (PROs) can be interpreted as pain, function or patient satisfaction. To be able to interpret clinical relevance of a PRO, the structural validity and internal consistency is tested. The Dutch version of the DASH has not yet been validated.
The aim of this study was to evaluate the structural validity and the internal consistency of the existing Dutch version of the DASH. The relevance of reporting subscale scores was investigated.

Methods: This study was a retrospective analysis of cross-sectional data of 370 patients with an isolated hand or wrist injury. Adult patients aged 18 to 65 years treated conservatively or surgically were included. Patients unable to understand or read the Dutch language were excluded. Confirmatory factor analysis was used to investigate the structural validity, while Cronbach's alpha and coefficient omega were used to assess internal consistency.

Results: All investigated models (a single factor model, a 3-correlated factor, and a bifactor model) were associated with a good model fit. Both the single factor and the 3-correlated factor model were associated with factor loadings of at least 0.70. In addition, the covariance between the factors in the 3-correlated factor model was positive (at least 0.89) and statistically significant ($p < 0.001$). In the bifactor model, the additional value of subscales was limited as the items loaded high on the general factor but low on the subscale factors.

Conclusion: This study indicates that the Dutch version of the DASH should be considered as an unidimensional trait. A single score should be reported.

Keywords: Disability arm shoulder hand, Hand, Wrist, Structural validity, Confirmatory factor analysis, Bifactor model

Background

Hand and wrist injuries are commonly seen in adults [1–4]. About 20% of all visits to the emergency departments are due to hand and wrist injuries [5, 6]. Considering the ageing of the population, the incidence for these injuries is going to grow [7, 8].

The prevalence of chronic pain following distal radius fractures is reported to be as high as 30%. Of these patients, 11% report moderate to very severe pain 1 year after the initial injury [9, 10]. Longterm disability largely affects elderly patients, of whom 46–95% report some degree of disability 1 year following the initial accident, and 7–16% even report moderate to very severe disability [9, 10]. Aforementioned complaints may result in patients' inability to perform daily activities.

The International Classification of Functioning, Disability and Health, the ICF, provides a standard language and framework for the description of functioning and

[*] Correspondence: m.el.moumni@umcg.nl
University of Groningen, University Medical Center Groningen, Department of Surgery, Groningen, The Netherlands

disability [11]. In the ICF, functioning problems are classified in three areas: Impairments, Activity limitations and Participation restrictions. The broad concept of disability can refer to any or all areas of functioning in the ICF. Patient reported outcomes (PROs) are one of the most common techniques to assess the different facets of functioning. These outcomes are reported by patients and not defined by an observer [12]. They may be used in clinical decisionmaking, as well as in health care policies and reimbursement decisions [13, 14]. To ensure a PRO can be used in clinical practice for these abovementioned functions, they have to be validated. [14]

Recently, recommendations for a core set of domains for standardized reporting in distal radius fractures have been published. [15] Pain and function were considered as primary domains.

In every day practice, mostly traditional outcome measures are used to determine results of treatment. For hand and wrist injuries these include physical examining, range of motion, grip strength and radiographic imaging. These examinations mainly reflect aspects of disability in bodily functions. However, the traditional outcome measures are "clinician based" and do not correlate well with aspects that patients find important, such as activity limitations [16]. Therefore, PROs are increasingly used to evaluate the result of treatment and rehabilitation, also in patients with hand and wrist injuries.

The American Academy of Orthopedic Surgeons, the Council of Musculoskeletal Specialty Societies and the Institute for Work and Health developed a questionnaire which reflects the impact of injury on function of a variety of upper extremity musculoskeletal disorders or injuries and developed the Disabilities of the Arm, Shoulder and Hand, questionnaire (the DASH) [17]. The DASH is a 30-item, self-report questionnaire to measure physical function and symptoms in people with musculoskeletal disorders of the upper limb [17]. The questionnaire consists of 3 subscales: a physical subscale, a symptoms subscale and the psychosocial subscale. The DASH has been translated and adapted into several languages [18–32].

In literature exploratory factor analyses (EFA) have been conducted by several authors in different languages to examine the underlying factors of the DASH questionnaire [22, 23, 33]. EFA is a data-driven method without making specifications about the number of and relationships between the latent factors. This approach is used as an exploratory technique. In contrast, confirmatory factor analysis (CFA) requires strong empirical or conceptual grounds to guide the specification and evaluation of the structure of the model in advance [34]. To date, only two studies reported on CFA of the DASH, which were performed on the Italian and American version of the DASH [35, 36].

In this study, the structural validity of the existing translated Dutch version of the DASH (DASH-DLV) was investigated in a patient population with hand and wrist injuries [37]. Particularly, a CFA was conducted, followed by an assessment of internal consistency. Because Veehof et al. already translated the DASH into a Dutch version, we chose not to translate the DASH again [33].

Methods

Patients
As described previously, adult patients who sustained an isolated hand or wrist injury in 2012 and 2013 were requested to participate in this cross-sectional study [38]. All patients were treated at a level I traumacenter in the Netherlands, either conservatively or surgically. Included patients had to be 18–65 years of age at the time of injury. Exclusion criteria were unability to speak or read Dutch. All of these patients were invited and sent a paper version of the DASH-DLV, and a reminder after 2 weeks, if needed. The local institutional review board (the Medical Ethics Committee of the University Medical Center Groningen) has reviewed the study protocol and waived further need for approval. In addition, the study was performed in compliance with the principles outlined in the Declaration of Helsinki on ethical principles for medical research involving human subjects [39].

Disability of arm, shoulder and hand questionnaire
In 1993, the need for a PRO that reflected the impact of a variety of musculoskeletal diseases and injuries of the upper limb on function was independently identified by researchers from the American Academy of Orthopaedic Surgeons' Outcomes Studies Committee and the Institute for Work & Health [40]. The goal was to develop a self-administered tool that would assess symptoms and physical function at the level of disability, with a focus on physical function, of any or multiple joints or conditions of the upper limb [41]. Item generation and item reduction based on clinimetric and psychometric principles resulted in a 30-item questionnaire [42, 43]. The final 30-item DASH questionnaire includes 21 physical function items, six symptom items and three social/role function items, plus the optional four-item work and sports/performing arts modules.

Structural validity and internal consistency
Structural validity, defined as the degree to which scores of an instrument are an adequate reflection of the dimensionality of the construct to be measured, of the DASH-DLV was assessed by CFA [44]. A single factor model of the DASH-DLV (Fig. 1), and a correlated 3-factor model (*Physical Function, Symptom and Psychosocial* subscale, Fig. 2) were explored. In addition, a bifactor model was investigated (Fig. 3). A bifactor model

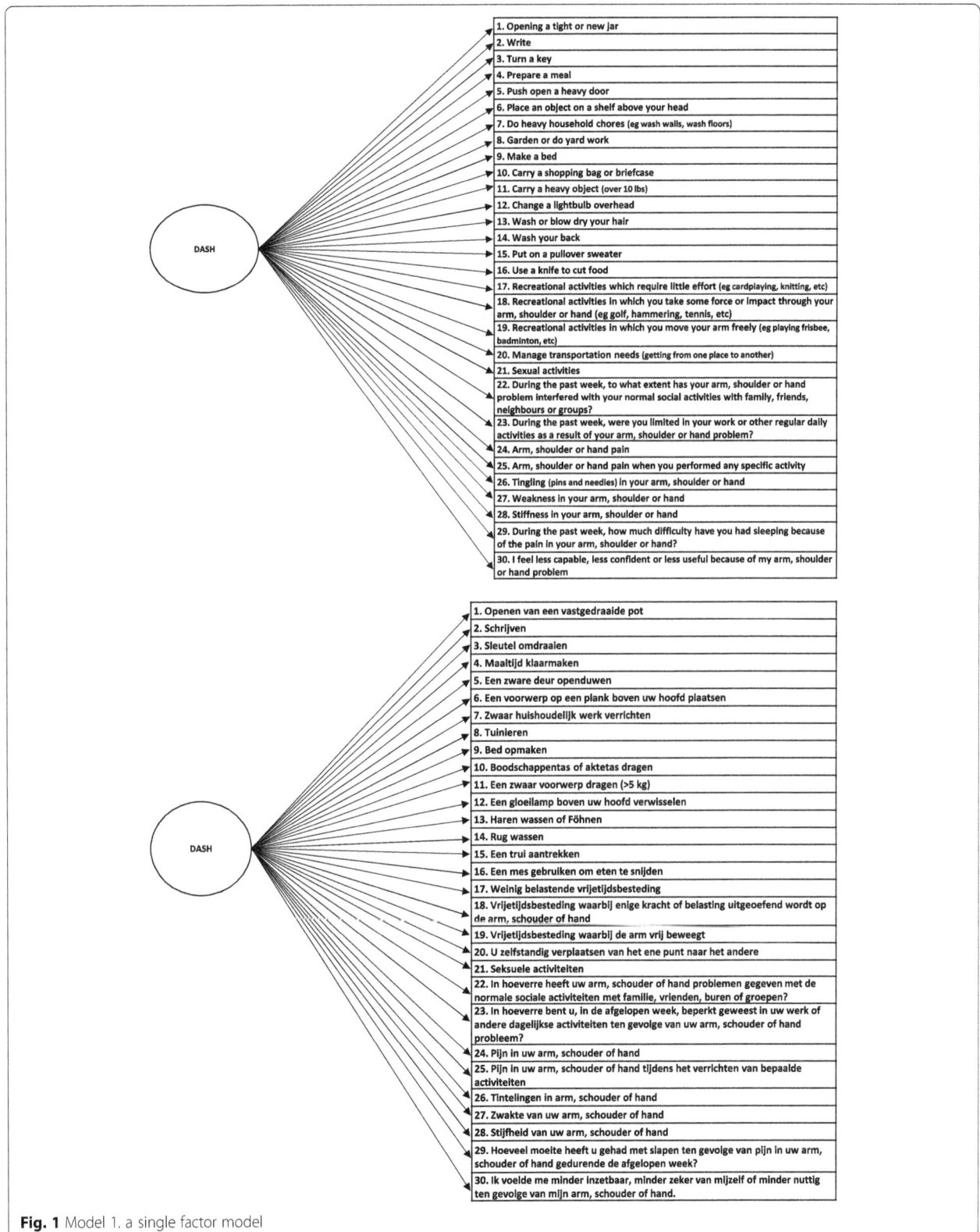

1. Opening a tight or new jar
2. Write
3. Turn a key
4. Prepare a meal
5. Push open a heavy door
6. Place an object on a shelf above your head
7. Do heavy household chores (eg wash walls, wash floors)
8. Garden or do yard work
9. Make a bed
10. Carry a shopping bag or briefcase
11. Carry a heavy object (over 10 lbs)
12. Change a lightbulb overhead
13. Wash or blow dry your hair
14. Wash your back
15. Put on a pullover sweater
16. Use a knife to cut food
17. Recreational activities which require little effort (eg cardplaying, knitting, etc)
18. Recreational activities in which you take some force or impact through your arm, shoulder or hand (eg golf, hammering, tennis, etc)
19. Recreational activities in which you move your arm freely (eg playing frisbee, badminton, etc)
20. Manage transportation needs (getting from one place to another)
21. Sexual activities
22. During the past week, to what extent has your arm, shoulder or hand problem interfered with your normal social activities with family, friends, neighbours or groups?
23. During the past week, were you limited in your work or other regular daily activities as a result of your arm, shoulder or hand problem?
24. Arm, shoulder or hand pain
25. Arm, shoulder or hand pain when you performed any specific activity
26. Tingling (pins and needles) in your arm, shoulder or hand
27. Weakness in your arm, shoulder or hand
28. Stiffness in your arm, shoulder or hand
29. During the past week, how much difficulty have you had sleeping because of the pain in your arm, shoulder or hand?
30. I feel less capable, less confident or less useful because of my arm, shoulder or hand problem

1. Openen van een vastgedraaide pot
2. Schrijven
3. Sleutel omdraaien
4. Maaltijd klaarmaken
5. Een zware deur openduwen
6. Een voorwerp op een plank boven uw hoofd plaatsen
7. Zwaar huishoudelijk werk verrichten
8. Tuinieren
9. Bed opmaken
10. Boodschappentas of aktetas dragen
11. Een zwaar voorwerp dragen (>5 kg)
12. Een gloeilamp boven uw hoofd verwisselen
13. Haren wassen of Föhnen
14. Rug wassen
15. Een trui aantrekken
16. Een mes gebruiken om eten te snijden
17. Weinig belastende vrijetijdsbesteding
18. Vrijetijdsbesteding waarbij enige kracht of belasting uitgeoefend wordt op de arm, schouder of hand
19. Vrijetijdsbesteding waarbij de arm vrij beweegt
20. U zelfstandig verplaatsen van het ene punt naar het andere
21. Seksuele activiteiten
22. In hoeverre heeft uw arm, schouder of hand problemen gegeven met de normale sociale activiteiten met familie, vrienden, buren of groepen?
23. In hoeverre bent u, in de afgelopen week, beperkt geweest in uw werk of andere dagelijkse activiteiten ten gevolge van uw arm, schouder of hand probleem?
24. Pijn in uw arm, schouder of hand
25. Pijn in uw arm, schouder of hand tijdens het verrichten van bepaalde activiteiten
26. Tintelingen in arm, schouder of hand
27. Zwakte van uw arm, schouder of hand
28. Stijfheid van uw arm, schouder of hand
29. Hoeveel moeite heeft u gehad met slapen ten gevolge van pijn in uw arm, schouder of hand gedurende de afgelopen week?
30. Ik voelde me minder inzetbaar, minder zeker van mijzelf of minder nuttig ten gevolge van mijn arm, schouder of hand.

Fig. 1 Model 1. a single factor model

includes a general factor associated with all test items and one or more group factors associated with a limited number of items [45] The general factor and group factors are assumed to be uncorrelated. Bifactor models may be used when subscores are expected. Bifactor models are valuable in determining the contribution of subscale scores over and

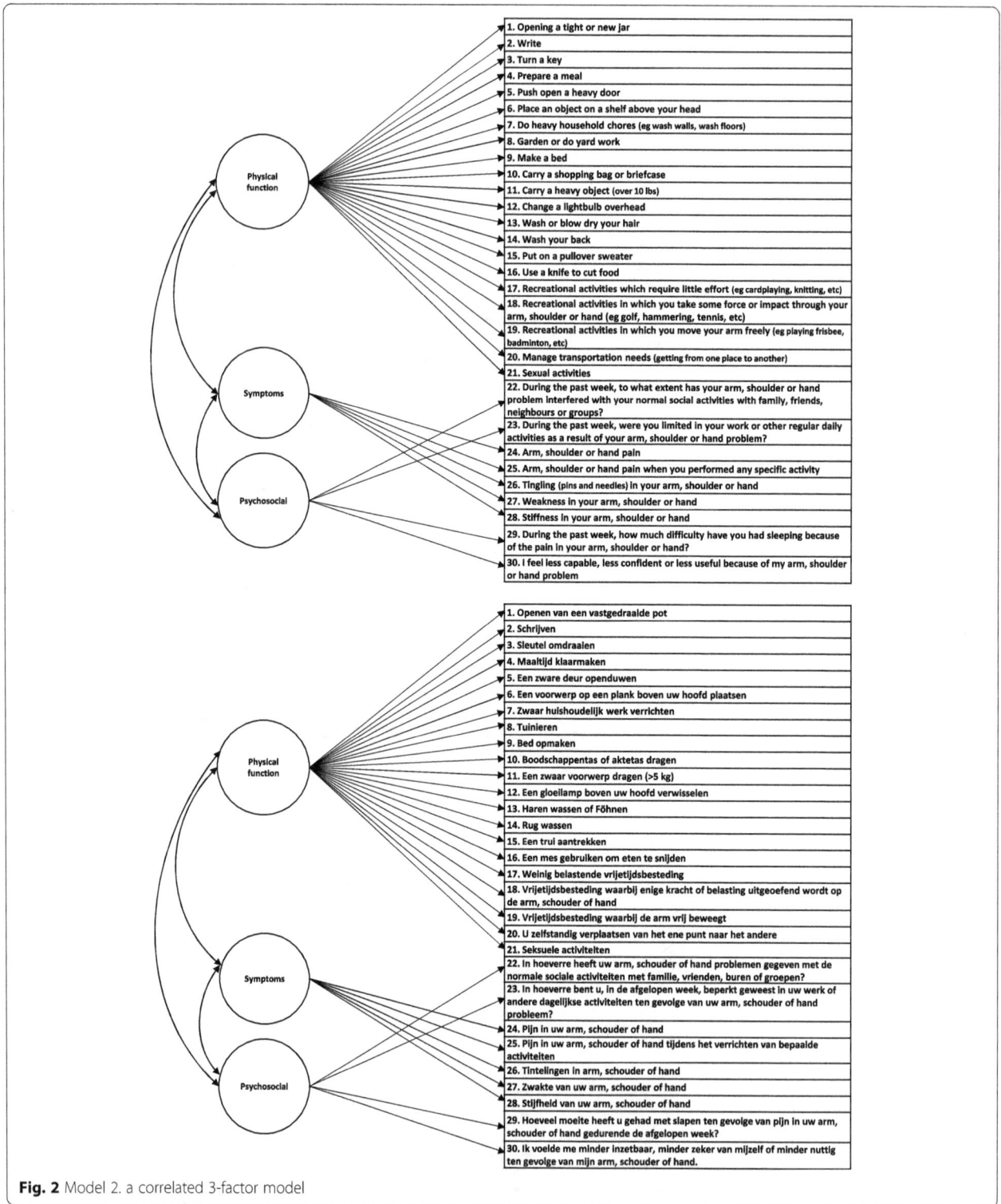

Fig. 2 Model 2. a correlated 3-factor model

above the general factor [46]. All the investigated DASH-DLV models are presented in Figs. 1, 2 and 3.

Internal consistency examines to what degree the items in a questionnaire are interrelated, and measure the same construct [47]. In this study, the internal consistency was determined after conducting a factor analysis to verify the dimensionality. Two approaches were used. First, Crohnbach's α was calculated for each (sub) scale. It represents a ratio between the true score variance and the total variance. [47] However, Crohnbach's

Physical function

1. Opening a tight or new jar
2. Write
3. Turn a key
4. Prepare a meal
5. Push open a heavy door
6. Place an object on a shelf above your head
7. Do heavy household chores (eg wash walls, wash floors)
8. Garden or do yard work
9. Make a bed
10. Carry a shopping bag or briefcase
11. Carry a heavy object (over 10 lbs)
12. Change a lightbulb overhead
13. Wash or blow dry your hair
14. Wash your back
15. Put on a pullover sweater
16. Use a knife to cut food
17. Recreational activities which require little effort (eg cardplaying, knitting, etc)
18. Recreational activities in which you take some force or impact through your arm, shoulder or hand (eg golf, hammering, tennis, etc)
19. Recreational activities in which you move your arm freely (eg playing frisbee, badminton, etc)
20. Manage transportation needs (getting from one place to another)
21. Sexual activities
22. During the past week, to what extent has your arm, shoulder or hand problem interfered with your normal social activities with family, friends, neighbours or groups?
23. During the past week, were you limited in your work or other regular daily activities as a result of your arm, shoulder or hand problem?
24. Arm, shoulder or hand pain
25. Arm, shoulder or hand pain when you performed any specific activity
26. Tingling (pins and needles) in your arm, shoulder or hand
27. Weakness in your arm, shoulder or hand
28. Stiffness in your arm, shoulder or hand
29. During the past week, how much difficulty have you had sleeping because of the pain in your arm, shoulder or hand?
30. I feel less capable, less confident or less useful because of my arm, shoulder or hand problem

Symptoms · Psychosocial · General

Physical function

1. Openen van een vastgedraaide pot
2. Schrijven
3. Sleutel omdraaien
4. Maaltijd klaarmaken
5. Een zware deur openduwen
6. Een voorwerp op een plank boven uw hoofd plaatsen
7. Zwaar huishoudelijk werk verrichten
8. Tuinieren
9. Bed opmaken
10. Boodschappentas of aktetas dragen
11. Een zwaar voorwerp dragen (>5 kg)
12. Een gloeilamp boven uw hoofd verwisselen
13. Haren wassen of Föhnen
14. Rug wassen
15. Een trui aantrekken
16. Een mes gebruiken om eten te snijden
17. Weinig belastende vrijetijdsbesteding
18. Vrijetijdsbesteding waarbij enige kracht of belasting uitgeoefend wordt op de arm, schouder of hand
19. Vrijetijdsbesteding waarbij de arm vrij beweegt
20. U zelfstandig verplaatsen van het ene punt naar het andere
21. Seksuele activiteiten
22. In hoeverre heeft uw arm, schouder of hand problemen gegeven met de normale sociale activiteiten met familie, vrienden, buren of groepen?
23. In hoeverre bent u, in de afgelopen week, beperkt geweest in uw werk of andere dagelijkse activiteiten ten gevolge van uw arm, schouder of hand probleem?
24. Pijn in uw arm, schouder of hand
25. Pijn in uw arm, schouder of hand tijdens het verrichten van bepaalde activiteiten
26. Tintelingen in arm, schouder of hand
27. Zwakte van uw arm, schouder of hand
28. Stijfheid van uw arm, schouder of hand
29. Hoeveel moeite heeft u gehad met slapen ten gevolge van pijn in uw arm, schouder of hand gedurende de afgelopen week?
30. Ik voelde me minder inzetbaar, minder zeker van mijzelf of minder nuttig ten gevolge van mijn arm, schouder of hand.

Symptoms · Psychosocial · General

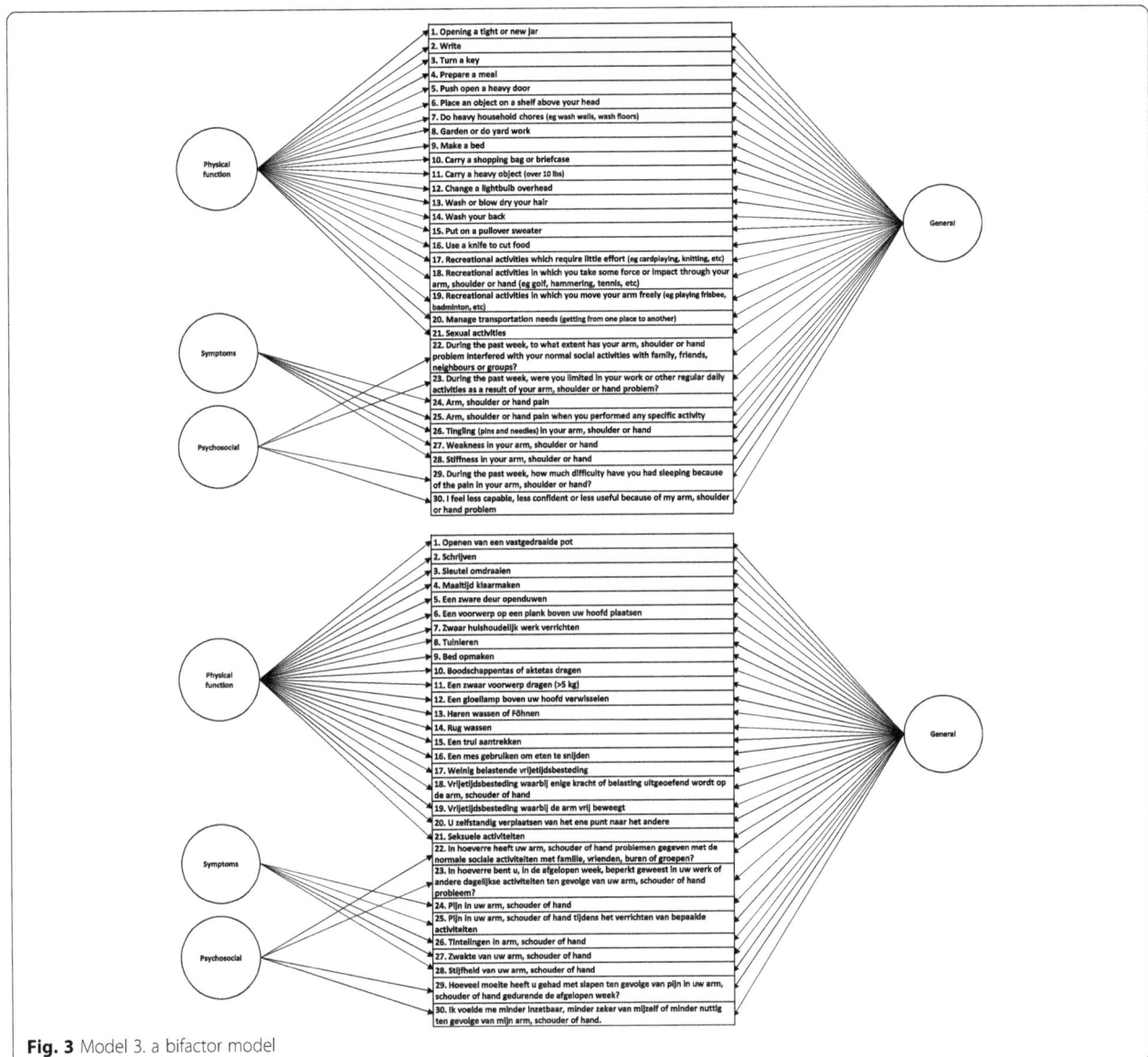

Fig. 3 Model 3. a bifactor model

α tends to overestimate the reliability of the general factor in a multidimensional data structure and can therefore be misleading in bifactor models [48–50]. Preferably, the coefficient omega total (ω_T), and omega hierarchical (ω_H) are used to estimate the internal consistency in a bifactor model [48, 51].

Omega total (ω_T) is an estimation of the reliability of a factor combining the general factor and the group factor variance. Omega hierarchical (ω_H) coefficient gives the proportion of variance in scale scores accounted for by a general factor [51]. The coefficient ω_H can be extended to estimate the reliability of the group factors, controlling for that part of the reliability due to the general factor in a bifactor model, termed omega subscale (ω_S) [49, 50]. These coefficients provide useful information to judge whether scores for a group factor can be interpreted with confidence or only the total score (general factor) should be reported. A Cronbach's α, coefficient omega total, omega hierarchical, or omega subscale of 0.70–0.95 were considered an appropriate reliability.

To evaluate whether our data is 'unidimensional enough', two 'factor strength' indices were calculated. [50] First, we used coefficient omega hierarchical. [51] A high ω_H value indicates that a composite score is reflected by a single common source, i.e. one common factor underlies item responses. In addition, we calculated the Explained Common Variance (ECV), which is the ratio of the variance explained by the general factor, divided by the variance explained by the general factor and the group factors. There are no criteria for ECV to determine whether the data is unidimensional enough, but a higher ECV is seen as a stronger indication for unidimensionality [52].

Statistical analyses

For validating a questionnaire, there are numerous ways to determine the sample size [53]. In this study, a sample size of 300 cases was chosen, as Comrey and Lee recommend for conducting a factor analysis [54]. Confirmatory factor analyses were conducted using the R's package *lavaan* [55, 56].

The robust weighed least squares means and variance (WLSMV) estimator with mean- and variance-adjustment was used to fit the models. Completely standardized results were used to report the factor loadings and covariances.

For each model, the χ^2 goodness-of-fit statistic was computed as the test of global fit. However, this statistic calculation is sensitive to the sample size. Four other commonly used fit indices were calculated as well to evaluate model fit. These indices included the comparative fit index (CFI), the Tucker-Lewis Index (TLI), the root mean square error of approximation (RMSEA), and the standardized root mean square residual (SRMR). A CFI and TLI close to 0.95 or higher, a RMSEA close to or less than 0.06, and a SRMR close to or less than 0.08 were considered as adequate model fit [57].

Results

As described previously, a cohort of 466 patients who sustained isolated hand or wrist injury were eligible, of which 370 (79.4%) patients (188 males and 182 females) participated in the current study, with a mean age of 43.6 (SD = 14.2) years [38]. The majority of the hand and wrist injuries (82%) were treated conservatively. A large proportion of the injuries were fractures, mainly of distal radius (130/334) (Table 1). The follow-up time ranged from 1 to 25 months. The DASH-DLV questionnaire was completely filled in by 329 of the responders (88.9%). Sixteen patients (4.3%) had a missing response on the item "sexual activities". The rest of the items were missing in less than 3%. Total scores could be calculated according to the DASH manual for all patients [40].

The 3 CFA models with corresponding fit statistics are presented in Table 2, the standardized factor loadings are presented in Table 3. Although associated with a

Table 1 Frequencies of hand and wrist injuries

Injury	Frequency (%)
Distal radius fractures	132 (35.7)
Carpal fractures	44 (11.9)
Metacarpal fractures	61 (16.5)
Phalangeal fractures	99 (26.8)
Finger joint dislocations	31 (8.4)
Others	3 (0.8)
Total	370

significant χ^2 goodness-of-fit (584.83, df = 405, $p < 0.001$) adequate levels of absolute (RMSEA and SRMR) and incremental fit indexes (CFI and TLI) were calculated for Fig. 1. All factor loadings for this model were higher than 0.70 (Table 3).

Figure 2 also yielded a significant χ^2 goodness-of-fit value (498.12, df = 402, $p = 0.001$), but satisfactory absolute and incremental fit indexes. In Fig. 2, all items loaded high on one of the three correlated subscale factors *Physical*, *Symptoms* and *Psychosocial*. The factor loadings ranged from 0.75 to 0.95. Only 5 and 4 items loaded on subscale factors *Symptoms* and *Psychosocial*, respectively. The covariance between the correlated factors was positive and statistically significant (*Physical* versus *Symptoms* = 0.89, *Physical* versus *Psychosocial* = 0.94, *Symptoms* versus *Psychosocial* = 0.92, all p-values< 0.001).

The bifactor Fig. 3 was associated with good levels of model fit indexes: χ^2 value of 419.96 (df = 375, $p = 0.054$), RMSEA = 0.018, SRMR = 0.041, CFI = 0.998, TLI = 0.998.

However, in Fig. 3, many items loaded high (ranging from 0.69 to 0.93) on the general factor, but low on the subscale factors (Table 3). As an example, the correlated model (Fig. 2) suggests that item 8 'Garden or do yard work' was a strong indicator of the *Physical* subscale (i.e. a factor loading of 0.93). In contrast, Fig. 3 (the bifactor model) indicated that item 8 was a weak indicator (i.e. a factor loading of 0.06).

The ECV is 0.92 in Fig. 3. The factor strength indexes are also presented in Table 3. The coefficient ω_H was high for the general factor (0.96), but ω_S was low for the group factors (*Phyical*, *Symptoms* and *Psychosocial*; which were 0.01, 0.26 and 0.11 respectively). These results indicate that a large portion of the total variance is explained by the general factor, and only a very small portion of the total variance is explained by subscale factors. Regarding internal consistency, Crohnbach's α of the single and the 3-correlated factor models (Figs. 1 and 2) were high, ranging from 0.88 to 0.97. These findings suggest that the DASH-DLV measures a single factor model and that it is not beneficial to report subscale scores.

Discussion

The various CFA models were used to clarify how the items of the DASH-DLV relate to each other, and to explore if there were any subscale scores that should be used when scoring the questionnaire. This study suggests that the DASH-DLV reflects a unidimensional trait, and thus reporting subscale scores in the Dutch translation of the DASH is of very limited value and should be avoided.

The Upper Extremity Collaboration Group used principle component analysis to determine the dimensionality of the DASH. Although a two-factor model explained more variance and the scree plot suggested two

Table 2 Fit statistics for the 3 CFA models

	Chi-squared goodness of fit	df	p	RMSEA (90% confidence interval)	SRMR	CFI	TLI
Model 1	584.83	405	0.000	0.035 (0.028–0.041)	0.055	0.993	0.992
Model 2	498.12	402	0.001	0.026 (0.017–0.033)	0.050	0.996	0.996
Model 3	419.96	375	0.054	0.018 (0.000–0.027)	0.041	0.998	0.998

df degrees of freedom, *p* = *p* value, *RMSEA* root mean square error of approximation, *CFI* comparative fit index, *TLI* tucker-Lewis index, *SRMR* standardized root mean square residual

factors, a one-factor model is recommended given its simplicity [40].

While principal component analysis aims to explain all variance in the data set, making it most appropriately applied as a data reduction technique, EFA is used to only explain the common variance of all items, discovering a set of yet unknown latent variables based on the data. In contrast, confirmatory factor analysis makes it possible to test whether the data fit a prehypothesized factor structure based on empirical data or theory, making this technique more appropriate to confirm the factor structure (i.e. dimensionality) of a questionnaire. The choice for a particular method of factor analysis is crucial, because the different techniques have different assumptions about the data and answer different research questions [58].

In this study, we used CFA since our reseach question was to confirm the factor structure of the DASH-DLV. To our knowledge, only two studies have conducted CFA to examine the DASH questionnaire [35, 36]. Franchignoni et al. investigated the factor structure of the Italian version of the DASH [35]. After an exploratory approach, the 3-factor structure showed adequate fit, nonetheless with some misfitting items. A 1-factor model of the DASH was not confirmed as indicated by poor fit statistics.

In the American version, Lehman et al. also tested a 3-factor model after excluding item 20 and 21 because of their unacceptably low factor loadings [36]. Although the TLI and SRMR values indicated good fit, the CFI and RMSEA do not. In addition, they found high inter-factor correlations (> 0.83).

All models in our study yielded adequate fit to the data (Table 2). Both Fig. 1 (one-factor) and Fig. 2 (3-correlated factors) showed high and statistically significant factor loadings. However, the subscales *Symptoms* and *Psychosocial* of Fig. 2 included only 3 and 2 items, respectively, potentially compromising the coverage of the construct's theoretical domain. All items in the bifactor model (Fig. 3) were associated with high factor loadings on the general factor, but low on the group factors. Bifactor analysis allows researchers to empirically examine the appropriateness of using subscales. To date, research in assessing the structural validity of DASH has not included bifactor models.

Several important findings support that the DASH-DLV is sufficiently unidimensional. First, the covariance between the 3 correlated factors in Fig. 2 were all positive and significant, indicating unidimensionality. Second, the factor loadings of the general factor in the bifactor model (Fig. 3) are very similar to the loadings in the single factor model (Fig. 1). Furthermore, the factor loadings are high and statistically significant on the general factor, but substantially lower on the group factors. This suggests that the subscale factor contribution 'over and above' the general factor is very limited. [46] Third, the general factor of Fig. 3 accounted for more than 90% (ECV = 0.92) of the common variance, indicating a high degree of unidimensionally. Finally, although the coefficient omega total values estimated in the bifactor model showed very good reliability for the general and subscale factors, the values of omega hierarchical of the general factor differed significantly from the omega subscale of the subscale factors. Omega hierarchical (ω_H) coefficient gives the proportion of variance in scale scores accounted for by a general factor, whereas the omega subscale represents the reliability estimate of the subscales, accounting for the effects of the reliability due to the general factor in bifactor models [51, 59]. The coefficient omega hierarchical therefore provides useful information on whether scores for subscale factors can be interpreted with confidence, or that only the general factor score should be used. In this study, ω_S was very low for the subscale factors (ranging 0.01–0.26), but ω_H was high (0.96) for the general factor. This indicates that the subscale factors account for only 1 to 26%, while the general factor accounts for 96% of the variance. This implies that reporting subscale scores in the DASH-DLV is of extremely limited value.

This study has some limitations. The patients who were included mainly experienced distal radius fractures, and were mostly treated non-surgically. This distribution of patients may limit the generalizability of the results. For this study, we only included trauma cases and no elective cases. This may have caused a selection bias towards elderly females. In addition, an existing Dutch translation of the DASH questionnaire was used without employing a translation and culturally adaptation process. However, this Dutch version is widely used and supported by the Institute for Work & Health [37]. Despite these limitations, the response rate was sufficiently high and an adequate sample size was included. There was only a small number of missing values, from which total scores for all patients could still be calculated according to the DASH manual. [40] Finally, future studies should assess

Table 3 Factorloadings of the 3 different confirmatory factor models

	Correlated factor model				Bifactor model			
	Model 1 1-factor	Model 2 3-factor			Model 3 Bifactor (3-factor)			
Item	λ_1	λ_1	λ_2	λ_3	λ_G	λ_{g1}	λ_{g2}	λ_{g3}
	DASH	Physical	Symptoms	Psychosocial				
1	0.84	0.85			0.84	0.13[a]		
2	0.78	0.79			0.79	−0.13[a]		
3	0.82	0.83			0.83	−0.04[a]		
4	0.88	0.89			0.88	−0.17[a]		
5	0.85	0.85			0.85	0.24[a]		
6	0.90	0.90			0.90	−0.05[a]		
7	0.91	0.92			0.91	0.12		
8	0.92	0.93			0.93	0.06[a]		
9	0.90	0.90			0.90	−0.07[a]		
10	0.93	0.94			0.89	0.36		
11	0.91	0.92			0.88	0.40		
12	0.88	0.88			0.88	−0.10[a]		
13	0.85	0.85			0.83	−0.34[a]		
14	0.85	0.85			0.85	−0.18[a]		
15	0.89	0.90			0.88	−0.38[a]		
16	0.85	0.85			0.86	−0.17[a]		
17	0.88	0.90			0.89	−0.16[a]		
18	0.89	0.90			0.90	0.03[a]		
19	0.91	0.92			0.92	0.07[a]		
20	0.88	0.89			0.87	−0.25[a]		
21	0.80	0.81			0.80	−0.12[a]		
22	0.86			0.89	0.86			0.08[a]
23	0.90			0.94	0.89			0.37[a]
24	0.90		0.93		0.83		0.57	
25	0.91		0.95		0.86		0.37	
26	0.71		0.75		0.69		0.25	
27	0.89		0.95		0.88		0.22	
28	0.80		0.84		0.78		0.30	
29	0.86			0.89	0.86			0.09[a]
30	0.91			0.94	0.90			0.36[a]
$(\Sigma\lambda^2)$	25.10	16.28	3.94	3.35	22.31	0.88	0.66	0.28
ECV					0.92			
α	0.97	0.96	0.91	0.88				
ω_T					0.98†	0.97†	0.91†	0.90†
ω_H					0.96†			
ω_s						0.01†	0.26†	0.11†

Factor loadings are completely standardized estimates. All factor loadings were statistically significant except those marked with [a]. G general factor, g group factor, λ factor loading, ECV explained common variance, a cronbach's alpha, ω_T omega total, and ω_H omega hierarchical, ω_S omega subscale. †$p < 0.001$

validity in more detail, and other measurement properties of the DASH, such as test-retest reliability and responsiveness, should be evaluated.

Conclusions

In conclusion, this study suggests that the DASH-DLV reflects a unidimensional trait, and thus reporting subscale scores in the Dutch translation of the DASH is of very limited value and should be avoided. Further studies should assess the validity of the DASH-DLV in more detail, as well as other measurement properties, such as test-retest, reliability, measurement error and responsiveness, to ensure reliable interpretation of this patient reported outcome measure in clinical practice.

Abbreviations

CFA: Confirmatory factor analysis; CFI: Comparative fit index; DASH: Disability of arm shoulder and hand questionnaire; DASH-DLV: Disability of arm shoulder and hand questionnaire Dutch language version; df: Degrees of freedom; ECV: Explained common variance; EFA: Exploratory factor analysis; ICF: The International Classification of Functioning, Disability and Health; PRO: Patient rated outcome; RMSEA: Root mean square error of approximation; SD: Standard deviation; SRMR: Standardized root mean square residual; TLI: Tucker Lewis index; WLSMV: Weighed least squares means and variance

Authors' contributions

ME, CM and MM have contributed substantially to the conception and design of the study, acquisition of data, analysis and interpretation of the data. They all have approved the final version of this manuscript.

Competing interests

The authors declare that they have no competing interests.

References

1. Nellans KW, Kowalski E, Chung KC. The epidemiology of distal radius fractures. Hand Clin. 2012;28(2):113–25. https://doi.org/10.1016/j.hcl.2012.02.001.
2. Feehan L, Sheps S. Incidence and demographics of hand fractures in British Columbia, Canada: a population-based study. J Hand Surg Am. 2006;31(7):1068–74.
3. Ootes D, Lambers KT, Ring DC. The epidemiology of upper extremity injuries presenting to the emergency department in the United States. Hand. 2012;7(1):18–22. https://doi.org/10.1007/s11552-011-9383-z.
4. van Onselen E, Karim R, Hage J, Ritt M. Prevalence and distribution of hand fractures. J Hand Surg Br. 2003;28(5):491–5.
5. Larsen CF, Mulder S, Johansen AMT, Stam C. The epidemiology of hand injuries in the Netherlands and Denmark. Eur J Epidemiol. 2004;19(4):323–7. https://doi.org/10.1023/B:EJEP.0000024662.32024.e3.
6. Angermann P, Lohmann M. Injuries to the hand and wrist. A study of 50,272 injuries. J Hand Surg Am. 1993;18(5):642–4. https://doi.org/10.1016/0266-7681(93)90024-A.
7. Shauver MJ, Yin H, Banerjee M, Chung KC. Current and future National Costs to Medicare for the treatment of distal radius fracture in the elderly. J Hand Surg Am. 2011;36:1282–7. https://doi.org/10.1016/j.jhsa.2011.05.017.
8. De Putter CE, Selles RW, Polinder S, et al. Epidemiology and health-care utilisation of wrist fractures in older adults in the Netherlands, 1997-2009. Injury. 2013;44(4):421–6. https://doi.org/10.1016/j.injury.2012.10.025.
9. MacDermid JC, Roth JH, Richards RS. Pain and disability reported in the year following a distal radius fracture: a cohort study. BMC Musculoskelet Disord. 2003;4:24. https://doi.org/10.1186/1471-2474-4-24.
10. Moore CM, Leonardi-Bee J. The prevalence of pain and disability one year post fracture of the distal radius in a UK population: a cross sectional survey. BMC Musculoskelet Disord. 2008;9:129. https://doi.org/10.1186/1471-2474-9-129.
11. WHO. How to use the ICF: a practical manual for using the International Classification of Functioning, Disability and Health (ICF). http://www.who.int/classifications/icf/en/. Published 2013.
12. Calvert M, Blazeby J, Altman DG, et al. Reporting of patient-reported outcomes in randomized trials: the CONSORT PRO extension. JAMA. 2013;309(8):814–22.
13. Greenhalgh J, Dalkin S, Gooding K. Functionality and feedback: a realist synthesis of the collation, interpretation and utilisation of patient-reported outcome measures data to improve patient care. Heal Serv Deliv Res. 2017; 5(2) https://doi.org/10.3310/hsdr05020

14. Holmes MM, Lewith G, Newell D, Field J, Bishop FL. The impact of patient-reported outcome measures in clinical practice for pain: a systematic review. Qual Life Res. 2016;26(2):1–13. https://doi.org/10.1007/s11136-016-1449-5.
15. Goldhahn J, Beaton D, Ladd A, Macdermid J, Hoang-Kim A. Recommendation for measuring clinical outcome in distal radius fractures: a core set of domains for standardized reporting in clinical practice and research. Arch Orthop Trauma Surg. 2014;134(2):197–205.
16. Lameijer C, ten Duis H, van Dusseldorp I, Dijkstra P, van der Sluis C. Prevalence of posttraumatic arthritis and the association with outcome measures following distal radius fractures in young non-osteoporotic patients. A systematic review. Arch Orthop Trauma Surg. 2017;137(11):1499–513.
17. Hudak PL, Amadio PC, Bombardier C. Development of an upper extremity outcome measure: the DASH (disabilities of the arm, shoulder and hand) [corrected]. The upper extremity collaborative group (UECG). Am J Ind Med. 1996;29(6):602–8. https://doi.org/10.1002/(SICI)1097-0274(199606)29:6<602::AID-AJIM4>3.0.CO;2-L.
18. Atroshi I, Gummesson C. The Disabilities of the Arm , Shoulder and Hand (DASH) outcome questionnaire. Acta Orthop Scand. 2000;6:613–8.
19. Cheng H, Sampaio R, Mancini M. Disabilities of the arm, shoulder and hand (DASH): factor analysis of the version adapted to Portuguese/Brazil. Disabil Rehabil. 2008;30(25):1901–9.
20. Chen H, Ji X, Zhang W, Zhang Y, Zhang L, Tang P. Validation of the simplified Chinese (mainland) version of the disability of the arm, shoulder, and hand questionnaire (DASH-CHNPLAGH). J Orthop Surg Res. 2015;10(5):76.
21. Haldorsen B, Svege I, Roe Y, Bergland A. Reliability and validity of the Norwegian version of the disabilities of the arm, shoulder and hand questionnaire in patients with shoulder impingement syndrome. BMC Musculoskelet Disord. 2014;15(5):78.
22. Fayad F, Lefevre-Colau M, Mace Y. Validation of the French version of the disability of the arm, shoulder and hand questionnaire (F-DASH). Joint Bone Spine. 2008;75:195–200.
23. Lee EWC, Chung MMH, Li APS, Lo SK. Construct validity of the Chinese version of the disabilities of the arm, shoulder and hand questionnaire (DASH-HKPWH). J Hand Surg Am. 2005;30(1):29–34. https://doi.org/10.1016/j.jhsb.2004.09.010.
24. Lee JY, Lim JY, Oh JH, Ko YM. Cross-cultural adaptation and clinical evaluation of a Korean version of the disabilities of arm, shoulder, and hand outcome questionnaire (K-DASH). J Shoulder Elb Surg. 2008;17(4):570–4.
25. Liang HW, Wang HK, Yao G, Horng YS, Hou SM. Psychometric evaluation of the Taiwan version of the disability of the arm, shoulder, and hand (DASH) questionnaire. J Formos Med Assoc. 2004;103(10):773–9.
26. Mousavi SJ, Parnianpour M, Abedi M, et al. Cultural adaptation and validation of the Persian version of the disabilities of the arm, shoulder and hand (DASH) outcome measure. Clin Rehabil. 2008;22(8):749–57.
27. Mulero-Portela AL, Colón-Santaella CL, Cruz-Gómez C. Cross-cultural adaptation of the disability of arm, shoulder, and hand questionnaire: Spanish for Puerto Rico version. Int J Rehabil Res. 2009;32(4):287–93.
28. Offenbacher M, Ewert T, Sanga O, Stucki G. Validation of a German version of the "disabilities of arm, shoulder and hand" questionnaire (DASH-G). Z Rheumatol. 2003;62:168–77.
29. Orfale AG, Araújo PM, Ferraz MB, Natour J. Translation into Brazilian Portuguese, cultural adaptation and evaluation of the reliability of the disabilities of the arm, shoulder and hand questionnaire. Braz J Med Biol Res. 2005;38(2):293–302.
30. Padua R, Padua L, Ceccarelli E. Italian version of the disability of the arm, shoulder and hand (DASH) questionnaire. Cross-cultural adaptation and validation. J Hand Surg Am. 2003;28(2):179–86.
31. Themistocleous GS, Goudelis G, Kyrou I, et al. Translation into Greek, cross-cultural adaptation and validation of the disabilities of the arm, shoulder, and hand questionnaire (DASH). J Hand Ther. 2006;19(3):350–7.
32. Tongprasert S, Rapipong J, Buntragulpoontawee M. The cross-cultural adaptation of the DASH questionnaire in Thai (DASH-TH). J Hand Ther. 2014; 27(1):49–54. https://doi.org/10.1016/j.jht.2013.08.020.
33. Veehof M, Sleegers E, van Veldhoven N. Psychometric qualities of the Dutch language version of the disabilities of the arm, shoulder and hand questionnaire (DASH-DLV). J Hand Ther. 2002;15:347–54.
34. Streiner DL. Figuring out factors: the use and misuse of factor analysis. Can J Psychiatr. 1994;39(3):135–40.
35. Franchignoni F, Giordano A, Sartorio F, Vercelli S, Pascariello B, Ferriero G. Suggestions for refinement of the disabilities of the arm, shoulder and hand

outcome measure (DASH): a factor analysis and Rasch validation study. Arch Phys Med Rehabil. 2010;91:1370–7.

36. Lehman LA, Woodbury M, Velozo CA. Examination of the factor structure of the disabilities of the arm, shoulder, and hand questionnaire. Am J Occup Ther. 2011;65(2):169–78. https://doi.org/10.5014/ajot.2011.000794.

37. Schuurman A, Sleegers E. The DASH-DLV: Institute for Work & Health. http://www.dash.iwh.on.ca/available-translations?field_language_tid=dutch. Published; 2003.

38. El Moumni M, Van Eck ME, Wendt KW, Reininga IHF, Mokkink LB. Structural validity of the Dutch version of the patient-rated wrist evaluation (PRWE-NL) in patients with hand and wrist injuries. Phys Ther. 2016;96(6):908–16. https://doi.org/10.2522/ptj.20140589.

39. WMA Declaration of Helsinki - Ethical Principles for Medical Research Involving Human Subjects. World Medical Association. https://www.wma.net/policies-post/wma-declaration-of-helsinki-ethical-principles-for-medical-research-involving-human-subjects/. Published 1964.

40. Kennedy CA, Beaton DE, Solway S, McConnell S, Bombardier C. Disabilities of the Arm, Shoulder and Hand (DASH). The DASH and QuickDASH outcome measure User's manual. Third Edition. Toronto: Institute for Work & Health; 2011. http://www.dash.iwh.on.ca/dash-manual.

41. Beaton D, Bombardier C, Guillemin F. Guidelines for the process of cross-cultural adaptation of self-report measures. Spine (Phila Pa 1976). 2000;25(24):3186–91.

42. Marx RG, Bombardier C, Hogg-Johnson S, Wright JG. Clinimetric and psychometric strategies for development of a health measurement scale. J Clin Epidemiol. 1999;52(2):105–11.

43. Wright JG, Feinsten AR. A comparative contrast of clinimetric and psychometric methods for constructing indexes and rating scales. J Clin Epidemiol. 1992;45(11):1201–18.

44. Mokkink LB, Terwee CB, Patrick DL, et al. The COSMIN study reached international consensus on taxonomy, terminology, and definitions of measurement properties for health-related patient-reported outcomes. J Clin Epidemiol. 2010;63(7):737–45. https://doi.org/10.1016/j.jclinepi.2010.02.006.

45. Babyak MA, Green SB. Confirmatory factor analysis: an introduction for psychosomatic medicine researchers. Psychosom Med. 2010;72(6):587–97. https://doi.org/10.1097/PSY.0b013e3181de3f8a.

46. Chen FFF, West SGSSG, Sousa KKH. A comparison of Bifactor and second-order models of quality of life. Multivariate Behav Res. 2006;41(2):189–225. https://doi.org/10.1207/s15327906mbr4102_5.

47. Cortina JM. What is coefficient alpha? An examination of theory and applications. J Appl Psychol. 1993;78(1):98–104. https://doi.org/10.1037/0021-9010.78.1.98.

48. Zinbarg RE, Revelle W, Yovel I, Li W. Cronbach's alpha, Revelle's beta and McDonald's omega-H: their relations with each other and two alternative conceptualizations of reliability. Psychometrika. 2005;70(1):123–33. https://doi.org/10.1007/s11336-003-0974-7.

49. Gignac GE, Palmer BR, Stough C. A confirmatory factor analytic investigation of the TAS-20: corroboration of a five-factor model and suggestions for improvement. J Pers Assess. 2007;89(3):247–57. https://doi.org/10.1080/00223890701629730.

50. Reise SP. The rediscovery of Bifactor measurement models. Multivariate Behav Res. 2012;47(5):667–96. https://doi.org/10.1080/00273171.2012.715555.

51. McDonald RP. Test theory: a unified treatment. Test theory A unified Treat. 1999:485.

52. Berge JMF, Sočan G. The greatest lower bound to the reliability of a test and the hypothesis of unidimensionality. Psychometrika. 2004;69(4):613–25. https://doi.org/10.1007/BF02289858.

53. Hogarty KY. The quality of factor solutions in exploratory factor analysis: the influence of sample size, communality, and Overdetermination. Educ Psychol Meas. 2005;65(2):202–26. https://doi.org/10.1177/0013164404267287.

54. Comrey A, Lee HA. First Course in Factor Analysis. 2nd ed. Hillsdale. New Jersey: Lawrence Erlbaum Associates, Inc; 1992.

55. Rosseel Y. Lavaan: an R package for structural equation modeling. J Stat Softw. 2012;48(2):1–36. https://doi.org/10.18637/jss.v048.i02.

56. R Core Team. R. A language and environment for statistical computing. Vienna, Austria. https://www.r-project.org. Published: R Foundation for statistical Computing; 2016.

57. Hu L, Bentler PM. Cutoff criteria for fit indexes in covariance structure analysis: conventional criteria versus new alternatives. Struct Equ Model A Multidiscip J. 1999;6(1):1–55. https://doi.org/10.1080/10705519909540118.

58. De Vet H. Are factor analytical techniques used appropriately in the validation of health status questionnaires? A systematic review on the quality of factor analysis of the SF-36. Qual Life Res. 2005;14(5):1203–18.

59. Revelle W, Wilt J. The general factor of personality: a general critique. J Res Pers. 2013;47(5):493–504. https://doi.org/10.1016/j.jrp.2013.04.012.

18

What factors impact on the implementation of clubfoot treatment services in low and middle-income countries?: a narrative synthesis of existing qualitative studies

Sarah Drew[1*], Rachael Gooberman-Hill[2,3] and Christopher Lavy[1]

Abstract

Background: Around 100,000 children are born annually with clubfoot worldwide and 80% live in low and middle-income counties (LMICs). Clubfoot is a condition in which children are born with one or both feet twisted inwards and if untreated it can limit participation in everyday life. Clubfoot can be corrected through staged manipulation of the limbs using the Ponseti method. Despite its efficacy and apparent availability, previous research has identified a number of challenges to service implementation. The aim of this study was to synthesise these findings to explore factors that impact on the implementation of clubfoot services in LMICs and strategies to address them. Understanding these may help practitioners in other settings develop more effective services.

Methods: Five databases were searched and articles screened using six criteria. Articles were appraised using the Critical Appraisal Skills Programme (CASP) checklist. 11 studies were identified for inclusion. A thematic analysis was conducted.

Results: Thematic analysis of the included studies showed that a lack of access to resources was a challenge including a lack of casting materials and abduction braces. Difficulties within the working environment included limited space and a need to share treatment space with other clinics. A shortage of healthcare professionals was a concern and participants thought that there was a lack of time to deliver treatment. This was exacerbated by the competing demands on clinicians. Lack of training was seen to impact on standards, including the nurses and midwives attending to the child at birth that were failing to diagnose the condition. Financial constraints were seen to underlie many of these problems. Some participants identified failures in communication and cooperation within the healthcare system such as a lack of awareness of clinics. Strategies to address these issues included means of increasing resource availability and the delivery of targeted training. The use of non-governmental organisations to provide financial support and methods to disseminate best practice were discussed.

Conclusions: This study identified factors that impact on the implementation of clubfoot services in LMIC settings. Findings may be used to improve service delivery.

Keywords: Clubfoot, Ponseti, Narrative synthesis, Qualitative

* Correspondence: sarah.drew@ndorms.ox.ac.uk
[1]Oxford NIHR Musculoskeletal Biomedical Research Unit, Nuffield Department of Orthopaedics, Rheumatology and Musculoskeletal Sciences, University of Oxford, Windmill Road, Headington, Oxford OX3 7LD, UK
Full list of author information is available at the end of the article

Background

Around 100,000 children are born annually with clubfoot worldwide and of these, 80% live in middle-income counties (LMICs) [1]. Clubfoot is a condition in which children are born with one or both feet twisted inwards. Although it is not initially painful, if left untreated or 'neglected', clubfoot can significantly impair function and in some cases, lead to exclusion in the community [2]. Clubfoot can be corrected through staged manipulation of the limbs with plaster of Paris, a technique known as the Ponseti method. In this, approximately five manipulations are carried out on a weekly basis. This is then followed by a tenotomy, a small operation under local anesthetic to release a tight Achilles tendon. A final cast is then applied for two weeks. Correction is then maintained using foot abduction braces which must be worn full time for 2–3 months, and then nightly for 3–4 years [3]. The Ponseti technique is one of the most widely used methods to treat clubfoot throughout the world [4–6]. High numbers of treatment centers exist in LMICs [7].

Despite the efficacy of the Ponseti method and its apparent availability, previous research has identified a number of challenges to eradicating clubfoot. It has been suggested that a high proportion of children in LMICs fail to present at clinics and of those that do, many do not complete treatment [8–10]. Reasons for this have been explored in a recent meta-synthesis exploring treatment seeking behavior for clubfoot in LMICs [11]. Research has also highlighted a number of challenges to service delivery, including a lack of resources [9, 12, 13] and insufficient training for service providers [8, 12, 14]. Understanding factors that impact on the implementation of clubfoot treatment may help practitioners in other settings develop more effective services.

Qualitative studies enable researchers to explore views and experiences of service delivery [15]. Furthermore, it is thought that synthesising related qualitative studies provides findings that are relevant across multiple settings [16]. A growing body of literature aims to explore factors that impact on the implementation of clubfoot services across a range of LMICs. This literature contains findings that may relevant to providers working in similar settings.

A number of methods have been developed to synthesise qualitative research studies [17, 18]. Narrative synthesis has been chosen here to enable us to integrate findings and combine studies using a range of methodological approaches [18]. Narrative syntheses can be distinguished from traditional, narrative reviews by their systematic approach to study identification, quality appraisal and transparent methods of synthesis [18].

The aim of this study is to use a narrative synthesis to synthesise findings from existing qualitative research to explore factors that impact on the implementation of clubfoot services in LMICs and strategies to address them. This is intended to complement existing work that explores factors that impact on patient access to services across a range of LMICs, along with strategies to address them [11]. It is hoped that this will provide further information to healthcare professionals about how to develop services to better meet the needs of patients.

Methods

A narrative synthesis was conducted in four stages: identifying studies for inclusion, appraising quality, data extraction and synthesis and reporting findings. Methods correspond to our previous meta-synthesis exploring treatment-seeking behaviour for clubfoot [11].

Identifying studies for inclusion

Articles were identified by searching five databases: Ovid MEDLINE, PsycINFO, Embase, Global Health and CINAHL. Search criteria were broad in order to capture the highest number of publications. A combination of keyword searches and thesaurus terms or subject headings (Table 1) were applied to each database. A search filter to identify qualitative studies was then applied [19]. Databases were searched in December 2016.

Articles were manually screened to identify studies which fulfilled the following criteria:

1. The study related only to clubfoot services or treatments
2. The population was healthcare professionals involved in the organisation or delivery of clubfoot treatment
3. The study was conducted in a low or middle income country as defined by the World Bank [20]
4. The study explored factors that impacted on the implementation of services
5. The study was published in the last 10 years
6. Issues were explored using qualitative research methods
7. The research output was either an article or a report

Additional records were identified by searching the bibliographies of relevant articles.

Appraising quality

To appraise study quality, the Critical Appraisal Skills Programme (CASP), a 10 point tool to help guide the evaluation of qualitative studies was used [21]. As in our previous review, items of the CASP framework were grouped into three domains: 1) study's aims and appropriateness of methodology (items 1 and 2); 2) study design and conduct, including research design, recruitment, data collection, relationship with researcher, ethics and analysis

Table 1 Search terms to explore factors that impact on the implementation of clubfoot treatment services

Patient	"Idiopathic clubfoot"	Clubfoot	"Club-foot"	Equinovarus	Talipes		
Service or intervention	Ponseti	Correction	Treatment	Tenotomy	Therapy	Service*	Surg*/Surgic*

(items 3–8); and 3) clarity of findings and value of the research (items 9–10). Each study was evaluated in relation to the three domains. Articles were then categorised into three groups. These were: 'fully addresses CASP items', 'mainly addresses CASP items' or 'partially addresses CASP items' [11].

Articles were independently appraised by two members of the study team (SD and RGH) andthr same judgements were reached about each article. Of these, one study was deemed to fully address CASP items, six mainly address items and four partially address items. Nevertheless all studies were included in the final review since it was thought they all provided insights into the implementation of services [22]. Table 2 details the characteristics of each study in relation to the three CASP groups and the extent to which we felt they addressed CASP items.

Data extraction and synthesis
Articles were imported into NVivo qualitative analysis software [23] and analysed using an inductive thematic analysis. That is, by identifying themes and subthemes in the articles [24]. Analysis was limited to the secondary interpretations of authors on account of the lack of primary data included.

Reporting findings
The review was presented in accordance with ENTREQ guidelines, a 21 item list to improve the transparency of qualitative syntheses [16].

Results
One hundred one articles were initially identified from the search criteria and 11 included in the review. The process of identifying studies for inclusion is detailed in a PRISMA flow chart in Fig. 1.

Of the 22 included studies, four were part of a mixed methods study. Studies explored the implementation of clubfoot treatment settings in the following care settings: Nigeria (1), Latin America (2), India (1), Sri Lanka (1), Kenya (1), China (1), Brazil (1), Peru (1) and Vietnam (1). One study explored implementation across 12 LMICs (Democratic Republic Congo, Rwanda, Dominican Republic, Haiti, Honduras, Ethiopia, Laos, Malawi, Nepal, Paraguay, Tanzania, Zambia). A summary of the characteristics of the studies are presented in Table 2. This includes the aims, country, methods, characteristics in relation to the three CASP domains and extent it addresses the CASP items.

Below we explore factors impacting on the implementation of clubfoot services in LMICs. We also identify strategies to address these challenges.

Resources and working space
Across the studies, a lack of access to resources was identified as a barrier to service delivery, including a lack of casting materials [14, 25, 26] and poor quality materials [26, 27]. Acquiring abduction braces was difficult for some [8, 26–28] and healthcare professionals in Brazil were concerned that there were a lack of stores that could manufacture them to the required standard [8]. There were also challenges with the working environment and in some settings practitioners felt they had limited space to work [13, 27, 28]. In Vietnam, clinics had to share the space with patients with different conditions and the clinics were considered to provide an unpleasant environment to work due to a lack of air conditioning and overcrowding [13]. Others in Sri Lanka were concerned that they could not access a sterile environment for performing tenotomies [27].

Staffing levels
Participants felt that there was a shortage of healthcare personnel to treat patients [28, 29]. They also thought that there was a lack of time available for delivery of treatment in clinics [9, 13, 27, 28]. Conflicting demands on healthcare professionals such as dealing with trauma cases exacerbated this problem [25, 27, 28]. In two settings children were treated in general orthopaedic clinics rather than organised clubfoot clinics. This meant they had to compete with other patients for treatment time [25, 28].

Training and education
Participants felt there was a lack of training and education about the treatment amongst healthcare professionals [8, 9, 12–14, 25, 26, 28, 29]. It was felt that the nurses and midwives attending to the child at birth and in the early years were failing to diagnose the condition or were unaware about the existence of the method. As a result referrals were missed and treatment was delayed [12, 13, 26, 28, 29]. Some physicians were concerned that their training had lapsed since they had seen very few cases and that they were no longer equipped to deliver the treatment effectively [9, 12–14, 25]. Senior members of staff in two settings were keen to delegate more responsibilities to lab technicians and nurses but were unable to do so due to the lack of availability of

Table 2 Summary of the characteristics of papers included in the review

First author	Aims	Country	Methods	Characteristics in relation to three CASP domains	Extent it addresses CASP items
Akintayo, O. A., 2012 [1]	To explore the dissemination of the Ponseti method, inlcuding barriers and facilitators to its implementation.	Nigeria	Semi-structured interviews and focus groups with 25 healthcare providers practising the method, 6 newly trained practitioners, 42 parents of children with clubfoot	1) Aims and appropriateness Aims of the research clearly explained. 2) Design and conduct Triangulation used such that semi-structured interviews and focus groups were used to strengthen findings. Ethical considerations were not outlined. Little information given about how thematic analysis was conducted. 3) Clarity and value Grouping of themes provided clarity to presentation. Srengths and weakenesses were not discussed. Article makes clear how findings may be applied in the future.	Partially
Boardman, A., 2011 [2]	To explore the implementation of the Ponseti method, including barriers and facilitators.	Chile, Peru, Guatemala	Semi-structured interviews with 30 healthcare providers practising the Ponseti method.	1) Aims and appropriateness Aims of research clearly outlined. 2) Design and conduct Methods appropriate and ethical issues outlined. 3) Clarity and value Ambiguity in presentation of findings since primary data and author interpretations are integrated. Relationship of study to existing literature is discussed, along with the potential application of the research.	Mainly
Gadhok, K., 2012 [3]	To explore the implementation of Ponseti method, including barriers and facilitators.	India	Semi-structured interviews with 15 orthopaedic surgeons practising Ponseti method and 15 guardians of children receiving treatment. [As part of a mixed methods study]	1) Aims and appropriateness Objectives of research clearly outlined. 2) Design and conduct Range of methods used to strengthen findings, although it is unclear what each contributed. There is no description of how patients were sampled. Reasons for study setting are clea. Ethical issues have been discussed. There is ambiguity in how data analysis has been conducted. 3) Clarity and value Study findings are clear. The presentation of findings under dominant themes and outlined in a table contributed to this. Strengths and weaknesses are considered. However, there is a lack of discussion about how the work may be used to inform practice.	Mainly
Jayawardena, A., 2013 [4]	To explore the implementation of a 'Train the Trainer' approach to educating practitioners about the Ponseti method.	Sri Lanka	Interviews, focus groups and observations with 162 patients and healthcare providers involved with clubfoot care.	1) Aims and appropriateness Study aims clearly outlined. 2) Design and conduct Methods used appropriate for addressing study aims. No discussion of why participants or study setting were selected. Methods of data collection discussed in detail, along with ethical considerations. However, it is unclear why the study	Mainly

Table 2 Summary of the characteristics of papers included in the review (*Continued*)

First author	Aims	Country	Methods	Characteristics in relation to three CASP domains	Extent it addresses CASP items
				was exempt from ethics review. Methods of analysis are not fully outlined. 3) Clarity and value Study findings are clear. The presentation of findings under dominant themes and outlined in a table contributes to this. Strengths and weaknesses are considered. However, there is a lack of discussion about how work may be used to inform practice.	
Jayawardena, A., 2011 [5]	To explore the implementation of low bandwidth webconferencing to educate practitioners about the Ponseti method.	Guatemala, Peru and Chile	Semi-structured interviews and observations with 33 healthcare providers participating in webconferencing sessions.	1) Aims and appropriateness Study aims clear. 2) Design and conduct Methods used appropriate for addressing study aims although there is no discussion of why participants or the study setting were selected. Processes of collecting observational data are not described. Ethical issues are discussed and details of the ethical review board provided. Methods of analysis are clearly outlined. 3) Clarity and value Organisation of methods into key themes provides clarity. However, there is no discussion on strengths and weaknesses or how study contributes to existing literature. Areas of future research are not outlined.	Mainly
Kingau, N. W., 2015 [6]	To explore the implementation of the Ponseti method, including those faced by guardians a nd healthcare professionals.	Kenya	Semi-structured interviews with 10 service providers and 10 guardians involved in clubfoot care.	1) Aims and appropriateness Study aims clear. 2) Design and conduct Methods are described in detail including how data were collected and data saturation is discussed. Ethical considerations are not outlined. Data analysis is described in detail 3) Clarity and value Themes are clear and primary data is used to enhanced the presentation of findings. There is a consideration of strengths and weaknesses. The contribution of study to exisiting literature is discussed, along with a consideration of its potential application.	Fully
Lu, N., 2010 [7]	To explore the implementation of the Ponseti method, including the experiences of guardians and healthcare providers.	China	Semi-structured interviews and focus groups with 39 healthcare providers practising the Ponseti method and 8 sets of parents of children receiving Ponseti treatment.	1) Aims and appropriateness Study aims clearly outlined. 2) Design and conduct Methods appropriate to aims and objectives of the research. Reasons for selecting participants outlined, although there is no justification for research setting. Ethical issues are discussed, including informed consent and the ethical review board. Methods of data analysis have been outlined and	Mainly

Table 2 Summary of the characteristics of papers included in the review (*Continued*)

First author	Aims	Country	Methods	Characteristics in relation to three CASP domains	Extent it addresses CASP items
				independent coding has been undertaken by two members of the study team to enhance confidence in the findings. 3) Clarity and value. Presentation of study findings is clear. There is no consideration of strengths and weaknesses. The potential application of findings is discussed.	
Nogueira, M. P., 2013 [8]	To evaluate barriers to bracing compliance.	Brazil	Semi-structured interviews with 45 orthopaedists delivering the Ponseti method.	1) Aims and appropriateness. Study aims clearly outlined. 2) Design and conduct. No justification of sampling strategy or why study setting was selected. Processes of data collection and analysis not discussed. 3) Clarity and value. Study findings clearly outlined and weaknesses of study design considered. How the study contributes to wider literature has not been discussed but suggestions for service improvements based on study findings are presented.	Partially
Owen, R. M., 2012 [9]	Evaluation of implementation of 10 clubfoot treatment progammes.	Democratic Republic Congo, Rwanda, Dominican Republic, Haiti, Honduras, Ethiopia, Laos, Malawi, Nepal, Paraguay, Tanzania, Zambia	Semi-structured interviews and observations of clinics with 10 clubfoot programme coordinators, 7 programme planners, regional coordinators or trainers, 10 sets of parents attending clinics and 10 trained practitioners in Ethiopia or Laos. [As part of a mixed methods study]	1) Aims and appropriateness. Clear statement of study aims. 2) Design and conduct. Research methods appropriate for addressing research aims. Justification for choosing semi-structured interviews and advantages of triangulation of data included. However, unclear why Ethiopia and Laos were selected for observations. No discussion of the strategy used to recruit participants. Lack of detail on how interviews and observations carried out. Ethical considerations have been dicussed including anonymisation, data storage and informed consent. Processes of data analysis clearly outlined. 3) Clarity and value. Findings clear and discussion included about the strengths and limitations of the study. Researcher discusses value of research and transferability of findings to other settings.	Mainly
Palma, M., 2013 [10]	To explore barriers to the implementation of the Ponseti method.	Peru	Semi-structured interviews with 25 healthcare providers practising the Ponseti method.	1) Aims and appropriateness. Aims of study are clearly outlined in the main body of the text although they are not as clear in the abstract. 2) Design and conduct. Methods of data collection are appropriate although the sampling strategy and justification of study setting are not discussed. Ethical issues are outlined including the ethical review board and	Partially

Table 2 Summary of the characteristics of papers included in the review (Continued)

First author	Aims	Country	Methods	Characteristics in relation to three CASP domains	Extent it addresses CASP items
				anonymisation of participants. There is a lack of detail about processes of data analysis. 3) Clarity and value Presentation of findings is clear and divided into themes. Strengths and weaknesses are not discussed althoug the potential application of research findings is considered.	
Wu, V., 2012 [11]	To explore the impact of the Ponseti method and challenges to its implementation, including the use of web-conferencing to educate practitioners.	Vietnam	Semi-structured interviews, focus groups and observations with 12 healthcare providers delivering Ponseti treatment and 99 parents of children with clubfoot and their extended family. [As part of a mixed methods study]	1) Aims and appropriateness Aims of research clearly outlined. 2) Design and conduct Methods chosen are appropriate for addressing research questions. Use of multiple methods of data collection to increase confidence in study findings discussed. Sampling strategy outlined although reasons for selecting participants or the choice of study setting are not discussed. Processes of data collection are not outlined. There is no discussion of ethical issues. 3) Clarity and value Presentation of findings clear and strengths and weaknesses discussed. There is a consideration of how findings may be used to inform service delivery, including a series of recommendations.	Partially

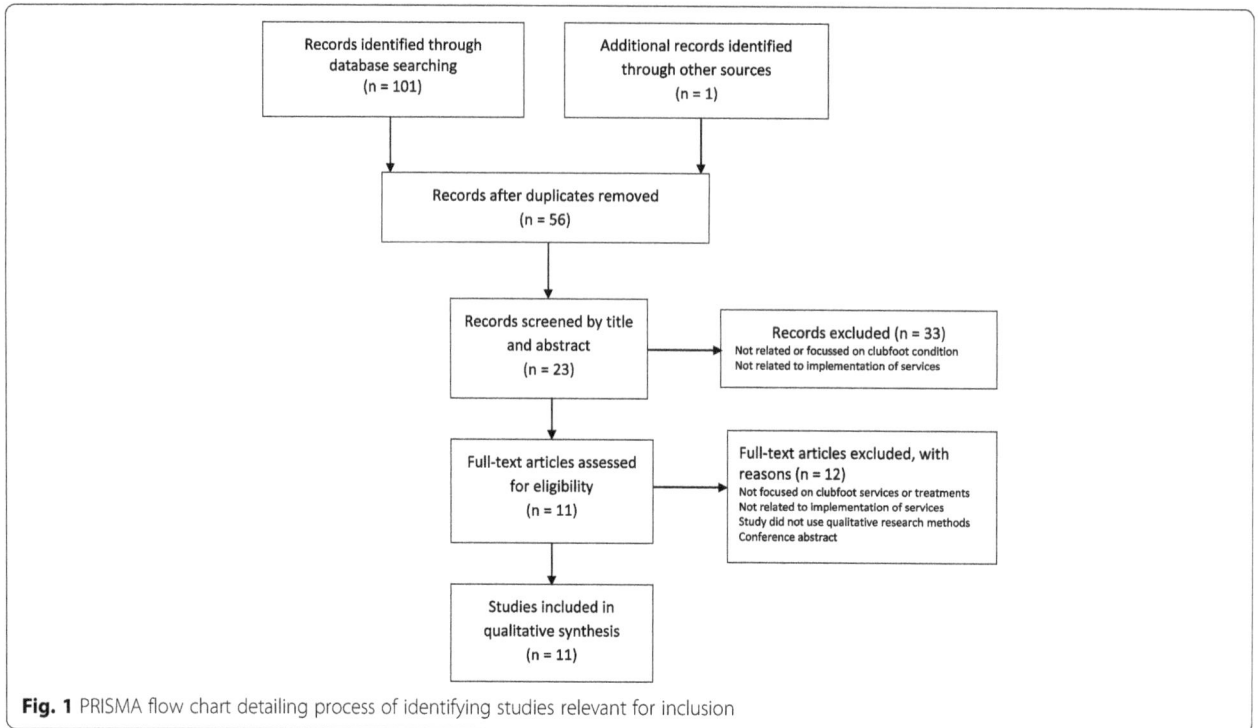

Fig. 1 PRISMA flow chart detailing process of identifying studies relevant for inclusion

training [13, 28]. In a number of settings it was found that professionals were departing from Ponseti protocols, rendering the method less or even ineffective [8, 9, 12–14, 27, 29]. This included combining the Ponseti method with massaging of the limbs [9, 13], departing from casting protocols [9, 13, 27] and prescribing abduction braces for insufficient lengths of time [8].

Financial constraints

Underlying many of these problems were the financial constraints of the hospitals and by implication, the healthcare systems [9, 12, 25, 26, 28]. In Nigeria and Latin America, practitioners who attended the Ponseti training course had to pay for it themselves [14, 28]. To compound this difficulty, in some settings hospitals and orthopaedic surgeons received higher reimbursements for performing surgery rather than using the Ponseti treatment, discouraging the uptake of the method [9, 12, 13].

Communication and cooperation

Some participants identified failures in communication and cooperation within the healthcare system [12, 13, 25, 28, 29]. Failures to identify the condition at birth, as identified above, meant referrals were delayed [28]. In Kenya guardians were sometimes referred to practitioners without experience in the method [29]. Referrers were often unaware of nearby Ponseti clinics, meaning carers faced unnecessarily long journeys to treatment centres, a potential barrier to treatment seeking [13]. Inter-disciplinary disagreements also

hindered treatment delivery [26, 28], as did a lack of local leadership [26]. In Africa where services were delivered in collaboration with non-governmental organisations (NGOs), the level of support from the Ministry of Health was variable. Where support was low, programmes tended to develop more slowly [26].

Lack of difficulty in delivering services

A small number of participants in China did not experience difficulties [12] and there were high levels of support amongst professionals for the method in Vietnam [13].

Strategies to address issues identified

Strategies were suggested to address some of the issues identified. To increase the availability of abduction braces, participants in Kenya thought that local cobblers could make them to help manage costs [28]. It was also felt that training in the method should be made more widely available [13, 14, 26, 28], including a desire to train midwives and nurses in the community to identify clubfoot [13, 26, 28, 29], train more physicians [26, 28] and introduce refresher courses for those that lacked confidence in delivering the treatment [28]. 'Hands on' sessions, rather than ones that were more theoretical in orientation, were considered important [13]. Introducing specialised clinics or training those most likely to practice the method rather than wide-scale training programmes, was suggested as a means of ensuring high standards of treatment [9, 12, 14]. Educating support staff such as nurses and lab technicians in specific aspects of treatment was viewed as a way of 'freeing up' more highly qualified members of staff, enabling them to treat more children [9]. Some also felt that working with the Ministry of Health to introduce the Ponseti method into the medical curricula could facilitate its dissemination [12–14, 28]. National protocols for treatment may also help to deliver standardised care [13, 26]. Building strong and effective partnerships between NGOs and Ministries of Health was advocated [26].

In order to address the lack of funding available, it was suggested that NGOs could be used to provide support [26, 28]. There was a recognition that communication between practitioners working within the same country should be improved [13, 14]. It was also suggested that communication with other countries could also be facilitated as a means of sharing best practice. Suggested strategies for this were through virtual clinics, meetings and international conferences [13, 30]. Practitioners felt that this would give them the opportunity to discuss difficult cases, patient follow-up and experiences of establishing clinics [30]. However, the use of these was constrained by a lack of access to equipment,the internet, funding and time to attend these opportunities [30].

Discussion

The study has identified a range of factors that impact on the successful implementation of clubfoot treatment services in LMIC settings. These were focussed on five areas: resources and working space, staffing levels, training and education, financial constraints and communication and cooperation between healthcare professionals. A lack of access to resources was identified as a challenge across the majority of settings. Difficulties with the working environment included limited space, unpleasant working conditions and a need to share treatment space with other clinics. A shortage of healthcare professionals was also a major concern, along with competing demands on clinicians. Lack of training and education was seen to impact on standards of service delivery. There was a desire for more training for midwives and nurses attending the children at birth to help aid identification, as well as those delivering treatment. Financial constraints were seen to underlie many of these problems. Only a small number of participants in China did not experience any difficulties. Strategies to address these issues included means of increasing resource availability and delivering targeted training for healthcare professionals. The use of non-governmental organisations to provide financial support and methods to disseminate best practice were discussed. Although treatment was delivered across a range of settings, there was little difference between factors impacting on implementation or on strategies to address them. Findings also support those from a recent review that has highlighted the lack of physical resources and training for healthcare providers delivering the Ponseti method in of LMICs [31]. This study complements existing work that has explored factors that impact on patient access to clubfoot treatment, along with strategies to address them [11].

Strengths and weaknesses

We undertook a systematic and exhaustive search to identify studies. Although we cannot say with certainty that all literature was captured, by refining search terms with the study team, including a clinician with experience of delivering these services, meant this was probably the case. Using the ENTREQ guidelines, a 21 item list for improving the transparency of qualitative syntheses [16], also enhanced the presentation of our study.

The quality of the studies identified was variable and may have limited the findings of the review. According to our CASP quality appraisal [21], one study was deemed to fully address items, six mainly address items and four partially address items. To enhance confidence in these assessments, all 11 articles were independently appraised by two members of the study team and both arrived at the same judgements. However, a decision was made to include all the articles in the synthesis since they were all seen to provide valuable information about the issues under study.

We made the decision to limit our review to published qualitative studies that were more likely to be of higher quality and provide more systematic exploration of issues than grey or unpublished literature.

Further research

Further research is now needed to evaluate the implementation of clubfoot services in other LMIC settings, along with suggested strategies to improve service delivery. Doing so would provide additional information about how best to deliver clubfoot treatment services.

Conclusions

This study has identified factors that impact on the implementation of clubfoot services in LMICs and strategies to address them. These findings may help professionals across a range of LMICs implement services more effectively in the future.

Abbreviations
CASP: Critical Appraisal Skills Programme; LMICs: Low and middle-income countries

Acknowledgements
We could like to acknowledge the contribution of Elinor Harriss from The Knowledge Centre, Bodleian Health Care Libraries at Oxford University for providing advice and guidance on developing a search strategy for this review.

Funding
The study was jointly funded by CURE International UK and the COSECSA Oxford Orthopaedic Link (COOL) programme which is funded by the UK Department for International Development (Health Partnership Scheme). This study was supported by the NIHR Biomedical Research Centre at the University Hospitals Bristol NHS Foundation Trust and the University of Bristol. The views expressed in this publication are those of the author(s) and not necessarily those of the NHS, the National Institute for Health Research or the Department of Health.

Authors' contributions
SD, RGH and CL all contributed to the design of this research, analysis and interpretation of data. All authors contributed to drafting this work and revising it for important intellectual content and gave final approval for the version to be submitted.

Consent for publication
Not applicable.

Competing interests
SD and CL and have no conflicts of interest to report. RGH is a member of the Editorial Board for BMC Musculoskeletal Disorders.

Author details
[1]Oxford NIHR Musculoskeletal Biomedical Research Unit, Nuffield Department of Orthopaedics, Rheumatology and Musculoskeletal Sciences, University of Oxford, Windmill Road, Headington, Oxford OX3 7LD, UK. [2]School of Clinical Sciences, University of Bristol, Learning and Research Building, Level 1, Southmead Hospital, Bristol BS10 5NB, UK. [3]National Institute for Health Research Bristol Biomedical Research Centre, University of Bristol, Bristol, UK.

References
1. Harmer L, Rhatigan J. Clubfoot Care in Low-Income and Middle-Income Countries: From Clinical Innovation to a Public Health Program. World J Surg. 2014;38(4):839–48.
2. Alavi Y, et al. Indignity, exclusion, pain and hunger: the impact of musculoskeletal impairments in the lives of children in Malawi. Disabil Rehabil. 2012;34(20):1736–46.
3. IV, P., Congenital Clubfoot. Fundamentals of Treatment. 1966, Oxford: Oxford University Press.
4. Radler C. The Ponseti method for the treatment of congenital club foot: review of the current literature and treatment recommendations. Int Orthop. 2013;37(9):1747–53.
5. Zionts LE, et al. Has the rate of extensive surgery to treat idiopathic clubfoot declined in the United States? J Bone Joint Surg Am. 2010;92(4):882–9.
6. Zionts LE, et al. The current management of idiopathic clubfoot revisited: results of a survey of the POSNA membership. J Pediatr Orthop. 2012;32(5):515–20.
7. Shabtai L, Specht SC, Herzenberg JE. Worldwide spread of the Ponseti method for clubfoot. World J Orthop. 2014;5(5):585–90.
8. Nogueira MP, et al. The Ponseti method of treatment for clubfoot in Brazil: barriers to bracing compliance. Iowa Orthop J. 2013;33:161–6.
9. Gadhok K, et al. Qualitative assessment of the challenges to the treatment of idiopathic clubfoot by the Ponseti method in urban India. Iowa Orthop J. 2012;32:135–40.
10. McElroy T, et al. Understanding the barriers to clubfoot treatment adherence in Uganda: a rapid ethnographic study. Disability & Rehabilitation. 2007;29(11–12):845–55.
11. Drew S, Lavy C, Gooberman-Hill R. What factors affect patient access and engagement with clubfoot treatment in low- and middle-income countries? Meta-synthesis of existing qualitative studies using a social ecological model. Tropical Med Int Health. 2016;21(5):570–89.
12. Lu N, et al. From cutting to casting: impact and initial barriers to the Ponseti method of clubfoot treatment in China. Iowa Orthop J. 2010;30:1–6.
13. Wu V, et al. Evaluation of the progress and challenges facing the Ponseti method program in Vietnam. Iowa Orthop J. 2012;32:125–34.
14. Boardman A, et al. The Ponseti method in Latin America: initial impact and barriers to its diffusion and implementation. Iowa Orthop J. 2011;31:30–5.
15. Gooberman-Hill R. Qualitative approaches to understanding patient preferences. The Patient. 2012;5(4):215–23.
16. Tong A, et al. Enhancing transparency in reporting the synthesis of qualitative research: ENTREQ. BMC Med Res Methodol. 2012;12:181.
17. Popay, J., Guidance on the conduct of narrative synthesis on systematic reviews. 2006: ESRC Methods Programme.
18. Campbell R, et al. Evaluating meta-ethnography: systematic analysis and synthesis of qualitative research. Health Technol Assess. 2011;15(43):164.
19. Search filters for various databases. Available from: http://libguides.sph.uth.tmc.edu/ovid_medline_filters.
20. Bank, T.W. Country and lending groups. 2015.
21. CASP. qualitative checklist: 10 questions to help you make sense of qualitative research. 2013. Critical Appraisal Skills Programme.
22. Campbell R, et al. Evaluating meta-ethnography: systematic analysis and synthesis of qualitative research. Health Technol Assess. 2011;15(43):1–164.
23. Smyth, R., NVivo (Software). The Sage Encyclopedia of Qualitative Research Methods. SAGE Publications, Inc. Thousand Oaks, CA: SAGE Publications, Inc. 564–566.
24. SAGE Publications, I., Thematic Coding and Analysis. The SAGE Encyclopedia of Qualitative Research Methods. SAGE Publications, Inc. Thousand Oaks, CA: SAGE Publications, Inc.
25. Palma M, et al. Barriers to the Ponseti method in Peru: a two-year follow-up. Iowa Orthop J. 2013;33:172–7.
26. Owen RM, et al. A collaborative public health approach to clubfoot intervention in 10 low-income and middle-income countries: 2-year outcomes and lessons learnt. J Pediatr Orthop B. 2012;21(4):361–5.
27. Jayawardena A, et al. Early effects of a 'train the trainer' approach to Ponseti method dissemination: a case study of Sri Lanka. Iowa Orthop J. 2013;33:153–60.
28. Akintayo OA, et al. Initial program evaluation of the Ponseti method in Nigeria. Iowa Orthop J. 2012;32:141–9.
29. Kingau NW, Rhoda A, Mlenzana N. Barriers experienced by service providers and caregivers in clubfoot management in Kenya. Trop Dr. 2015;45(2):84–90.
30. Jayawardena A, et al. Diffusion of innovation: enhancing the dissemination of the Ponseti method in Latin America through virtual forums. Iowa Orthop J. 2011;31:36–42.
31. Johnson RR, et al. The Ponseti Method for Clubfoot Treatment in Low and Middle-Income Countries: A Systematic Review of Barriers and Solutions to Service Delivery. J Pediatr Orthop. 2017;37(2):e134–9.

19

Pharmacological effects of *N*-[2-[[2-[2-[(2,6-dichlorophenyl)amino]phenyl]acetyl]oxy]ethyl]hyaluronamide (diclofenac Etalhyaluronate, SI-613), a novel sodium hyaluronate derivative chemically linked with diclofenac

Keiji Yoshioka*, Tomochika Kisukeda, Ryoji Zuinen, Yosuke Yasuda and Kenji Miyamoto

Abstract

Background: Osteoarthritis (OA) is the most common joint disorder worldwide and one of the leading causes of disability in the elderly. We have investigated the novel sodium hyaluronate derivative chemically linked with diclofenac (DF), diclofenac etalhyaluronate (SI-613), which is a potentially safer and more effective treatment for OA knee pain. In this study, we evaluated the pharmacological effects of SI-613 in experimental arthritis models.

Methods: We compared the analgesic and anti-inflammatory effects of intra-articularly administered SI-613, hyaluronic acid (HA), and of orally administered diclofenac sodium (DF-Na) in rat silver nitrate-induced arthritis model and rabbit antigen-induced arthritis model.

Results: A single intra-articular (IA) administration of SI-613 significantly suppressed pain responses in rats in a dose-dependent manner. The analgesic effects were greater than those of HA, a mixture of DF-Na and HA, or an oral once-daily administration of DF-Na. In the rabbit arthritis model, SI-613 significantly reduced knee joint swelling compared with that in the control group on day 1 after a single IA injection. This significant anti-inflammatory effect was observed until day 28. In the pharmacokinetic study, the DF concentration in the synovium after SI-613 administration reached its maximum concentration of 311.6 ng/g on day 1, and gradually declined to 10 ng/g by day 28. It fell below the lower limit of quantification on day 35. Thus, a clear correlation was found between pharmacokinetics and pharmacodynamics. These results demonstrate that SI-613 exerts its long-lasting and potent anti-inflammatory effect by sustainable release of DF in the knee joint tissues.

Conclusion: A single IA injection of SI-613 was shown to exert analgesic and anti-inflammatory effects for 28 days in non-clinical pharmacological studies, suggesting that SI-613 will be a promising candidate in the treatment of osteoarthritis pain.

Keywords: Osteoarthritis, Hyaluronan, Diclofenac etalhyaluronate, Sustained-release, Conjugate technology

* Correspondence: keiji.yoshioka@seikagaku.co.jp
Central Research Lab., Research & Development Div., Seikagaku Corporation,
1253, Tateno 3-chome, Higashiyamato-shi, Tokyo 207-0021, Japan

Background

Osteoarthritis (OA) is the most common joint disorder worldwide and one of the leading causes of disability in the elderly [1]. Treatment for knee OA aims to relieve pain and improve function, in order to mitigate reductions in physical activity. The mainstay of pharmacological therapy for OA includes acetaminophen, nonsteroidal anti-inflammatory drugs (NSAIDs) (oral and topical), cyclooxygenase-2 (COX-2) inhibitors, and IA therapies such as intra-articular sodium hyaluronate (IA-HA) injections and intra-articular-steroid (IA-steroid) injections.

Oral NSAIDs are widely prescribed for the treatment of OA pain. Nevertheless, upper gastrointestinal tract complications have been reported in patients who received long-term oral NSAIDs [2]. NSAIDs are also considered to have limited efficacy for OA pain relief. In the 1990s, a number of selective COX-2 inhibitors were developed to reduce the adverse events of NSAIDs. However, most of them were withdrawn from the market after the cardiovascular adverse effects of COX-2 inhibitors were reported in 2004 [3]. Meanwhile, oral NSAIDs including diclofenac sodium (DF-Na) were also reported to have the same concerns as COX-2 inhibitors [4, 5]. Thereafter, a few topical NSAIDs formulations were developed and launched for the relief of OA pain. Topical NSAIDs formulations, such as diclofenac sodium 1% gel, have equivalent efficacy and fewer adverse events compared with oral NSAIDs [6–8]. The intra-articular (IA) injection of hyaluronic acid (HA) is a recognized treatment for pain associated with symptomatic knee OA [9–11]. The pain relief afforded by IA-HA injections is long lasting and often lasts longer than 13 weeks [12, 13]. However, the efficacy of IA-HA injections is moderate compared to that of IA-steroids or oral NSAIDs. Therefore, the profiles of the next generation of OA therapeutics should be potent and longer lasting with higher safety, which will improve the quality of life for OA patients.

In the pursuit of the next generation of OA therapeutics, we developed a novel conjugated compound, SI-613. It is a novel derivative of high-molecular-weight fermented HA (600,000 to 1,200,000 Da), which tethers the NSAID diclofenac (DF) via a 2-aminoethanol linker extended from glucuronic acid moieties (Fig. 1). SI-613 gradually releases DF by hydrolytic cleavage of the ester linkage in a pH-dependent manner. Furthermore, SI-613 releases DF locally in a sustained manner and remains in the joint for a long period, similar to the existing IA-HA injection. It is expected to be more advantageous compared to IA-HA injections and NSAIDs in terms of efficacy and duration.

In the present study, we investigated the pharmacological effects of the IA administration of SI-613 and compared them with those of p.o. DF-Na and IA-HA administration. Furthermore, we investigated the pharmacokinetics of intra-articularly administered SI-613.

Methods

Animals

Male Sprague-Dawley (SD) rats (5 weeks old) were obtained from Charles River Laboratories Japan Inc. (Tokyo, Japan). Male New Zealand White rabbits (12–15 weeks old) were obtained from Oriental Yeast Co., Ltd. (Tokyo, Japan). Animals were maintained under specific pathogen free conditions at a room temperature of 23 ± 3 °C and air humidity of $50 \pm 20\%$ on a 12-h/12-h light/dark cycle. Animals were quarantined and acclimatized to the environmental conditions for 1 week.

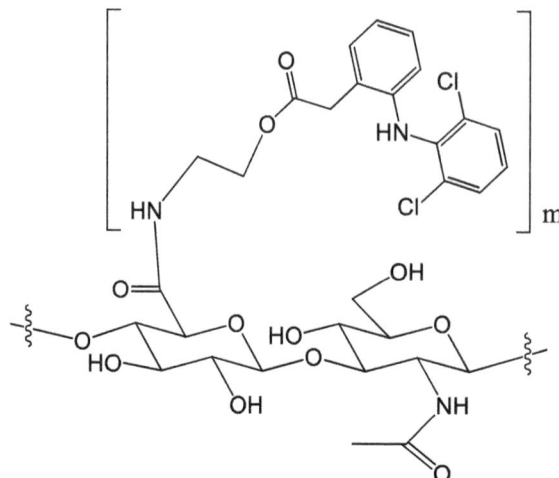

Fig. 1 Chemical structure of *N*-[2-[[2-[2-[(2,6-dichlorophenyl)amino]phenyl]acetyl]oxy]ethyl]hyaluronamide (diclofenac etalhyaluronate, SI-613)

Rat model of silver nitrate-induced arthritic pain

The silver nitrate-induced arthritic pain model is known as a subacute arthritis model, in which the inflammatory response and pain last for at least 3 days following injury. This model involves the activation of prostaglandin pathways and has been used for evaluating the analgesic effects of various NSAIDs or kappa-opioid receptor agonist [14–18]. Overall, 136 male Sprague-Dawley (SD) rats were obtained from Charles River Laboratories Japan Inc. General anesthesia was maintained by the inhalation of isoflurane (Forane; Dainippon Sumitomo Pharma Co., Ltd., Osaka, Japan). Silver nitrate solution (1%, Wako Pure Chemical Industries, Ltd., Osaka, Japan) at a volume of 50 μL/joint was injected in the knee joint cavity of the left hindlimbs of rats. Animals with no abnormalities were allocated to four groups in each study based on the weight-bearing rate of the inflamed joints and pain score at the time of allocation, by using stratified continuous randomization. Test substances were administered on the day following the arthritis induction. In the first study, SI-613 (contents of DF; 11.8% (w/w), manufactured by Seikagaku Corporation, Tokyo, Japan) at doses of 0.05, 0.15, and 0.5 mg/50 μL/joint (5.9, 17.7, and 59 μg/joint in DF equivalent) or phosphate-buffered saline (PBS) was once injected into the joint cavities of the left hindlimbs for the dose-response assessments.

In the second study, SI-613 (0.5 mg/joint, 59 μg/joint in DF equivalent), HA (0.5 mg/joint, Seikagaku Corporation), a mixture of DF-Na (59 μg/joint, Wako Pure Chemical Industries, Ltd.) and HA (0.5 mg/joint) (DF-Na + HA), or PBS was administered in the same manner for the proof of concept. The doses of DF-Na and HA were set at those of respective components in SI-613 formulation. The DF-Na solution (1 mg/mL) was prepared using the Water for Injection (Otsuka Pharmaceutical Factory, Inc., Tokyo, Japan) and administered orally at a dose of 2 mg/kg (approximately 0.3 mg/body) once daily for 3 days. The oral DF-Na dose, 2 mg/kg, was set in accordance with the dose for adult humans with a body weight of 50 kg, on the assumption that the maximum daily dose in clinical practice administered to patients with OA or rheumatoid arthritis would be 100 mg. It has been reported that DF-Na exerted anti-inflammatory effects in rats when administered at this dose [19].

Pain was assessed under blinded conditions by scoring pain-related behaviors based on the following criteria and measuring the weight-bearing rates of hindlimbs with a load-measuring device (Tokken Inc., Chiba, Japan) at a same time each day for 3 days after the injection of the test materials.

The criteria for assigning pain scores were as follows: 0; normal, 1; mild claudication with lifting the foot, 2; severe claudication with completely closing the toe, 3;

walking on three legs. The weight-bearing rate was calculated using the following formula:

Weight-bearing rate (%) = Mean weight-bearing load on inflamed leg (g) / Body weight (g) × 100.

In addition, the prostaglandin E_2 (PGE$_2$) content, which plays a critical role in inducing inflammation and pain associated with arthritis, was determined in the synovial fluid (SF). Briefly, SI-613 (0.5 mg/joint) or PBS was administered into the joint cavity of the left hindlimb. After assessing the severity of pain, animals were sacrificed by exsanguination under 2% isoflurane anesthesia 1, 2 and 3 days after administration, respectively. The SF was collected by washing the joint cavity with saline (Otsuka Pharmaceutical Factory, Inc.) containing indomethacin (Indacin, MSD K. K., Tokyo, Japan), which was effective to prevent joint puncturing-induced production of PGE$_2$ (unpublished result). The PGE$_2$ content in the SF was measured with a High Sensitivity PGE$_2$ Correlate-EIA kit (Assay Designs Inc., Ann Arbor, MI).

Effect of SI-613 on the PGE$_2$ content in the SF of rabbits with antigen-induced arthritis

The anti-inflammatory effects of SI-613 were evaluated in a rabbit arthritis model induced by ovalbumin (OVA) [20–22], and compared with those of orally-administered DF-Na or the active chemical compositions of SI-613. To prepare the anesthetic, saline (2 mL), midazolam (1 mL, 5 mg/mL, Astellas Pharma Inc., Tokyo, Japan), xylazine (2 mL, 0.02 g/mL, Bayer Medical Ltd., Tokyo, Japan), and butorphanol tartrate (1 mL, 5 mg/mL, Meiji Seika Kaisha, Ltd., Tokyo, Japan) were mixed. The anesthetic was administered intravenously to each animal at a volume of 1 mL/body. OVA (Sigma-Aldrich Co., St. Louis, MO) emulsion with Freund's complete adjuvant (FCA; CAPPEL Laboratories Inc., Cochranville, PA) was injected intradermally into the backs of 80 male rabbits at a dose of 5 mg/animal twice at an interval of 13 or 14 days. Twenty-three days after the first immunization, 1% OVA solution was injected in the joint cavities of the left hindlimb at a volume of 500 μL/joint to induce arthritis. Two days after the induction of arthritis, test materials of 5 mg/joint SI-613, a mixture of 0.59 mg/joint DF-Na and 5 mg/joint HA (DF-Na + HA), or PBS (control) were administered at a volume of 500 μL/joint in the knee joint cavity. DF-Na was orally administered at a dose of 2 mg/kg. Animals were sacrificed by exsanguination under 2% isoflurane anesthesia 3 and 72 h after administration, respectively. The SF was collected by washing the joint cavity twice with saline (Otsuka Pharmaceutical Factory, Inc.) containing 20 μg/mL of indomethacin (Indacin, MSD K. K.) at 3 or 72 h after the administration of the test materials. The PGE$_2$ content in the SF was determined as a mechanism biomarker for the anti-inflammatory effect using a High Sensitivity Prostaglandin E_2 Enzyme Immunoassay Kit (Assay Designs Inc.).

Long-lasting anti-inflammatory effect of SI-613 on antigen-induced arthritis in rabbits

The duration and efficacy of the anti-inflammatory effect of SI-613 was studied in OVA-induced arthritis rabbits [20–22]. Two days after the arthritis induction, the knee joint diameter in all 60 rabbits was measured with a digital thickness gauge (Teclock Corp., Nagano, Japan). The joint swelling was expressed as the difference in millimeters between the inflamed (left) and non-inflamed (right) knee joint diameters. The same researcher evaluated the knee joint swelling on all groups on all days. Fifteen animals (knee joint swelling was not more than 7.30 mm) and 5 animals (knee joint swelling was not less than 10.40 mm) were excluded. Forty animals were divided into two groups of 20 animals each by the stratified random sampling method based on the knee joint swelling and body weight of the day, and were administered with 5 mg/joint SI-613 or PBS at a volume of 500 μL/joint into the joint cavities. The knee joint swelling was evaluated the day before (day 0), and on days 1, 3, 7, 14, 21, 28, 35, and 42 after a single injection of the test materials. The knee joint swelling was expressed as the difference in the width of the right and left knee joint.

Distribution of DF in knee tissues after a single IA administration of SI-613 and its chemical compositions in rabbits: Short-term study

Arthritis was induced in the 12 rabbits as described above. Two days after the induction of arthritis, 5 mg/joint SI-613, a mixture of 0.59 mg/joint DF-Na and 5 mg/joint HA (DF-Na + HA), or PBS was administered to the knee joint cavity at a volume of 500 μL/joint. DF-Na was orally administered at a dose of 2 mg/kg. The concentrations of free DF in the synovium and synovial lavage fluid were measured by high performance liquid chromatography coupled with tandem mass spectrometry (LC-MS/MS) at 3 and 72 h after a single IA administration and after a single oral administration of the test materials, respectively. Moreover, plasma concentrations of DF were determined to compare the systemic exposure of DF after the administration of SI-613 with that of the other compounds. The synovium was homogenized in 40-fold volume (40 mL for 1 g tissue) of 10 mM ammonium formate (pH 6.0)/methanol (3:2, v/v) on an ice bath. Then, free DF in the homogenate was extracted with tert-butyl methyl ether-1% acetic acid (6:1, v/v). Free DF in the synovial fluid or plasma was adsorbed to an Oasis HLB cartridge (30 mg/1 cm^3, Waters Corporation, Milford, MA) and eluted with methanol.

The internal standard of deuterium-labeled diclofenac (diclofenac-d7) was added to each sample. The extract was loaded onto a CAPCELL PAK C18 MG HPLC column (Shiseido Co. Ltd., Tokyo, Japan, column size: 4.6 mm × 35 mm, particle size: 5 μm) at 40 °C, and eluted with 10 mM ammonium formate (pH 6.0)/methanol (2:3, v/v) at a flow rate of 0.5 mL/minute. For mass detection, we used a QTRAP 5500 System (AB SCIEX, Framingham, MA) equipped with an electrospray ionization (ESI) source in positive ions in multiple reaction monitoring (MRM) mode. Linear calibration ($r > 0.999$) was attained at 5–1000 ng/g for the synovium and at 1–200 ng/mL for the synovial fluid and plasma. The extraction efficiencies of diclofenac were 84.2–92.9% for the synovium, 95.2–100.3% for the synovial fluid, and 94.2–96.5% for the plasma.

Evaluation of DF in knee tissues after a single IA administration of SI-613 in rabbits: long-term study

Arthritis was induced in the 24 rabbits as described above. Two days after the induction of arthritis in the rabbits [20–22], 5 mg/joint SI-613 or PBS was administered at a volume of 500 μL/joint into the knee joint cavity. Concentrations of DF in the synovium and synovial lavage fluid were measured by LC-MS/MS on days 1, 3, 7, 14, 21, 28, 35, and 42 after a single IA administration.

Statistical analyses

Statistical analyses were performed using the Statistical Analysis System, SAS (SAS Institute Inc., Cary, NC). Direct effects from treatment with SI-613 were assessed using two-way analyses of variance followed by Williams' or Tukey's test for the analgesic assessment of the joint pain model in rats. A Student's t-test, Welch's t-test, or Tukey's test was performed for the assessment of the PGE$_2$ content in the SF. A Student's t-test with Holm's correction was used for the assessment of long-lasting anti-inflammatory effects. Results of the measurements in each group were represented as the mean and 95% confidence intervals (CI) for the pharmacological study or standard deviations (SD) for the pharmacokinetic study; p values of < 0.05 were considered statistically significant.

Results

Analgesic effects of SI-613 on silver nitrate-induced arthritic pain in rats

SI-613 improved the pain behavioral scores significantly at doses of 0.05, 0.15, and 0.5 mg/joint in a dose-dependent manner (Fig. 2a and c). In addition, SI-613 at 0.15 and 0.5, but not at 0.05 mg/joint significantly increased the weight-bearing rates in a dose-dependent manner compared with those in the control group (Fig. 2b and d). Furthermore, compared with PBS, HA, or

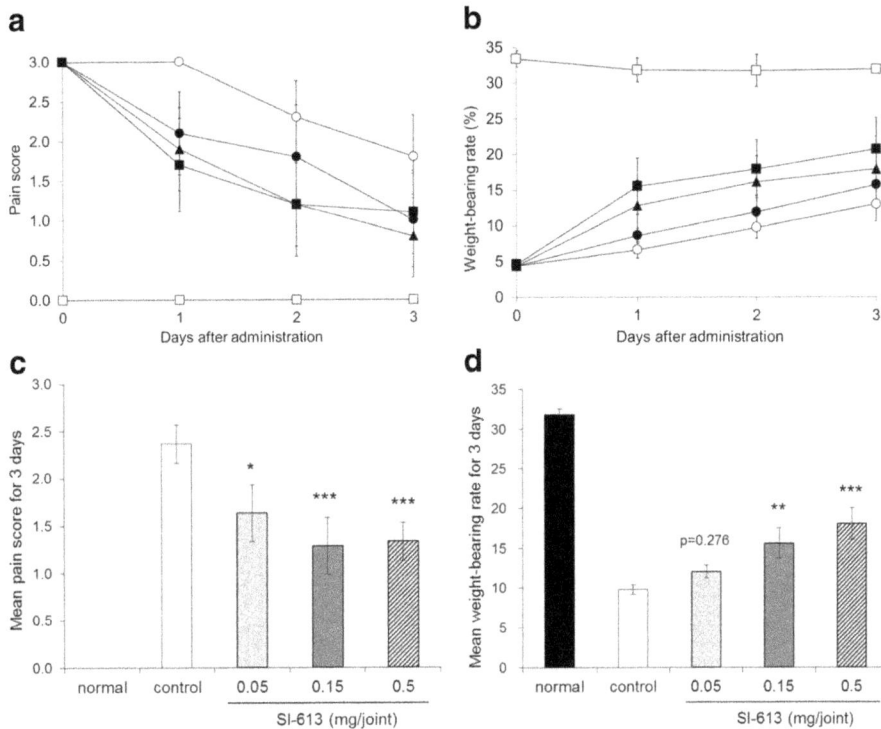

Fig. 2 Analgesic effect of SI-613 in silver nitrate-induced arthritic pain model in rats. Silver nitrate-induced arthritic rats given 0.05 mg (closed circle), 0.15 mg (closed triangle), 0.5 mg (closed square) SI-613, or vehicle (open circle) intra-articularly, and non-treated normal rats (open square) were evaluated for pain score (**a**) and weight-bearing rate (**b**) over time. Mean values of pain scores (**c**) and weight-bearing rate (**d**) for 3 days were calculated and subjected to statistical analysis: two-way analyses of variance followed by Williams' test. ***$p < 0.005$, **$p < 0.01$, *$p < 0.05$ (vs. control, significant level at 5%, two-tailed). Values represent the means ±95% confidence intervals ($n = 9$ per group, except for the normal group $n = 3$)

DF-Na + HA, or the repeated oral administration of DF-Na, SI-613 significantly improved the pain behavioral score (Fig. 3a and c) and increased the weight-bearing rate (Fig. 3b and d). On day 1, the pain score in the DF-Na + HA group was lower than that in the control group; however, this analgesic effect was not observed on and after day 2. It is concluded that a single IA administration of SI-613 exerts a more efficacious and longer-lasting analgesic effect for arthritic pain than that exerted by individual chemical compositions.

In addition, the anti-inflammatory effect of SI-613 was assessed by measuring the PGE$_2$ content in the SF. The PGE$_2$ content decreased over time, but high values were maintained for 3 days in this animal model. SI-613 group showed lower PGE$_2$ content than the control group (Fig. 4b). The analgesic effect was confirmed each day (Fig. 4a).

Effect of SI-613 on the PGE$_2$ content in the SF of rabbits with antigen-induced arthritis

At 3 h after administration, the mean PGE$_2$ content in the SF was 27,651 pg/joint (95% CI = 17,844–37,458 pg/joint) in the control group, whereas that in the DF-Na group was 3767 pg/joint (95% CI = 847–6687 pg/joint) (Fig. 5a). Orally administered DF-Na significantly

suppressed the production of PGE$_2$ in the SF compared with the control group, suggesting that this model was appropriate for measuring PGE$_2$. At 72 h after the injection, the mean PGE$_2$ content in the SF was 8267 pg/joint (95% CI = 6535–9999 pg/joint) in the control group. In the DF-Na, DF-Na + HA, and SI-613 groups, the PGE$_2$ content was 8873 pg/joint (95% CI = 6464–11,282 pg/joint), 6378 pg/joint (95% CI = 4319–8437 pg/joint), and 106 pg/joint (95% CI = 70–142 pg/joint), respectively. SI-613 significantly suppressed the production of PGE$_2$ in the SF compared with that of DF-Na, DF-Na + HA, and the control group (Fig. 5b). No significant differences were observed between the DF-Na, DF-Na + HA, and control groups. A single IA administration of SI-613 was shown to exert a longer-lasting effect compared with DF-Na or DF-Na + HA.

Long-lasting anti-inflammatory effect of SI-613 on antigen-induced arthritis in rabbits

SI-613 significantly decreased the knee joint swelling compared with the control on day 1 after the injection, and exerted an anti-inflammatory effect continuously until day 28 (Fig. 6). However, on day 35 and day 42, there was no significant difference in the joint swelling of SI-613-treated and control animals.

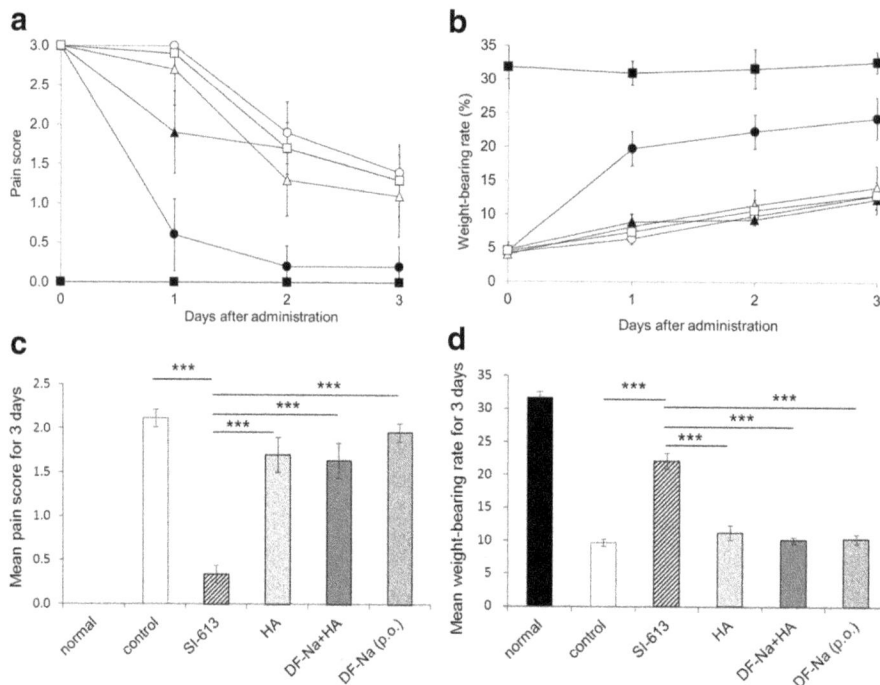

Fig. 3 Analgesic effects of SI-613 and its chemical compositions in silver nitrate-induced arthritic pain model in rats. Silver nitrate-induced arthritic rats given SI-613 (closed circle), HA (open triangle), DF-Na + HA (closed triangle), or vehicle (open circle) intra-articularly; those given DF-Na orally once daily for 3 days (open square); and non-treated normal rats (closed square) were evaluated for pain score (**a**) and weight-bearing rate (**b**) over time. Mean values of pain scores (**c**) and weight-bearing rate (**d**) for 3 days were calculated and subjected to statistical analysis: two-way analyses of variance followed by Tukey's test. ***$p < 0.001$ (vs. SI-613, significant level at 5%, two-tailed). Values represent the means ±95% confidence intervals ($n = 9$ per group, except for the normal group $n = 3$)

Distribution of DF in knee tissues after a single administration of SI-613 and its chemical compositions in rabbits: short-term study

In the antigen-induced arthritis model, the DF concentrations in the synovium and synovial lavage fluid were determined at 72 h after a single IA administration of SI-613 or a mixture of DF-Na and HA. In addition, the DF concentrations at 3 and 72 h after the oral administration of DF-Na were determined. As shown in Table 1, the SI-613-treated group showed higher DF concentrations in the synovium and synovial lavage fluid than the other groups at 72 h after the injection.

Time for calculation of area under the DF plasma concentration-time curve (AUC_{0-t}), t (day), was the latest time point at which DF was quantifiable. The half-life ($T_{1/2}$) was determined by semi-log plotting the data of at least three time points after T_{max}. $T_{1/2}$, $AUC_{0-\infty}$, and AUC_{0-t} were not obtained for one animal in the DF-Na + HA group and all animals in the SI-613 group, both of which did not provide a required number of effective time points after T_{max}, and shown as NC (not calculated). The maximum plasma concentration (C_{max}) of DF in the SI-613 group (IA) was 462 and 94 times lower than those of the DF-Na group (oral) and DF-Na + HA group (IA), respectively. Similarly, the AUC_{0-t} of

the SI-613 group (IA) was 187 and 16 times smaller than that of the DF-Na group (oral) and DF-Na + HA group (IA), respectively (Table 2).

Evaluation of DF in knee tissues after a single IA administration of SI-613 in rabbits: long-term study

Concentrations of DF in the synovium and synovial lavage fluid of antigen-induced arthritis rabbits were determined after a single IA injection of 5 mg of SI-613 by LC-MS/MS. The mean concentration in the synovium was 9.754 ng/g on day 28 and decreased below the lower limit of quantification (< 5 ng/g) on day 35 (Fig. 7a). The mean amount of DF in the joint cavity lavage fluid was 5.940 ng/joint on day 21 and decreased below the lower limit of quantification (< 1 ng of DF per mL of synovial lavage fluid) on day 28 (Fig. 7b). The pharmacokinetic parameters of DF are listed in Table 3.

Discussion

We have investigated the novel HA derivative chemically linked with DF, SI-613, which is a potentially safer and more effective treatment for OA knee pain. In the present study, the pharmacological effects of SI-613 were comprehensively evaluated by comparing the pain response, weight-bearing rate on the inflamed legs, joint

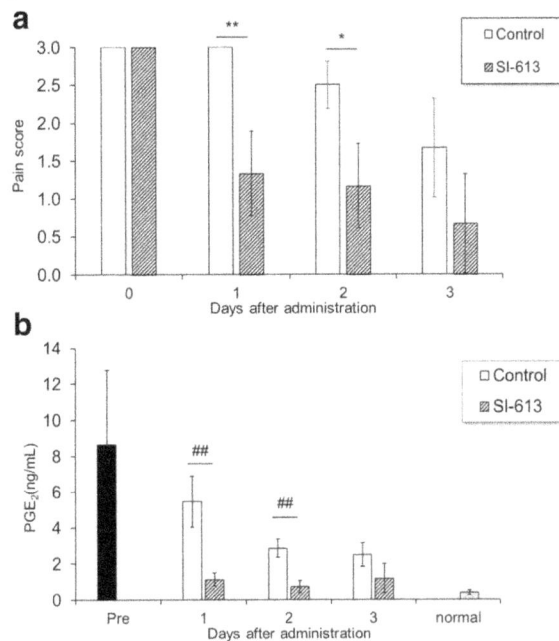

Fig. 4 Effects of SI-613 on PGE_2 content in the synovial fluid of silver nitrate-induced arthritic rats. Silver nitrate-induced arthritic rats given 0.5 mg SI-613 or vehicle intra-articularly were evaluated for pain score (**a**), and sacrificed for measurement of the prostaglandin E_2 (PGE_2) content in the SF (**b**) on days 1, 2, and 3. For statistical analysis of pain score, Wilcoxon test was used. **$p < 0.01$, *$p < 0.05$ (vs. control, significant level at 5%, two-tailed). For statistical analysis of the PGE_2 content, Welch's t-test was used. ##$p < 0.01$ (vs. control, significant level at 5%, two-tailed). Values represent the means ±95% confidence intervals [$n = 6$ per group, except for the normal group (PGE_2 content) $n = 7$]

swelling, and PGE_2 content in the SF as an indicator of hydrarthrosis using rat and rabbit arthritis models. In the arthritic pain model, it was shown that a single IA injection of SI-613 exerted an analgesic effect more effectively than orally administered DF-Na in a dose-dependent manner. The analgesic effect of SI-613 was most probably due to inhibition of PGE_2 production, although the effect on it was slightly varying depending on the model. The PGE_2-inhibitory effect was statistically significant at 72 h after SI-613 administration in the rabbit model but not in the rat model. This can be attributed to the difference of the dynamic range between the models. In the rabbit models, the difference of normal and control groups was sufficiently large even at 72 h. On the other hand, the PGE_2 level of the control group in the rat model was only about 6 times larger than that of the normal group, and then there was no statistically significant difference between the SI-613 and control groups. Moreover, the effect of SI-613 was long-lasting, which was never achieved with the DF-Na + HA mixture. The unstable analgesic effect of uncombined-DF-Na (without HA) is probably due to the fact that it is not well retained in the synovium, which is a therapeutic target tissue for OA. In contrast, it is most likely that intra-articularly administered SI-613 is retained in the synovium for a prolonged period and sustainably releases DF in the inflamed region. The relevance of this notion is supported by other studies that found that HA

administered intra-articularly to the joint cavity penetrated into the synovium and remained in the synovium for a longer period [23, 24]. Furthermore, this efficient retention in the synovium might benefits from the high affinity of HA and its cell surface receptor, CD44 [25], expressed in the synovium [26]. SI-613, thus, delivered efficacious concentrations of DF to synoviocytes. Therefore, we consider that HA is an indispensable component for the analgesic effect of SI-613.

The superiority of SI-613 was supported by its inhibitory effect on the production of PGE_2. This effect resulted from DF being sustainably released from SI-613. The relationship between the pharmacological effects and pharmacokinetics of SI-613 was investigated using a rabbit antigen-induced arthritis model. SI-613 showed a sustainable anti-inflammatory effect for 72 h after administration, whereas the mixture of DF and HA or oral DF-Na did not. The concentration of DF in the synovium and SF at 72 h after the administration of SI-613 was higher than that after the administration of the mixture of DF and HA or oral DF-Na. SI-613 exerted a long-lasting analgesic effect, for 28 days. However, no significant difference was observed on day 35 and 42. The DF concentration in the synovium reached its maximum level of 311.6 ng/g on day 1 after the injection and this gradually declined to 10 ng/g by day 28. It fell below the lower limit of quantification (< 5 ng/g) on day 35. Therefore, there is a clear correlation between the

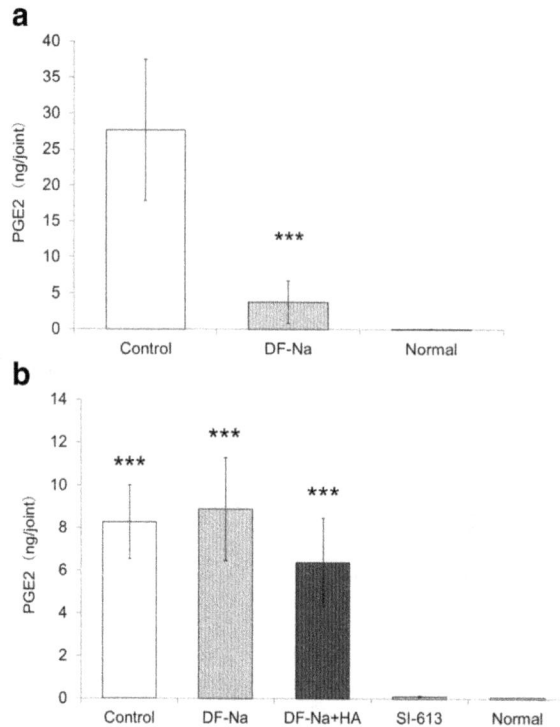

Fig. 5 Effects of SI-613 on PGE$_2$ content in the synovial fluid of antigen-induced arthritis in rabbits. Two days after the induction of arthritis, the test materials were administered. The synovial fluid (SF) was collected at 3 (**a**) or 72 (**b**) hours after the administration of the test materials. The prostaglandin E$_2$ (PGE$_2$) content in the SF was measured with a PGE$_2$ enzyme-linked immunosorbent assay (ELISA) kit. For statistical analysis, a Student's t-test and Tukey's test were used for the 3 h and 72 h data, respectively. **a** ***$p < 0.001$ (vs. control, significant level at 5%, two-tailed). Values represent the means ±95% confidence intervals. ($n = 10$ per group, except for the normal group $n = 5$) (**b**) ***$p < 0.001$ (vs. SI-613, significant level at 5%, two-tailed). Values represent the means ±95% confidence intervals. ($n = 10$ per group, except for the normal group $n = 5$)

analgesic effect and the retention period of DF. The DF concentrations at 28 days after the SI-613 administration were at comparable levels with those in humans after repeated administration of DF preparations. In the clinical studies of current DF preparations, the DF concentrations in the synovium ranged from 5 to 35 ng/g after repeated oral administration of DF tablets and hard capsules or repeated topical administration of DF gel ointments and cataplasms [27, 28]. These findings suggest that SI-613 exerted an analgesic effect via the sustained release of DF, and this pharmacological effect lasted for at least 28 days.

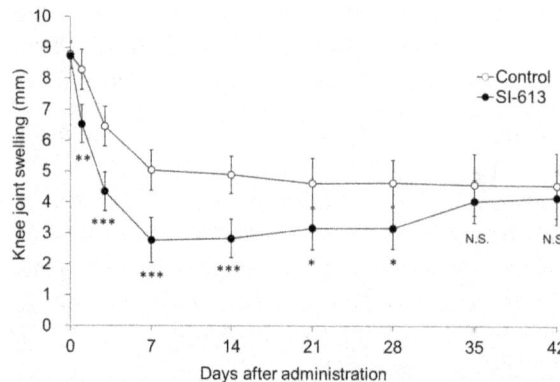

Fig. 6 Long-lasting anti-inflammatory effect of SI-613 on the knee joint swelling of antigen-induced arthritic rabbits. Two days after the induction of arthritis, 1% SI-613 or PBS was administered at a volume of 500 µL/joint into the joint cavities. The knee joint swelling was evaluated on the day before (day 0), and on days 1, 3, 7, 14, 21, 28, 35, and 42 after the injection of test materials. For statistical analysis, a Student's t-test with Holm's correction was used. ***$p < 0.001$, **$p < 0.01$, *$p < 0.05$ (vs. control, significant level at 5%, two-tailed). N.S., not significant. Values represent the means ±95% confidence intervals. ($n = 20$ per group)

Table 1 DF concentrations in the synovium and synovial joint cavity of rabbits with antigen-induced arthritis

Group	Sampling point	Animal Number	Concentration of DF	
			Synovium (ng/g tissue)	Synovial lavage fluid (ng/mL fluid)
DF-Na (oral)	3 h	1	155.8	124.6
		2	52.88	58.23
		3	75.83	45.66
	72 h	4	BLQ1	BLQ2
		5	BLQ1	BLQ2
		6	BLQ1	BLQ2
A mixture of DF-Na and HA (IA)	72 h	1	BLQ1	BLQ2
		2	BLQ1	BLQ2
		3	48.02	21.70
SI-613 (IA)	72 h	1	15.23	60.64
		2	45.47	38.82
		3	351.1	1540

BLQ1: below limit of quantification, < 5 ng/g
BLQ2: < 1 ng of DF per mL of synovial lavage fluid

It has been reported that HA inhibits the phosphorylation of p38 mitogen-activated protein kinase (MAPK) via its principal receptor CD44 and exerts an anti-inflammatory effect [29]. Furthermore, HA inhibits the production of PGE_2, and pretreatment with OS/37, a monoclonal antibody specific for the hyaluronate-binding epitope on CD44, reversed the inhibitory effects of HA [30]. The inhibition of the production of PGE_2 by HA was also confirmed in a clinical study [31]. In addition, it was reported that HA exerted an analgesic effect by covering free nerve endings in articular tissues such as the synovial membranes, menisci, and ligaments [32]. This suggests that SI-613 exerts a clearly superior analgesic effect than DF or HA, or co-administered DF + HA.

Oral NSAIDs are widely prescribed for the relief of OA pain, however, upper gastrointestinal tract complications have been reported in patients who received long-term oral NSAIDs [2]. NSAIDs are also considered to have limited efficacy for OA pain relief. In 1990s, a number of selective COX-2 inhibitors were developed to reduce the adverse events of NSAIDs. However, most of them were withdrawn from the market after the cardiovascular adverse effects of COX-2 inhibitor were reported in 2004 [3]. Meanwhile, oral NSAIDs including DF-Na were also reported to have the same concerns as COX-2 inhibitors [4, 5]. In the present study, the C_{max} of DF (1.343 ng/mL) in the animals given a single IA effective dose of SI-613 was 462 times lower than that in the animals given a single oral effective dose of DF-Na. The AUC_{0-t} (25.11 ng·h/mL) of the SI-613-treated group was 187 times lower than that of the oral DF-Na-treated group. Moreover, the DF concentrations after the SI-613 injection were lower than the reported values of DF-Na after oral administration to humans at the clinical dose (3 × 50 mg/day) [33]. Additionally, the pharmacokinetics of Voltaren* Gel (1% diclofenac sodium topical gel) has been assessed in healthy volunteers following repeated applications to 1 knee [4 × 4 g per day (= 160 mg DF-Na per day)] for 7 days [33]. The C_{max} of DF was 15 ± 7.3 ng/mL, and the value is comparable with those of SI-613-treated animals. These results indicate that systemic toxicities are unlikely to be

Table 2 Plasma DF concentrations of rabbits with antigen-induced arthritis

Group	C_{max} (ng/mL)	T_{max} (h)	AUC_{0-t} (ng·h/mL)	$AUC_{0-\infty}$ (ng·h/mL)	$t_{1/2}$ (h)
DF-Na (oral)	621.0 ± 371.6	2.4 ± 3.2	4693 ± 1905	4132[b]	12.8[b]
Mixture[a]	125.9 ± 68.5	0.39 ± 0.53	393.4 ± 167.6	423.2 ± 154.5	3.4 ± 2.0
SI-613 (IA)	1.343 ± 0.050	24 ± 0	25.11[b]	NC	NC

Mean ± SD ($n = 3$ or $n = 2$) calculated from the individual PK parameters
NC Not calculated.
BLQ: < 1 ng/mL
[a] a mixture of DF-Na and HA (IA)
[b] $n = 2$

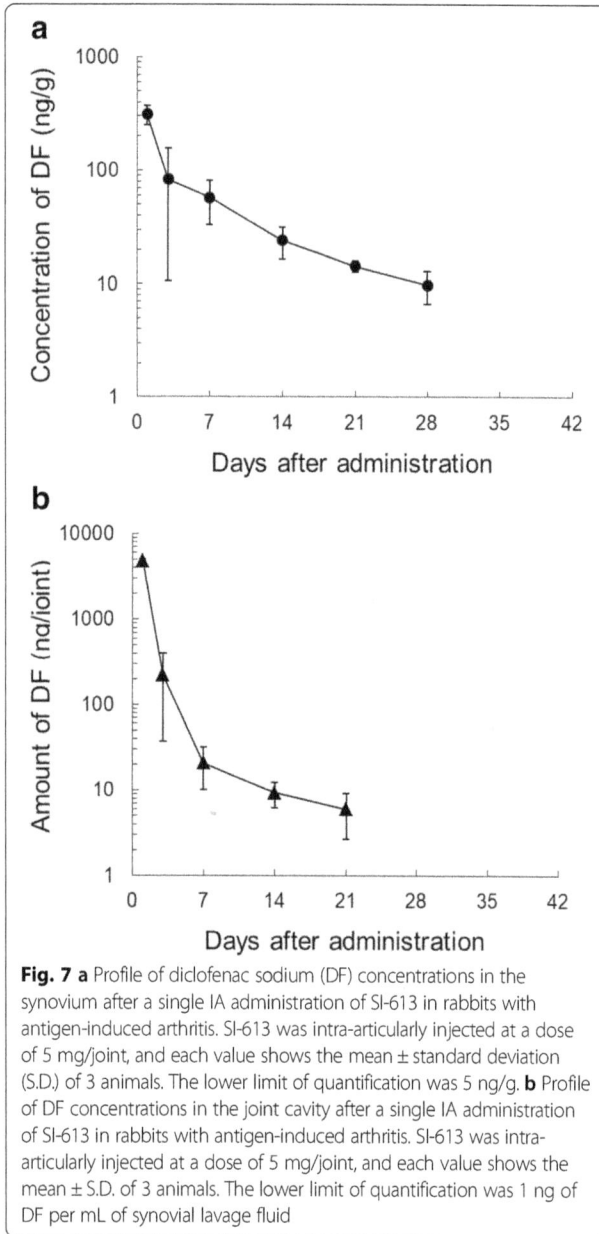

Fig. 7 a Profile of diclofenac sodium (DF) concentrations in the synovium after a single IA administration of SI-613 in rabbits with antigen-induced arthritis. SI-613 was intra-articularly injected at a dose of 5 mg/joint, and each value shows the mean ± standard deviation (S.D.) of 3 animals. The lower limit of quantification was 5 ng/g. **b** Profile of DF concentrations in the joint cavity after a single IA administration of SI-613 in rabbits with antigen-induced arthritis. SI-613 was intra-articularly injected at a dose of 5 mg/joint, and each value shows the mean ± S.D. of 3 animals. The lower limit of quantification was 1 ng of DF per mL of synovial lavage fluid

attributable to DF after a single IA administration of SI-613 to the knees.

OA is characterized by gradual cartilage degeneration. Although NSAIDs are effective in relieving OA pain and have been in use for decades, it remains controversial as to what effects NSAIDs have on the progression of OA. Reijman et al. made the observation that the chronic use of DF, but not ibuprofen, naproxen, or piroxicam, accelerated the progression of knee and hip OA in subjects aged over 55 years [34]. In another paper, Huskisson et al. reported that indomethacin increases the rate of radiological deterioration in the knee joint space of patients with OA [35]. However, the beneficial or neutral effects of NSAIDs have been reported in in vitro and in vivo studies [36–39]. de Boer et al. reported that celecoxib, a selective COX-2 inhibitor, has a chondroprotective effect [40]. Therefore, it is still unclear whether NSAIDs cause cartilage degeneration. IA-HA can protect against articular cartilage degeneration of the knee accelerated by NSAIDs (loxoprofen monosodium and indomethacin) via the inhibition of matrix metalloproteinase (MMP) production [41, 42]. MMPs are upregulated in the chondrocytes of human OA [43–45] and play a critical role in cartilage destruction by degrading collagen and aggrecan, the main proteoglycan of chondrocyte. SI-613, containing HA as a component, may inhibit the interleukin-1β-stimulated production of MMP-1, – 3 and – 13 in human chondrocytes as well as HA. Future research agendas on SI-613 should involve clarifying the pharmacological effect of HA moiety for SI-613.

Conclusion

In conclusion, our results show that a single IA administration of SI-613 provides an efficacious and safe treatment for OA pain with a potent and long-lasting analgesic effect compared to existing IA-HA injections or oral NSAIDs.

Table 3 PK parameters of DF after single IA administration of SI-613 in rabbits with antigen-induced arthritis

	C_{max} (ng/g)	T_{max} (day)	$AUC_{0-28day}$ (ng·day/g)	$AUC_{0-\infty}$ (ng·day/g)	$t_{1/2}$ (day)
Synovium	311.6	1	1336	1487	10.8[a]
	C_{max} (ng/joint)	T_{max} (day)	$AUC_{0-21day}$ (ng·day/joint)	$AUC_{0-\infty}$ (ng·day/joint)	$t_{1/2}$ (day)
Synovial lavage fluid	4726	1	7956	8018	7.7[b]

SI-613 was intra-articularly injected at a dose of 5 mg/joint. The PK parameters were calculated from mean concentrations of DF in synovium or mean amounts of DF in joint cavity (n = 3)
[a], Calculated from 14 to 28 days after administration
[b], Calculated from 7 to 21 days after administration

Abbreviations

CI: Confidence intervals; COX-2: Cyclooxygenase-2; DF: Diclofenac; FCA: Freund's complete adjuvant; HA: Hyaluronic acid; IA: Intra-articular; LC-MS/MS: High performance liquid chromatography coupled with tandem mass spectrometry; MAPK: Mitogen-activated protein kinase; MMP: Matrix metalloproteinase; NSAIDs: Nonsteroidal anti-inflammatory drugs; OA: Osteoarthritis; OVA: Ovalbumin; PBS: Phosphate-buffered saline; PGE_2: Prostaglandin E_2; SD: Standard deviations; SF: Synovial fluid

Acknowledgments

We wish to thank Dr. Tetsuya Ohtaki, Dr. Yoshitaka Tanaka and Takatoshi Kubo in Seikagaku Corporation for study support and assistance in the preparation of the manuscript.

Authors' contributions

KY, TK, RZ, and YY performed most experiments. KY, TK, RZ, and KM designed the study, interpreted the findings, and wrote the manuscript. All authors have read and approved the final manuscript.

Competing interests

All authors of this paper are employees of Seikagaku Corporation. The authors declare that they have no competing interests.

References

1. Buckwalter JA, Saltzman C, Brown T. The impact of osteoarthritis: implications for research. Clin Orthop Relat Res. 2004;427(Suppl):S6–15.
2. Schaffer D, Florin T, Eagle C, Marschner I, Singh G, Grobler M, et al. Risk of serious NSAID-related gastrointestinal events during long-term exposure: a systematic review. Med J Aust. 2006;185:501–6.
3. Tarone RE, Blot WJ, McLaughlin JK. Nonselective nonaspirin nonsteroidal anti-inflammatory drugs and gastrointestinal bleeding: relative and absolute risk estimates from recent epidemiologic studies. Am J Ther. 2004;11:17–25.
4. Bresalier RS, Sandler RS, Quan H, Bolognese JA, Oxenius B, Horgan K, et al. Cardiovascular events associated with rofecoxib in a colorectal adenoma chemoprevention trial. N Engl J Med. 2005;352:1092–102.
5. Trelle S, Reichenbach S, Wandel S, Hildebrand P, Tschannen B, Villiger PM, et al. Cardiovascular safety of non-steroidal anti-inflammatory drugs: network meta-analysis. BMJ. 2011;c7086:342.
6. Peniston JH, Gold MS, Wieman MS, Alwine LK. Long-term tolerability of topical diclofenac sodium 1% gel for osteoarthritis in seniors and patients with comorbidities. Clin Interv Aging. 2012;7:517–23.
7. Efe T, Sagnak E, Roessler PP, Getgood A, Patzer T, Fuchs-Winkelmann S, et al. Penetration of topical diclofenac sodium 4% spray gel into the synovial tissue and synovial fluid of the knee: a randomised clinical trial. Knee Surg Sports Traumatol Arthrosc. 2014;22:345–50.
8. Wadsworth LT, Kent JD, Holt RJ. Efficacy and safety of diclofenac sodium 2%topical solution for osteoarthritis of the knee: a randomized, double-blind,vehicle-controlled, 4 week study. Curr Med Res Opin. 2016;32:241–50.
9. Zhang W, Moskowitz RW, Nuki G, Abramson S, Altman RD, Arden N, et al. OARSI recommendations for the management of hip and knee osteoarthritis, part II: OARSI evidence-based, expert consensus guidelines. Osteoarthr Cartil. 2008;16:137–62.
10. Zhang W, Nuki G, Moskowitz RW, Abramson S, Altman RD, Arden NK, et al. OARSI recommendations for the management of hip and knee osteoarthritis part III: changes in evidence following systematic cumulative update of research published through January 2009. Osteoarthr Cartil. 2010; 18:476–99.
11. Recommendations for the medical management of osteoarthritis of the hip and knee: 2000 update. American College of Rheumatology Subcommittee on osteoarthritis guidelines. Arthritis Rheum. 2000;43:1905–15.
12. Strand V, Baraf HS, Lavin PT, Lim S, Hosokawa H. A multicenter, randomized controlled trial comparing a single intra-articular injection of Gel-200, a new cross-linked formulation of hyaluronic acid, to phosphate buffered saline for treatment of osteoarthritis of the knee. Osteoarthr Cartil. 2012;20:350–6.
13. Day R, Brooks P, Conaghan PG, Petersen M. Multicenter trial group. A double blind, randomized, multicenter, parallel group study of the effectiveness and tolerance of intraarticular hyaluronan in osteoarthritis of the knee. J Rheumatol. 2004;31:775–82.
14. Belle AL, Tislow R. A method of evaluating analgesics of the antiarthralgic type in the laboratory animal. J Pharm Exp Ther. 1950;98:19.
15. Nakamura H, Yokoyama Y, Motoyoshi S, Seto Y, Ishii K, Imazu C, et al. Anti-inflammatory and analgesic activities of a trans-cutaneous non-steroidal anti-inflammatory agent, etofenamate gel, in experimental animals.(in Japanese). Nippon Yakurigaku Zasshi. 1982;80:183–94.
16. Nakamura H, Yokoyama Y, Ishii K, Motoyoshi S, Seto Y, Shimizu M. Effect of a non-steroidal anti-inflammatory drug, tolmetin sodium on arthritic pain, traumatic edema and LPS-induced fever. (in Japanese). Yakugaku Zasshi. 1981;101:649–56.
17. Nakamura H, Yokoyama Y, Motoyoshi S, Ishii K, Imazu C, Seto Y, et al. The pharmacological profile of 2-(8-methyl-10,11-dihydro-11-oxodibenz[b, f]oxepin-2-yl)propionic acid (AD-1590), a new non-steroidal anti-inflammatory agent with potent antipyretic activity. Arzneimittelforschung. 1983;33(11):1555e69.
18. Tsukahara-Ohsumi Y, Tsuji F, Niwa M, Nakamura M, Mizutani K, Inagaki N, et al. SA14867, a newly synthesized kappa-opioid receptor agonist with antinociceptive and antipruritic effects. Eur J Pharmacol. 2010;647:62–7.
19. Tsurumi K, Hiramatsu Y, Yamaguchi A, Hayashi M, Shibuya T, Fujimura H. Anti-inflammatory action of N-(2,6-dichlorophenyl)-o-aminophenylacetic acid, its sodium salt, N-(2,6-dichlorophenyl)-anthranilic acid and its sodium salt. 2. On subacute inflammation. (in Japanese). Nippon Yakurigaku Zasshi. 1973;69:319–34.
20. Kiniwa M, Yamamoto N, Hashimoto Y, Miyake H, Masuda H. Anti-inflammatory effect of THS-201, a new intra-articular steroid. (in Japanese). Nippon Yakurigaku Zasshi. 1986;87:89–97.
21. Pettipher ER, Henderson B, Edwards JC, Higgs GA. Effect of indomethacin on swelling, lymphocyte influx, and cartilage proteoglycan depletion in experimental arthritis. Ann Rheum Dis. 1989;48:623–7.
22. Green KL, Foong WC. Treatment of antigen-induced arthritis in rabbits by the intra-articular injection of methylprednisolone, 90Y or chlorambucil. J Pharm Pharmacol. 1993;45:815–20.
23. Antonas KN, Fraser JR, Muirden KD. Distribution of biologically labelled radioactive hyaluronic acid injected into joints. Ann Rheum Dis. 1973;32: 103–11.
24. Jackson DW, Simon TM. Intra-articular distribution and residence time of Hylan a and B: a study in the goat knee. Osteoarthr Cartil. 2006;14:1248–57.
25. Aruffo A, Stamenkovic I, Melnick M, Underhill CB, Seed B. CD44 is the principal cell surface receptor for hyaluronate. Cell. 1990;61:1303–13.
26. Hale LP, Haynes BF, McCachren SS. Expression of CD44 variants in human inflammatory synovitis. J Clin Immunol. 1995;15:300–11.
27. Miyatake S, Ichiyama H, Kondo E, Yasuda K. Randomized clinical comparisons of diclofenac concentration in the soft tissues and blood plasma between topical and oral applications. Br J Clin Pharmacol. 2009;67: 125 9.
28. Mashima T, Kondo M, Sakiyama N. Concentrations of Voltaren (diclofenac sodium) SR capsule in serum and tissues of patients with rheumatoid arthritis. Japanese journal of inflammation (Japan). 1995;15:255–9.
29. Julovi SM, Ito H, Hiramitsu T, Yasuda T, Nakamura T. Hyaluronan inhibits IL-1β-stimulated collagenase production via down-regulation of phosphorylated p38 in SW-1353 human chondrosarcoma cells. Mod Rheumatol. 2008;18:263–70.
30. Mitsui Y, Gotoh M, Nakamura K, Yamada T, Higuchi F, Nagata K. Hyaluronic acid inhibits mRNA expression of proinflammatory cytokines and cyclooxygenase-2/prostaglandin E(2) production via CD44 in interleukin-1-stimulated subacromial synovial fibroblasts from patients with rotator cuff disease. J Orthop Res. 2008;26:1032–7.
31. Goto M, Hanyu T, Yoshio T, Matsuno H, Shimizu M, Murata N, et al. Intra-articular injection of hyaluronate (SI-6601D) improves joint pain and synovial fluid prostaglandin E_2 levels in rheumatoid arthritis: a multicenter clinical trial. Clin Exp Rheumatol. 2001;19:377–83.
32. Gotoh S, Miyazaki K, Onaya J, Sakamoto T, Tokuyasu K, Namiki O. Experimental knee pain model in rats and analgesic effect of sodium hyaluronate (SPH). (in Japanese). Nippon Yakurigaku Zasshi. 1988;92:17–27.

33. Prescribing Information for Voltaren 1% Gel (diclofenac sodium topical gel). (revised: Nov. 2011, NDA No. 022 122).

34. Reijman M, Bierma-Zeinstra SM, Pols HA, Koes BW, Stricker BH, Hazes JM. Is there an association between the use of different types of nonsteroidal antiinflammatory drugs and radiologic progression of osteoarthritis? The Rotterdam study. Arthritis Rheum. 2005;52:3137–42.

35. Huskisson EC, Berry H, Gishen P, Jubb RW, Whitehead J. Effects of antiinflammatory drugs on the progression of osteoarthritis of the knee. LINK study group. Longitudinal investigation of nonsteroidal Antiinflammatory drugs in knee osteoarthritis. J Rheumatol. 1995;22:1941–6.

36. Ding C. Do NSAIDs affect the progression of osteoarthritis? Inflammation. 2002;26:139–42.

37. Dingle JT. The effects of NSAID on the matrix of human articular cartilages. Z Rheumatol. 1999;58:125–9.

38. Smith RL, Kajiyama G, Lane NE. Nonsteroidal antiinflammatory drugs: effects on normal and interleukin 1 treated human articular chondrocyte metabolism in vitro. J Rheumatol. 1995;22:1130–7.

39. Dieppe P, Cushnaghan J, Jasani MK, McCrae F, Watt I. A two-year, placebo-controlled trial of non-steroidal anti-inflammatory therapy in osteoarthritis of the knee joint. Br J Rheumatol. 1993;32:595–600.

40. de Boer TN, Huisman AM, Polak AA, Niehoff AG, van Rinsum AC, Saris D, et al. The chondroprotective effect of selective COX-2 inhibition in osteoarthritis: ex vivo evaluation of human cartilage tissue after in vivo treatment. Osteoarthr Cartil. 2009;17:482–8.

41. Mihara M, Higo S, Uchiyama Y, Tanabe K, Saito K. Different effects of high molecular weight sodium hyaluronate and NSAID on the progression of the cartilage degeneration in rabbit OA model. Osteoarthr Cartil. 2007;15:543–9.

42. Hashizume M, Mihara M. Desirable effect of combination therapy with high molecular weight hyaluronate and NSAIDs on MMP production. Osteoarthr Cartil. 2009;17:1513–8.

43. Okada A, Okada Y. Progress of research in osteoarthritis. Metalloproteinases in osteoarthritis. Clin Calcium. 2009;19:1593–601.

44. Vincenti MP, Brinckerhoff CE. Transcriptional regulation of collagenase (MMP-1, MMP-13) genes in arthritis: integration of complex signaling pathways for the recruitment of gene-specific transcription factors. Arthritis Res. 2002;4:157–64.

45. Takaishi H, Kimura T, Dalal S, Okada Y, D'Armiento J. Joint diseases and matrix metalloproteinases: a role for MMP-13. Curr Pharm Biotechnol. 2008; 9:47–54.

20

Runners with patellofemoral pain demonstrate sub-groups of pelvic acceleration profiles using hierarchical cluster analysis

Ricky Watari[1,2], Sean T. Osis[1,3], Angkoon Phinyomark[4] and Reed Ferber[1,2,3,5*] (iD)

Abstract

Background: Previous studies have suggested that distinct and homogenous sub-groups of gait patterns exist among runners with patellofemoral pain (PFP), based on gait analysis. However, acquisition of 3D kinematic data using optical systems is time consuming and prone to marker placement errors. In contrast, axial segment acceleration data can represent an overall running pattern, being easy to acquire and not influenced by marker placement error. Therefore, the purpose of this study was to determine if pelvic acceleration patterns during running could be used to classify PFP patients into homogeneous sub-groups. A secondary purpose was to analyze lower limb kinematic data to investigate the practical implications of clustering these subjects based on 3D pelvic acceleration data.

Methods: A hierarchical cluster analysis was used to determine sub-groups of similar running profiles among 110 PFP subjects, separately for males ($n = 44$) and females ($n = 66$), using pelvic acceleration data (reduced with principal component analysis) during treadmill running acquired with optical motion capture system. In a secondary analysis, peak joint angles were compared between clusters ($a = 0.05$) to provide clinical context and deeper understanding of variables that separated clusters.

Results: The results reveal two distinct running gait sub-groups (C1 and C2) for female subjects and no sub-groups were identified for males. Two pelvic acceleration components were different between clusters (PC1 and PC5; $p < 0.001$). While females in C1 presented similar acceleration patterns to males, C2 presented greater vertical and anterior peak accelerations. All females presented higher and delayed mediolateral acceleration peaks than males. Males presented greater ankle eversion ($p < 0.001$), lower knee abduction ($p = 0.007$) and hip adduction ($p = 0.002$) than all females, and lower hip internal rotation than C1 ($p = 0.007$).

Conclusions: Two distinct and homogeneous kinematic PFP sub-groups were identified for female subjects, but not for males. The results suggest that differences in running gait patterns between clusters occur mainly due to sex-related factors, but there are subtle differences among female subjects. This study shows the potential use of pelvic acceleration patterns, which can be acquired with accessible wearable technology (i.e. accelerometers).

Keywords: Patellofemoral pain, Running kinematics, Pelvic acceleration, Gait analysis, Biomechanics, Principal component analysis, Cluster analysis

* Correspondence: rferber@ucalgary.ca
[1]Faculty of Kinesiology, University of Calgary, Calgary, Alberta, Canada
[2]Coordination for the Improvement of Higher Education Personnel (CAPES), Brasilia, Brazil
Full list of author information is available at the end of the article

Background

Patellofemoral pain (PFP) is the most common musculo-skeletal overuse injury in runners, regardless of sex and age [1] and it has been suggested that atypical gait kinematics may play a role in its etiology [2–4]. However, a general consensus on the pathomechanics of this injury has yet to be reached [4] possibly due to the existence of more than a single atypical gait pattern [5–8].

Distinct running kinematic sub-groups have been identified in PFP patients, with a sub-group presenting lower peak hip adduction; another with greater peak knee abduction angles [6]; and a sub-group that presented an attempt to compensate for a greater initial hip internal rotation with an external rotation during mid-stance [7], suggesting the existence of multiple kinematic pathomechanical pathways or motor adaptations associated with PFP. It also has been shown that kinematic differences are influenced by sex-related factors, wherein males with PFP present lower angles of hip adduction and knee abduction during running [8]. These findings should be interpreted with caution, as they are from relatively small sample sizes ($n = 16$–22) and were based on visual inspection of the data, approaches which may not fully describe the etiology of PFP and related sub-groups.

The consensus statement from the 3rd International Patellofemoral Pain Research [9] concluded that "identification of sub-groups remains the 'holy grail' for PFP research". Identification of sub-groups could provide insight into the pathomechanics associated with PFP as well as inform personalized treatment. One approach to identify homogenous sub-groups within a dataset is the use of cluster analyses. With the advance of technology and data science methods the use of machine learning techniques in gait analysis is growing and exploratory analysis of complex data such as gait kinematics is important to bring new insights in the field [10, 11]. Recent research from our laboratory [12] utilized a hierarchical cluster analysis (HCA) approach to successfully identify two distinct and homogeneous kinematic sub-groups among 121 healthy runners. However, because the acquisition of 3-dimensional (3D) kinematics data is time consuming, it usually relies on multiple assessors to collect data on larger sample sizes, introducing sources of imprecision into the data collection process, especially from marker placement errors [13–15]. Therefore, finding alternative methods for evaluating gait mechanics becomes important for clinical applications.

Recently, axial segment acceleration data has provided unique insight into running mechanics, discriminating between fatigue states [16] and training levels [17]. Therefore, the analysis of pelvic acceleration profiles could also be useful to identify sub-groups of runners with PFP, with the advantage of being less influenced by identification of anatomical landmarks when using optical motion capture systems. Furthermore, the study of segmental accelerations has the option to use wearable devices for data acquisition, which are becoming increasingly popular in both academia and industry, and there has been an effort to further investigate their potential applications in health systems [18–20]. Therefore, this approach may offer an accessible and objective method of assessment with clinical applicability.

The purpose of this exploratory study was to determine if running gait patterns in PFP runners could be clustered into homogeneous sub-groups using pelvic acceleration data, using a large dataset of males and females with PFP. Based on the results from previous studies, we hypothesized that more than one running gait pattern sub-group, or cluster, would be present in female PFP runners, since the studies suggesting the existence of sub-groups were mostly comprised of women [6, 7]. Furthermore, female runners with PFP would be different from their male counterparts, given that sex-related kinematic differences have been identified previously [8]. A secondary purpose was to analyze kinematic differences between the sub-groups, by comparing lower limb peak angles that are considered important in the pathomechanics of PFP, and thereby investigate the practical and clinical implications of clustering these subjects based on 3D pelvic acceleration data. Based on the kinematic sub-groups that has been described in the literature [6, 7], we expected female clusters to present differences in hip and knee frontal and transverse plane angles, and males to display lower peak angles of hip adduction and knee abduction [8].

Methods

Participants

Data from 110 physically active individuals with PFP with running as their primary exercise modality for at least 6 months, were analyzed in this cross-sectional study. The presence of PFP was confirmed by a licensed healthcare professional (i.e., athletic therapist, physical therapist or medical doctor) based on specific inclusion and exclusion criteria (Table 1). Subjects experiencing pain in other sites were also included in the study, however the primary complaint had to be PFP. Data was collected either at the University of Calgary or in clinical settings partnered with the Running Injury Clinic.

Data collection

The data collection methods are described in detail elsewhere [21, 22]. Briefly, 8 high-speed digital video cameras (MX3/Nexus, Vicon, Oxford, UK) were used to film treadmill-running at 200 Hz. Spherical retro-reflective markers (9 mm diameter, Mocap Solutions, Huntington Beach, USA) were attached to the specific lower extremity

Table 1 Inclusion and exclusion criteria[a]

Inclusion criteria

1. Insidious onset of symptoms unrelated to trauma and persistent for at least 4 wk

2. Pain in the anterior knee associated with at least 3 of the following:

  a. During or after activity (running and other physical activity modalities)

  b. Prolonged sitting

  c. Stair ascent or descent

  d. Squatting

3. Pain with palpation of the patellar facets or pain during step down from a 20-cm box or during a double-legged squat

Exclusion criteria

1. Meniscal or other intra-articular injury

2. Cruciate or collateral ligament laxity or tenderness

3. Positive patellar-apprehension sign

4. Evidence of effusion

5. History of recurrent patellar subluxation or dislocation

6. History of surgery to the knee joint

7. Nonsteroidal anti-inflammatory drug or corticosteroid use within 24 hours before testing

8. History of head injury or vestibular disorder within the last 6 months

9. Pregnancy

[a]adapted from Ferber et al. (2015) [3]

anatomical landmarks bilaterally along with technical marker clusters on rigid shells placed to represent the pelvis and bilateral foot, shank, and thigh segments. Each participant wore the same shoes (Pegasus, Nike, Beaverton, USA) to standardize the footwear condition.

Following placement of all the anatomical and segment markers, each participant stood on a motorized treadmill (Bertec Corporation, Columbus, OH, USA) for a 1 s static trial. Upon completion of the static trial, the markers on the anatomical landmarks were removed while the technical marker clusters remained. The participants were instructed to warm-up on the treadmill for 2–3 min, and then ran on the treadmill at a comfortable self-selected pace (2.61 ± 0.20 m/s) for 20 s, in which approximately 60–80 consecutive running steps were collected for processing and analysis. All participants were experienced treadmill users and were permitted as much time as they required to familiarize themselves with treadmill running before beginning the data collection.

Data processing
Ankle, knee and hip joint sagittal plane angular accelerations were used for defining ground contact, using previously published event detection methods [23]. The position of the pelvis was measured using the centroid

of the pelvic marker cluster [24] and pelvic acceleration was calculated by double differentiation of pelvis displacement using a modified Savitzky-Golay method [25]. Differentiation was performed at both stages using a time-window of 10 data points, and 4th order polynomial fitting. In order to emulate a wearable device, marker accelerations in the global coordinate frame were then converted to a local coordinate frame on the pelvis, using segment markers and rigid body transformations [26]. The local coordinate frame was aligned with the global frame during the static trial.

Each step cycle was normalized to 100 points, with 80 data points for stance and 20 data points for flight phase, since we are analyzing an axial segment. These normalized phases were then combined to represent 100% of the step cycle, averaged over all extracted steps, and standardized to zero mean and unit variance. The kinematic data (3 planes of motions × 100 time-normalized pelvic accelerations) were combined into one 300-dimensional row vector for each subject, creating a matrix of 110 subjects-by-300 data points.

Data analysis
The HCA method was used to identify homogeneous running gait patterns separately for males and females based on the pelvic acceleration time-series, by creating a cluster tree, or dendrogram for each sex-group. Agglomerative strategy or a "bottom up" approach was used, which consists of three steps: (1) a measure of dissimilarity between sets of subjects using the Euclidean distance, (2) subject linkage using the Ward's minimum variance method [27], and (3) cluster determination using the variance ratio criterion [28].

Following identification of homogeneous clusters (subgroups) of PFP runners, differences in demographics, injury characteristics, vertical displacement of the pelvic centroid and peak joint angles were examined using one-way ANOVA (Tukey test for post-hoc analyses) and chi-squared test ($\alpha = 0.05$), and effect sizes were calculated based on η^2 and Cramer's V indices, respectively. In case the data did not present a normal distribution (Shapiro-Wilk test) or a homogeneous variance between sub-groups (Levene test), the Kruskal-Wallis test was performed (Dunn's test for post-hoc analyses). Differences in pelvic acceleration patterns were examined after applying a principal component analysis (PCA) to the standardized data matrix, and they were identified based on the interpretation of principal components (PCs) that presented a large effect size ($\eta^2 > 0.14$) [12, 29], which were used to reconstruct the acceleration waveforms for a better mechanical interpretation [30]. The squared coefficients of correlations between the PC scores and the raw acceleration data (squared loading) [31] were used to calculate the relative loading of the PCs in the vertical (VT), antero-posterior (AP) and medio-lateral (ML) directions to aid in the interpretation of the PCs [32].

We also selected joint angles that are considered important in PFP pathomechanics and that have been suggested to differ between PFP sub-groups [6, 33], to compare between sub-groups. The analyzed peak joint angles were: ankle eversion; knee flexion, knee abduction and knee external rotation; and hip adduction and internal rotation.

A Pearson's correlation coefficient was calculated between the significant PCs and demographic, injury characterization and kinematic variables that presented differences between sub-groups to determine whether these latter factors were significantly correlated with the acceleration patterns. All data processing and statistical analysis were performed on MATLAB 9.1 (The Math-Works Inc., Natick, MA,USA).

Results

Identification of PFP sub-groups

For the female subjects, the variance ratio criterion determined the optimal number of clusters to be two sub-groups (C1 and C2) (Fig. 1a), whereas for the male subjects, no sub-groups could be identified (Fig. 1b) in the HCA.

Subject clinical and demographic characteristics for each cluster are presented in Table 2. There was a significant difference in height ($H = 49.9$; df = 2; $p < 0.001$; $\eta^2 = 0.32$), with male subjects being taller than both female clusters ($p < 0.001$ for males vs C1, and males vs C2); and also in mass ($H = 50.2$; df = 2; $p < 0.001$; $\eta^2 = 0.32$), with male subjects being heavier than both female clusters ($p < 0.001$ for males vs C1, and males vs C2). There were no significant differences between clusters with respect to age ($F = 2.4$; df = 2; $p = 0.095$; $\eta^2 = 0.04$), running speed ($H = 1.3$; df = 2; $p = 0.521$; $\eta^2 = 0.01$), years running ($H = 0.9$; df = 2; $p = 0.629$; $\eta^2 = 0.01$); ratio of unilateral to bilateral involvement ($\chi^2 = 1.7$; $p = 0.434$; $V = 0.12$) or subjects with multiple injury sites ($\chi^2 = 0.5$; $p = 0.781$; $V = 0.07$).

Table 3 presents descriptive statistics for each cluster regarding pelvic acceleration components, vertical displacement and lower limb kinematics. There were significant differences with large effect sizes between subgroups only for the following principal components of pelvic acceleration: PC1 ($F = 39.7$; df = 2; $p < 0.001$; $\eta^2 = 0.43$), with the distinct group being the females in C2 (p

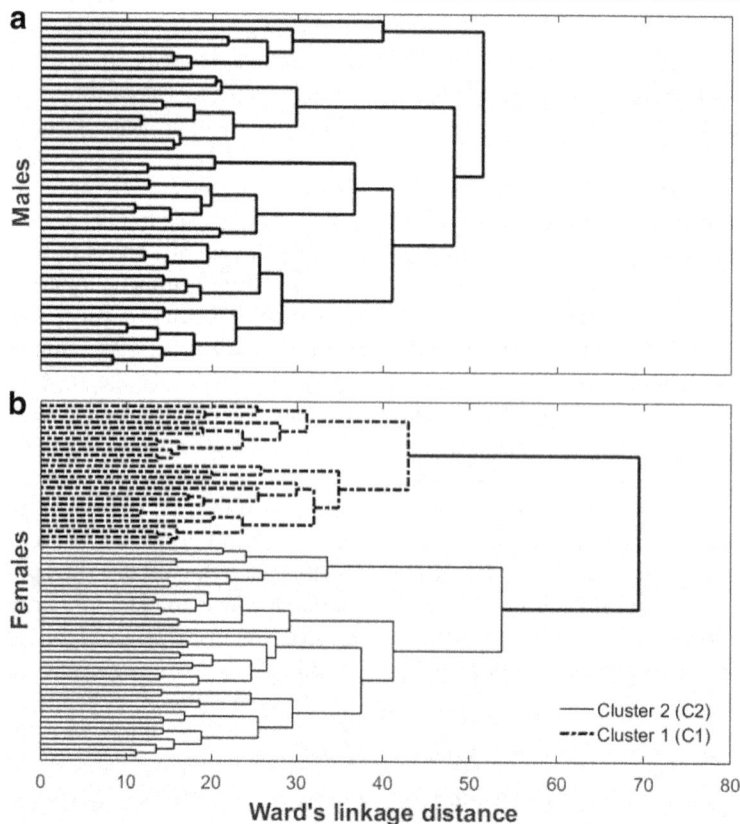

Fig. 1 Dendrogram of the hierarchical cluster analysis. Clustering of PFP patients produced by the hierarchical cluster analysis. **a** Male subjects; (**b**) Female subjects

Table 2 Number of PFP participants and subject specifications (Mean and (SD)) for the determined clusters

	Males (n = 44)	Females_C1 (n = 26)	Females_C2 (n = 40)
Age [years][a]	35.1 (1.5)	30.9 (2.0)	36.4 (1.6)
Height [m][b]	1.79 (0.01)*	1.66 (0.01)	1.66 (0.01)
Mass [kg][b]	77.2 (1.3)*	59.1 (1.7)	63.4 (1.4)
Running speed [m/s][b]	2.66 (0.03)	2.60 (0.04)	2.57 (0.03)
Years running [years][b]	8.6 (8.0)	7.0 (7.1)	9.0 (7.7)
Involvement [uni/bilateral][c]	20 / 24	13 / 13	14 / 26
Injury site [single/multiple][c]	33 / 11	19 / 7	32 / 8

[a]One-way ANOVA; [b] Kruskal-Wallis test; [c] chi-squared test; * significantly different from other 2 groups

< 0.001 for males vs C2, and C1 vs C2); and PC5 ($F = 19.8$; df = 2; $p < 0.001$; $\eta^2 = 0.27$), wherein C1 was the subgroup with significant difference ($p < 0.001$ for males vs C1, and C2 vs C1). However, these PCs explained less than 25% of the variance in the dataset (17.0% and 7.7%, respectively). Height presented a significant correlation with PC1 ($p = 0.016$), but not with PC5 ($p = 0.064$), and the correlation coefficients were weak ($r < 0.30$). Although, body mass was different between subgroups, it had no significant correlation ($p > 0.05$) with either of the selected PCs.

Differences in running kinematics between sub-groups
There was a significant difference in peak ankle eversion ($H = 15.1$; df = 2; $p < 0.001$; $\eta^2 = 0.12$), wherein male PFP subjects presented greater angles than C1 ($p = 0.003$) and C2 ($p = 0.004$), and this joint angle had a low but significant correlation with PC1 ($p < 0.036$, $r = -0.20$), but not with PC5. Peak knee abduction was also significantly different between clusters ($H = 12.3$; df = 2; $p = 0.002$; $\eta^2 = 0.09$), with males exhibiting lower angles when compared to C1 ($p = 0.019$) and C2 ($p = 0.005$), and this joint angle was also only correlated with PC1 ($p < 0.001$, $r = 0.38$). There were also differences in hip adduction ($\Gamma = 6.5$; df = 2; $p = 0.002$; $\eta^2 = 0.11$), with lower angles for male subjects in comparison to C1 ($p = 0.043$) and C2 ($p = 0.003$). The same tendency occurred

for hip internal rotation ($F = 5.2$; df = 2; $p = 0.007$; $\eta^2 = 0.09$), however the difference was only significant for males compared to women in C1 ($p = 0.006$). While peak hip adduction was correlated with PC1 ($p = 0.005$, $r = -0.27$), hip internal rotation demonstrated a correlation with PC 5 ($p = 0.014$, $r = -0.23$). There were no significant differences for knee flexion ($H = 2.2$; df = 2; $p = 0.331$; $\eta^2 < 0.01$) and external rotation ($F = 1.4$; df = 2; $p = 0.251$; $\eta^2 = 0.03$). Vertical displacement of the pelvis presented differences between sub-groups ($F = 11.1$; df = 2; $p < 0.001$; $\eta^2 = 0.17$), wherein females from C1 displayed lower magnitudes of displacement when compared to males ($p < 0.001$) and females in C2 ($p = 0.011$); and this variable was only correlated with PC5 ($p = 0.026$, $r = 0.21$).

PC1 presented a high relative loading in the VT direction (47.9%), representing variations in the peak acceleration and the magnitude at early stance phase (Fig. 2a). There was a lower relative loading of PC1 in the AP direction (28.9%), wherein it represented a phase shift of the posterior acceleration peak in early stance (Fig. 2b). In the ML direction, PC1 also represented phase shifts in ML peak accelerations towards the stance and swing limbs during the first half of stance phase (Fig. 2c), but it was the lowest relative loading (23.2%).

PC5 also had relatively high loadings in the VT axis (43.0%), denoting a difference in the rate of magnitude

Table 3 Mean and standard deviation of PC scores, vertical displacement and peak joint angles

	Males (n = 44)	Female C1 (n = 26)	Female C2 (n = 40)
PC 1 [a.u.] [a]	2.84 (0.8)	4.6 (1.1)	**−6.1 (0.9)***
PC 5 [a.u.] [a]	1.4 (0.6)	**−4.5 (0.8)***	1.4 (0.7)
Vertical displacement [mm] [a]	104.7 (2.1)	**88.8 (2.7)***	98.9 (2.2)
Ankle eversion [°] [b]	**7.2 (0.6)***	4.1 (0.8)	4.2 (0.7)
Knee flexion [°] [b]	44.6 (0.9)	43.2 (1.2)	44.2 (0.9)
Knee abduction [°] [b]	**9.3 (0.7)***	11.9 (0.9)	12.4 (0.7)
Knee external rotation [°] [a]	10.0 (1.4)	11.1 (1.8)	7.6 (1.4)
Hip adduction [°] [a]	**8.2 (0.7)***	10.9 (0.9)	11.6 (0.7)
Hip internal rotation [°] [a]	12.7 (1.1)[#]	18.3 (1.4)[#]	15.8 (1.1)

[a]One-way ANOVA; [b] Kruskal-Wallis test; * significantly different from the other 2 groups; [#] significant difference between the indicated groups
Bold number indicates a large effect size ($d > 0.8$)

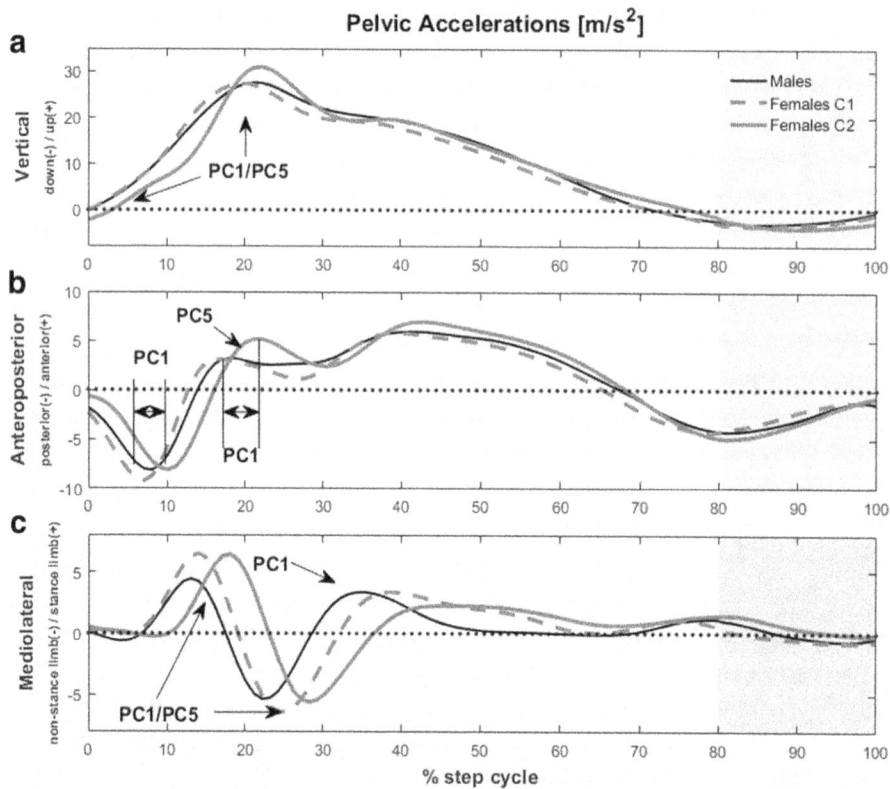

Fig. 2 Time-normalized pelvic accelerations. **a** Vertical acceleration, (**b**) Anteroposterior acceleration, and (**c**) Mediolateral acceleration for males and female sub-groups C1 and C2 during stance phase (1%–80%) and flight phase (81%–100%; gray area) of running. Regions represented by the significant principal components are indicated in the graphs

decrease after the peak acceleration (Fig. 2a), although these differences are subtle. The AP relative loading was the lowest for PC5 (25.0%) and it indicated a magnitude difference in the forward acceleration after weight acceptance (Fig. 2b). In the ML direction, there was a low relative loading (32.1%), representing a difference in magnitude variation during the first half of stance phase (Fig. 2c).

Overall, when comparing the pelvic acceleration patterns, males had similar acceleration patterns to females in C1 in the VT and AP directions, but the latter presented higher and delayed peaks ML accelerations. Females in C2 displayed lower acceleration magnitudes in early stance and a higher peak acceleration in the VT direction; a greater forward peak in early stance; and delayed peak accelerations in the AP and ML directions.

Discussion

PFP sub-groups based on pelvic acceleration

The first purpose of the present study was to determine if running gait patterns in individuals experiencing PFP at the time of testing could be clustered into homogeneous sub-groups based on combinations of pelvic acceleration components. In support of our hypothesis, two

distinct and homogenous sub-groups (clusters) were present in females with PFP, and these clusters were different when compared to PFP males. These results are similar to previous studies that also reported two to three different running patterns based on visual inspection of 3D kinematic data [6, 7] and mechanical differences between males and females with PFP [8].

There were no significant differences in running speed between sub-groups, which is a factor that has been shown to affect axial segment acceleration [34], especially in the ML axis [35]. Male subjects were significantly taller and heavier than females and these anthropometric differences are known to influence 3D kinematics during running [36]. However, there was a very weak correlation for height, and no correlation for body mass with the acceleration PCs that presented differences between sub-groups suggesting that the relationship with those factors was minimal.

The advantage of investigating pelvic acceleration as a measure of running mechanics is that it is less influenced by marker placement errors and is a much simpler method than a full 3D gait assessment, as it depends only on the trajectory of a single pelvic marker cluster. Additionally, these factors allow for the use of data from multiple research centres, allowing for the application of 'big data' analytics and a better understanding of the interaction between biomechanical factors and musculoskeletal injuries [10, 11]. Furthermore, the results of the present study opens the possibility for the use of wearable devices for data acquisition, such as a single triaxial accelerometer on the pelvis, an approach which is becoming increasingly popular in industry and health care [18, 20]. Therefore, the current work identifying sub-groups of PFP patients is a novel finding that can guide future studies in providing better context that can hopefully improve clinical practice.

Identification of differences in running gait patterns between sub-groups

A secondary purpose was to analyze peak joint angles between clusters to better understand the practical and clinical implications of clustering subjects with PFP based on 3D pelvic acceleration data. In general, differences in joint kinematics were sex-related, since there were no significant differences between female clusters, except for peak hip internal rotation. Moreover, the magnitude of mean differences were within the threshold for detectable kinematic changes reported by Osis et al. [15] for knee abduction (3.4°) and hip internal rotation (5.6°). However, the differences in ankle eversion and hip adduction between males and females are greater than the error margins caused by marker placement errors, confirming the findings of Willy et al. [8] who reported males with PFP to have less hip adduction than their female counterparts.

Phinyomark et al. [12] reported the existence of two different sub-groups of asymptomatic runners based on a HCA of lower limb joint kinematics, and when they compared the peak knee abduction angles of those clusters with a sample of subjects with PFP, group differences were dependent on the cluster of healthy individuals that was used as reference. Interestingly, all PFP sub-groups from the current study presented greater values of knee abduction when compared to the ones reported for healthy runners (healthy C1: 8.0°; healthy C2: 4.4°). However, there is a tendency for a progressively greater alteration in knee frontal plane angles when comparing males to females in C1 and C2, although there was no significant difference between the female clusters. This could be related with distinct pathomechanical pathways or differences in response to treatment. For example, in a previous work [37] we found that non-responders to exercise treatment protocol presented greater knee abduction angles during late stance and swing phases of running gait, and the current findings suggest that this could be identified by pelvic acceleration data.

To our knowledge, this is the first study to investigate pelvic acceleration profiles in runners with PFP, and the

identification of sub-groups could generate insights about differences in pathomechanics or adaptations to pain. Additionally, the analysis of segmental acceleration profiles minimizes measurement imprecisions originating from marker placement errors that propagate into the calculation of joint angles in 3D kinematics [14, 15]. Furthermore, the results of the current study suggest that accelerations acquired using wearable devices [24] may utilise this method in a clinical setting as an evidence-informed method to improve patient care and rehabilitation decisions.

The pelvic acceleration data can provide some clinical insight that can help clinicians make decisions regarding treatment options. For example, peak resultant pelvic acceleration is related to center of mass acceleration during 10 to 75% of stance phase [38]. Therefore, pelvic accelerations can provide some insights on shock absorption and lower limb stiffness. Nevertheless, this connection must be made with caution, since accelerations based on segmental measures overestimate the behavior of center of mass [38]. Women in C2 presented a higher VT peak acceleration, suggesting a diminished capacity for shock absorption. Since no differences in peak knee flexion angles were detected, this could be an indication of greater leg stiffness in these subjects, which is partially supported by the findings that women present higher leg stiffness during running [39] and drop jump landing tasks [40] when compared to males. In contrast, females in C1 were similar to males regarding VT acceleration patterns, which could be explained by the lower VT displacement.

Women also presented higher and delayed peak accelerations in the ML direction, suggesting differences in the control of side-to-side body movement during the first half of the stance phase, when these oscillations occur. This pattern could be related to the larger hip adduction angles exhibited during running, which led to increases in ML accelerations. In addition, females in C2 displayed a delay in peak AP accelerations in early stance, causing a prolonged period of deceleration. It is possible that this finding is related to strength differences between males and females [41, 42], as stronger individuals may be able to exert shorter impulses to achieve the same net change in momentum, however, strength differences were not quantified in the current study.

Although the identification of sub-groups among the female subjects with PFP did not coincide with significant differences in peak lower limb joint angles, there seems to be a progression of values in knee abduction and hip internal rotation depending on the cluster of female subjects. Specifically, there is a tendency for C1 to have lower knee abduction and higher hip internal rotation than C2. These factors could be related to symptom severity or differences in response to treatment, but would need further investigation.

Limitations

In addition to the differences in height and weight between males and females that were already discussed, other limitations to the current research study are acknowledged. First, this study included both subjects with uni- or bilateral involvement and with secondary pain symptoms besides PFP, which could have also modified running mechanics. However, there was no significant difference in the distribution of those variables between the two subgroups, leading us to believe that it was not an important factor for this clustering. Additionally, these types of patients are frequently seen in clinical practice, therefore these PFP patients are important to include in research studies.

Second, we did not have access to other clinical variables that could influence running mechanics and explain the differences that were found between subgroups. For example, Selfe et al. [43] has described 3 clusters of PFP patients that were grouped based on clinical measures of strength, flexibility and joint alignment and mobility. Additionally, experimental pain induction in the knee joint has been shown to cause reductions in peak torque in maximal voluntary contraction of knee flexors and extensors [44] and increased sway displacement during quiet stance [45], indicating that pain level could be a driver of changes in motor control. Therefore, future studies should include the aforementioned clinical variables to investigate whether they are related to the differences in running pattern found between sub-groups to have a better understanding in a clinical context.

Finally, this investigation used an HCA approach, which is an unsupervised machine learning technique suitable for exploratory analyses, to determine whether this type of data could be useful in the identification of subgroups within a cohort of runners with PFP. Overall, our hypothesis was supported by the findings and suggest that a supervised analysis could also be applied to identify specific subgroups with specific clinical relevance. For example, recent work from our laboratory used a supervised machine learning method to classify runners with PFP into responders or non-responders to exercise treatment based on running kinematic data, achieving 78% of classification accuracy [37]. Thus, a similar approach could be applied in this context, using pelvic acceleration data to develop an objective method for the identification of such subgroups with greater accessibility in a clinical setting. Regardless, the present study is an important first step to verify the utility of simple measures, like pelvic accelerations, for the objective assessment of gait biomechanics.

Conclusions

In conclusion, using a hierarchical cluster analysis, the present study is the first to identify distinct pelvic acceleration patterns during running gait in a large group of PFP runners. Two homogenous female sub-groups were identified based on pelvic accelerations with one sub-group demonstrating a delay in the posterior and mediolateral acceleration peaks compared to the other. However, both female sub-groups presented greater acceleration peaks than males in all directions. Further analysis of peak kinematic angles provided clinical context to these sub-groups and revealed that gender-differences hip internal rotation, an important factor related to PFP, is distinct among the female sub-group. These results suggest that the variability observed in running gait patterns for PFP runners occur mainly due to sex-related factors, but there are subtle differences among females that could influence the interpretation of kinematic data. The findings also highlight potential for the use of data acquired with accessible wearable technology in the identification of sub-groups in PFP patients. Future research can use this approach in order to classify PFP patients and develop targeted intervention and injury prevention strategies.

Abbreviations
3D: Three-dimensional; AP: Anteroposterior; HCA: Hierarchical cluster analysis; ML: Mediolateral; PCA: Principal component analysis; PCs: Principal components; PFP: Patellofemoral pain; VT: vertical

Funding
Funding for this research was provided by the Ministry of Education of Brazil, Coordination for the Improvement of Higher Education Personnel (CAPES) [grant #9408-13-4]. Funding was also provided by the National Athletic Trainers Association – Research and Education Foundation through the Outcomes Grant program [Grant #808OUT003R], Alberta Innovates: Health Solutions [Grant #200700478], and a Discovery Grant (Grant No. 1028495) and Accelerator Award (Award No. 1030390) through the Natural Sciences and Engineering Research Council of Canada (NSERC). The funders had no role in the study design, collection, analysis and interpretation of data; in the writing of the manuscript; or in the decision to submit the manuscript for publication.

Authors' contributions
RW was responsible for most of the data processing and analysis for the PCA and HCA, and interpretation of the results. SO manages the Running Injury Clinic database and devised methodologies for processing of the 3D gait kinematic data. AP contributed to the interpretation of the results. RF, along with the first author, was the idealizer of the study, participated in the interpretation of the results and was a major contributor in writing the manuscript. All authors read and approved the final manuscript.

Competing interests
There are no financial or personal relationships with other people or organizations that could potentially and inappropriately influence (bias) the submitted work and conclusions.

Author details
[1]Faculty of Kinesiology, University of Calgary, Calgary, Alberta, Canada. [2]Coordination for the Improvement of Higher Education Personnel (CAPES), Brasilia, Brazil. [3]Running Injury Clinic, University of Calgary, 2500 University

Drive NW, Calgary, Alberta T2N 1N4, Canada. [4]Institute of Biomedical Engineering, University of New Brunswick, Fredericton, New Brunswick, Canada. [5]Faculty of Nursing, University of Calgary, Calgary, Alberta, Canada.

References

1. Taunton JE. A retrospective case-control analysis of 2002 running injuries. Br J Sports Med. 2002;36:95–101.
2. Ferber R, Kendall KD, Farr L. Changes in knee biomechanics after a hip-abductor strengthening protocol for runners with patellofemoral pain syndrome. J Athl Train. 2011;46:142–9.
3. Ferber R, Bolgla LA, Earl-Boehm JE, Emery C, Hamstra-Wright K. Strengthening of the hip and core versus knee muscles for the treatment of patellofemoral pain: a multicenter randomized controlled trial. J Athl Train. 2015;50:366–77.
4. Barton CJ, Levinger P, Menz HB, Webster KE. Kinematic gait characteristics associated with patellofemoral pain syndrome: a systematic review. Gait Posture. 2009;30:405–16.
5. Dierks TA, Manal KT, Hamill J, Davis IS. Proximal and distal influences on hip and knee kinematics in runners with Patellofemoral pain during a prolonged run. J Orthop Sport Phys Ther. 2008;38:448–56.
6. Dierks TA, Manal KT, Hamill J, Davis I. Lower extremity kinematics in runners with patellofemoral pain during a prolonged run. Med Sci Sports Exerc. 2011;43:693–700.
7. Noehren B, Pohl MB, Sanchez Z, Cunningham T, Lattermann C. Proximal and distal kinematics in female runners with patellofemoral pain. Clin Biomech. 2012;27:366–71.
8. Willy RW, Manal KT, Witvrouw EE, Davis IS. Are mechanics different between male and female runners with patellofemoral pain? Med Sci Sports Exerc. 2012;44:2165–71.
9. Witvrouw E, Callaghan MJ, Stefanik JJ, Noehren B, Bazett-Jones DM, Willson JD, et al. Patellofemoral pain: consensus statement from the 3rd international patellofemoral pain research retreat held in Vancouver, September 2013. Br J Sports Med. 2014;48:411–4.
10. Ferber R, Osis ST, Hicks JL, Delp SL. Gait biomechanics in the era of data science. J Biomech. 2016;49:3759–61.
11. Phinyomark, A, Petri, G, Ibáñez-Marcelo, E, Osis ST, Ferber R. Analysis of Big Data in Running Biomechanics: Current Trends and Future Directions. Journal of Medical and Biological Engineering – Special Issue: Recent Advances in Biomedical Engineering. 2018;38:244–260.
12. Phinyomark A, Osis S, Hettinga BA, Ferber R. Kinematic gait patterns in healthy runners: a hierarchical cluster analysis. J Biomech. 2015;48:3897–904.
13. Della Croce U, Cappozzo A, Kerrigan DC. Pelvis and lower limb anatomical landmark calibration precision and its propagation to bone geometry and joint angles. Med Biol Eng Comput. 1999;37:155–61.
14. Gorton GE, Hebert DA, Gannotti ME. Assessment of the kinematic variability among 12 motion analysis laboratories. Gait Posture. 2009;29:398–402.
15. Osis ST, Hettinga BA, Macdonald S, Ferber R. Effects of simulated marker placement deviations on running kinematics and evaluation of a morphometric-based placement feedback method. PLoS One. 2016, 11:e0147111.
16. Schütte KH, Maas EA, Exadaktylos V, Berckmans D, Venter RE, Vanwanseele B. Wireless tri-axial trunk Accelerometry detects deviations in dynamic Center of Mass Motion due to running-induced fatigue. PLoS One. 2015;10:e0141957.
17. McGregor SJ, Busa MA, Yaggie JA, Bollt EM. High resolution MEMS accelerometers to estimate VO2 and compare running mechanics between highly trained inter-collegiate and untrained runners. PLoS One. 2009;4:e7355.
18. Chan M, Estève D, Fourniols J-Y, Escriba C, Campo E. Smart wearable systems: current status and future challenges. Artif Intell Med. 2012;56:137–56.
19. Li RT, Kling SR, Salata MJ, Cupp SA, Sheehan J, Voos JE. Wearable performance devices in sports medicine. Sports Health. 2016;8:74–8.
20. Haghi M, Thurow K, Stoll R. Wearable devices in medical internet of things: scientific research and commercially available devices. Healthc Inform Res. 2017;23:4.
21. Pohl MB, Lloyd C, Ferber R. Can the reliability of three-dimensional running kinematics be improved using functional joint methodology? Gait Posture. 2010;32:559–63.
22. Osis ST, Hettinga BA, Macdonald SL, Ferber R. A novel method to evaluate error in anatomical marker placement using a modified generalized Procrustes analysis. Comput Methods Biomech Biomed Engin. 2015;18:1108–16.
23. Osis ST, Hettinga BA, Ferber R. Predicting ground contact events for a continuum of gait types: an application of targeted machine learning using principal component analysis. Gait Posture. 2016;46:86–90.
24. Gullstrand L, Halvorsen K, Tinmark F, Eriksson M, Nilsson J. Measurements of vertical displacement in running, a methodological comparison. Gait Posture. 2009;30:71–5.
25. D'Errico J. Movingslope [Internet]. MATLAB Cent. File Exch. 2007 [cited 2016 Jun 15]. Available from: https://www.mathworks.com/matlabcentral/fileexchange/16997-movingslope.
26. Söderkvist I, Wedin PA. Determining the movements of the skeleton using well-configured markers. J Biomech. 1993;26:1473–7.
27. Ward JH. Hierarchical grouping to optimize an objective function. J Am Stat Assoc. 1963;58:236–44.
28. Calinski T, Harabasz J. A dendrite method for cluster analysis. Commun Stat Theory Methods. 1974;3:1–27.
29. Cohen J. Statistical power analysis for the behavioral sciences. 2nd ed. Hillsdale, NJ: Lawrence Erlbaum Associates; 1988.
30. Brandon SCE, Graham RB, Almosnino S, Sadler EM, Stevenson JM, Deluzio KJ. Interpreting principal components in biomechanics: representative extremes and single component reconstruction. J Electromyogr Kinesiol. 2013;23:1304–10.
31. Abdi H, Williams LJ. Principal component analysis. Wiley Interdiscip Rev Comput Stat. 2010;2:433–59.
32. Phinyomark A, Hettinga BA, Osis S, Ferber R. Do intermediate- and higher-order principal components contain useful information to detect subtle changes in lower extremity biomechanics during running? Hum Mov Sci. 2015;44:91–101.
33. Noehren B, Hamill J, Davis I. Prospective evidence for a hip etiology in patellofemoral pain. Med Sci Sports Exerc. 2013;45:1120–4.
34. Kawabata M, Goto K, Fukusaki C, Sasaki K, Hihara E, Mizushina T, et al. Acceleration patterns in the lower and upper trunk during running. J Sports Sci Routledge. 2013;31:1841–53.
35. Lin S-P, Sung W-H, Kuo F-C, Kuo TBJ, Chen J-J. Impact of center-of-mass acceleration on the performance of ultramarathon runners. J Hum Kinet De Gruyter Open. 2014;44:41–52.
36. Grau S, Maiwald C, Krauss I, Axmann D, Horstmann T. The influence of matching populations on kinematic and kinetic variables in runners with Iliotibial band syndrome. Res Q Exerc Sport. 2008;79:450–7.
37. Watari R, Kobsar D, Phinyomark A, Osis S, Ferber R. Determination of patellofemoral pain sub-groups and development of a method for predicting treatment outcome using running gait kinematics. Clin Biomech. 2016;38:13–21.
38. Nedergaard NJ, Robinson MA, Eusterwiemann E, Drust B, Lisboa PJ, Vanrenterghem J. The relationship between whole-body external loading and body-worn Accelerometry during team-sport movements. Int J Sports Physiol Perform. 2017;12:18–26.
39. Sinclair J, Shore HF, Taylor PJ, Atkins S. Sex differences in limb and joint stiffness in recreational runners. Hum Mov De Gruyter Open. 2015; 16:137 41.
40. Lyle MA, Valero-Cuevas FJ, Gregor RJ, Powers CM. Control of dynamic foot-ground interactions in male and female soccer athletes: females exhibit reduced dexterity and higher limb stiffness during landing. J Biomech. 2014;47:512–7.
41. Lephart SM, Ferris CM, Riemann BL, Myers JB, Fu FH. Gender differences in strength and lower extremity kinematics during landing. Clin Orthop Relat Res. 2002;(401):162-9.
42. Nakagawa TH, Moriya ÉTU, Maciel CD, Serrão FV. Trunk, pelvis, hip, and knee kinematics, hip strength, and gluteal muscle activation during a single-leg squat in males and females with and without Patellofemoral pain syndrome. J. Orthop. Sport. Phys. Ther. 2012;42:491–501.
43. Selfe J, Janssen J, Callaghan M, Witvrouw E, Sutton C, Richards J, et al. Are there three main subgroups within the patellofemoral pain population? A detailed characterisation study of 127 patients to help develop targeted intervention (TIPPs). Br. J. Sports Med. 2016;bjsports-2015-094792.
44. Henriksen M, Rosager S, Aaboe J, Graven-Nielsen T, Bliddal H. Experimental knee pain reduces muscle strength. J Pain Churchill Livingstone. 2011;12:460–7.
45. Hirata RP, Arendt-Nielsen L, Shiozawa S, Graven-Nielsen T. Experimental knee pain impairs postural stability during quiet stance but not after perturbations. Eur J Appl Physiol. 2012;112:2511–21.

Influence of surgery involving tendons around the knee joint on ankle motion during gait in patients with cerebral palsy

Seung Yeol Lee[1†], Soon-Sun Kwon[2†], Chin Youb Chung[3,4], Kyoung Min Lee[3], Ki Hyuk Sung[3], Sangwoo Kim[1] and Moon Seok Park[3*] (iD)

Abstract

Background: Simultaneous motion of the knee and ankle joints is required for many activities including gait. We aimed to evaluate the influence of surgery involving tendons around the knee on ankle motion during gait in the sagittal plane in cerebral palsy patients.

Methods: We included data from 55 limbs in 34 patients with spastic cerebral palsy. Patients were followed up after undergoing only distal hamstring lengthening with or without additional rectus femoris transfer. The patients' mean age at the time of knee surgery was 11.2 ± 4.7 years, and the mean follow-up duration was 2.2 ± 1.5 years (range, 0.9–6.0 years). Pre- and postoperative kinematic variables that were extracted from three-dimensional gait analyses were then compared to assess changes in ankle motion after knee surgery. Outcome measures included ankle dorsiflexion at initial contact, peak ankle dorsiflexion during stance, peak ankle dorsiflexion during swing, and dynamic range of motion of the ankle. Various sagittal plane knee kinematics were also measured and used to predict ankle kinematics. A linear mixed model was constructed to estimate changes in ankle motion after adjusting for multiple factors.

Results: Improvement in total range of motion of the knee resulted in improved motion of the ankle joint. We estimated that after knee surgery, ankle dorsiflexion at initial contact, peak ankle dorsiflexion during stance, peak ankle dorsiflexion during swing, and dynamic range of motion of the ankle decreased, respectively, by $0.4°$ ($p = 0.016$), $0.6°$ ($p < 0.001$), $0.2°$ ($p = 0.038$), and $0.5°$ ($p = 0.006$) per degree increase in total range of motion of the knee after either knee surgery. Furthermore, dynamic range of motion of the ankle increased by $0.4°$ per degree increase in postoperative peak knee flexion during swing.

Conclusions: Improvement in total knee range of motion was found to be correlated with improvement in ankle kinematics after surgery involving tendons around the knee. As motion of the knee and ankle joints is cross-linked, surgeons should be aware of potential changes in the ankle joint after knee surgery.

Keywords: Cerebral palsy, Gait analysis, Ankle kinematics, Distal hamstring lengthening, Rectus femoris transfer

Background

Stiff-knee gait and crouch gait are among the most common gait problems in ambulatory patients with cerebral palsy (CP) [1, 2]. Stiff-knee gait results in limited flexion and extension of the knee, and a restricted arc of motion during the swing phase [3]. Crouch gait, a major sagittal

plane deviation, is defined as excessive ankle dorsiflexion combined with knee and hip flexion during the stance phase [4]. To optimize knee function in CP patients with abnormal gait, various surgical treatments, such as rectus femoris transfer (RFT) for stiff knee gait, and distal hamstring lengthening (DHL) and distal femoral osteotomy for flexed knee gait, can be considered as part of single-event multilevel surgery (SEMLS).

Many patients with CP also undergo tendo-Achilles lengthening as part of SEMLS to release the tightness preventing suitable ankle dorsiflexion. However, some

---
* Correspondence: pmsmed@gmail.com
†Equal contributors
3Department of Orthopaedic Surgery, Seoul National University Bundang Hospital, 300 Gumi-Dong, Bundang-Gu, Seoungnam, Gyeonggi 463-707, South Korea
Full list of author information is available at the end of the article

patients with stiff- or flexed-knee gait show a relatively good ankle range of motion (ROM) [5, 6]. Thus, knee surgery procedures such as RFT or DHL without additional ankle surgery can be considered in these patients. Cross-linkage of the knee and ankle; however, still needs to be considered. Specifically, the gastrocnemius, a biarticular muscle that crosses the knee and ankle, acts as both a knee and ankle plantar flexor. The resultant simultaneous motion of the knee and ankle joints is required for many activities including standing, running, swimming, and cycling [7]. In addition, adequate coupling of plantar flexion and knee extension [8] regulates the direction and modulus of ground reaction force, which subsequently acts to optimize gait.

Given this relationship between the knee and ankle, we hypothesize that changes in the kinematics of the knee after knee surgery affect ankle motion during walking in patients with CP. For example, DHL- or DHL with RFT-induced improvement in knee motion during the swing phase may result in improved heel strike at initial contact in the gait cycle, which subsequently affects ankle motion during the stance phase. Indeed, many previous studies have reported improved ankle kinematics after knee surgeries in patients with CP, though these studies included patients who underwent concurrent surgeries that may have affected ankle kinematics [9–12]. In addition, changes in ankle motion during gait have not, to the best of our knowledge, been described in patients with CP who have undergone DHL or DHL with RFT specifically. Therefore, the present study aimed to evaluate the extent to which surgery involving tendons around the knee joint influences ankle motion during gait in the sagittal plane in patients with CP.

Methods
Ethical statement
This study was approved by the institutional board of our hospital, a tertiary referral center for CP. Informed consent was waived because of the retrospective nature of this study.

Patient recruitment
We reviewed the medical records of patients with spastic CP who were followed up after RFT or DHL, and who had undergone pre- and postoperative three-dimensional (3D) gait analysis between January 1995 and December 2015. Patients were included in this study if they did not meet the indications for tendo-Achilles lengthening or gastrocnemius recession (these indications are: the ankle is not correctable to more than a neutral position, as measured during knee extension; and increased plantar flexion in the stance phase of walking). Exclusion criteria were as follows: gross motor function classification system (GMFCS) level IV or V, any previous or concurrent surgeries as a part of

SEMLS, and incomplete or missing 3D gait analysis data. Age at the time of surgery, sex, anatomic type of CP, GMFCS level, and details of concomitant surgical procedures were obtained from patient medical records.

Operation protocol
RFT and DHL were performed by 2 orthopedic surgeons who had 27 and 11 years of experience in orthopedics. Both surgeons followed the same treatment approach. Indications for RFT were as follows: positive Duncan Ely test, knee flexion angle ≥15° less than the total range during the swing phase, and delayed peak knee flexion during the swing phase [13, 14]. When RFT was performed without DHL, the rectus femoris was transferred to the sartorius. In cases where RFT and DHL were performed concomitantly (DHT with RFT group), the gracilis tendon was used as the transfer site. Some patients also underwent DHL only (DHL only group). DHL was performed in patients who exhibited an increased popliteal angle and increased knee flexion at initial contact, as verified by preoperative 3D gait analysis. The procedure included gracilis lengthening, semitendinosus transfer to the adductor magnus, and aponeurotic lengthening of the semimembranosus.

Acquisition of kinematic data
3D gait analysis was performed pre- and postoperatively using a Vicon 370 motion capture system (Oxford Metrix, Oxford, UK) equipped with 7 cameras and 2 force plates (Advanced Medical Technology Incorporation, MA, USA). The Vicon Plug-in Gait marker model was used to place the markers. To obtain kinematic data, patients were recorded walking barefoot along a 9-m walkway 3 times, with an interval of approximately 30 s between each recording. The 3 trials were then averaged to determine the index variable values [13]. Next, pre- and postoperative kinematic variables were compared to assess changes in ankle motion after surgery involving tendons around the knee. Specifically, kinematic variables including knee flexion at initial contact, minimum knee flexion in the stance phase, peak knee flexion in the swing phase, total knee ROM, and knee flexion in the terminal swing phase were used to assess knee kinematics after DHL and RFT. On the other hand, ankle dorsiflexion at initial contact, peak ankle dorsiflexion in the stance phase, peak ankle dorsiflexion in the swing phase, and dynamic ROM were used as outcome measures for ankle motion changes after surgery.

Statistical analysis
The Kolmogorov-Smirnov test was used to verify the normal distribution of continuous variables, which were described using means, standard deviations, and frequencies. Changes in each gait parameter after surgery were analyzed using paired-t tests. A linear mixed model

(LMM) was then constructed to estimate changes in ankle motion between pre- and postoperative evaluations, with adjustment for multiple factors including sex and knee surgery type (i.e., DHL only or DHL with RFT). After univariate analysis, changes in the kinematics of the knee were considered fixed effects, whereas the interval between the 3D gait analyses, laterality (i.e., right or left), age, and each subject were considered random effects (Additional file 1).

Four LMMs were constructed for each ankle kinematic variable of interest (i.e., ankle dorsiflexion at initial contact, peak ankle dorsiflexion in the stance phase, peak ankle dorsiflexion in the swing phase, and dynamic ankle ROM), and the variance components covariance structure was used. The restricted maximum likelihood estimation method was used to produce an unbiased estimator. The adequacy of the models was determined using the Akaike information criterion (AIC) and Bayesian information criterion (BIC), with smaller values preferred for model selection. All models had low AIC/BIC scores (872.9/870.9 for peak ankle dorsiflexion at initial contact, 850.5/848.5 for peak ankle dorsiflexion during stance, 820.7/818.7 for peak ankle dorsiflexion during swing, and 883.0/881.0 for dynamic ankle ROM), and were thus accepted as valid representations of kinematic measurements.

Data were analyzed using SAS version 9.4 (SAS Institute, Cary, NC). All statistical tests were two-tailed. Confidence intervals (CIs) were considered significant when they did not include zero, and p-values < 0.05 were considered significant.

Results

Seventy-eight lower limbs from 50 patients met the inclusion criteria. After applying the exclusion criteria, a total of 55 limbs from 34 patients remained for inclusion in this study (Fig. 1). The patients' mean age at the time of knee surgery was 11.2 ± 4.7 years, and postoperative 3D gait analysis was performed at a mean of 0.9 ± 1.3 years after surgery (Table 1). The mean follow-up duration was $2.2 \pm$

Table 1 Patient demographics

Parameter	Value	
No. of patients (M / F)	34 (18/16)	
No. of limbs (M / F)	55 (29/26)	
Laterality (R / L)	27/28	
Anatomical type (hemi–/di–/quadriplegia)	27/2/26	
GMFCS level (patients /limbs)	I	13 (19)
	II	15 (25)
	III	6 (11)
Mean age at surgery (years)	11.2 (SD 4.7)	
Knee surgery (DHL / RFT/ both) (limbs)	27 / 2 / 26	
Interval between pre- and first postoperative 3D gait analysis (years)	0.9 ± 1.3	
Mean follow-up duration (years)	2.2 ± 1.5 (range, 0.9 to 6.0)	

M male, *F* female, *R* right, *L* left, *DHL* distal hamstring lengthening, *RFT* rectus femoris transfer

1.5 years (range, 0.9–6.0 years). Five patients (9 limbs) underwent postoperative 3D gait analysis twice, while 29 patients (46 limbs) underwent the examination once.

All knee kinematic variables improved between pre- and postoperative 3D gait analysis (Table 2). The mean total knee ROM increased from 38.9° to 50.2° overall (specifically, from 39.5° to 47.8° in the DHL group and from 38.8° to 52.2° in the DHL with RFT group) after surgery ($p < 0.001$) (Table 2) [14, 15].

LMM analysis showed that ankle kinematics were influenced by improvement in knee kinematics (Fig. 2), with improvement in total knee ROM resulting in decreased motion of the ankle joint. We estimated that ankle dorsiflexion at initial contact, peak ankle dorsiflexion in the stance phase, peak ankle dorsiflexion in the swing phase, and dynamic ankle ROM decreased by 0.4° ($p = 0.016$), 0.6° ($p < 0.001$), 0.5° ($p = 0.038$), and 0.2° ($p = 0.006$), respectively, per degree increase in total knee ROM after surgery (Table 3). Furthermore, dynamic ankle ROM increased by 0.4° per degree increase in postoperative peak

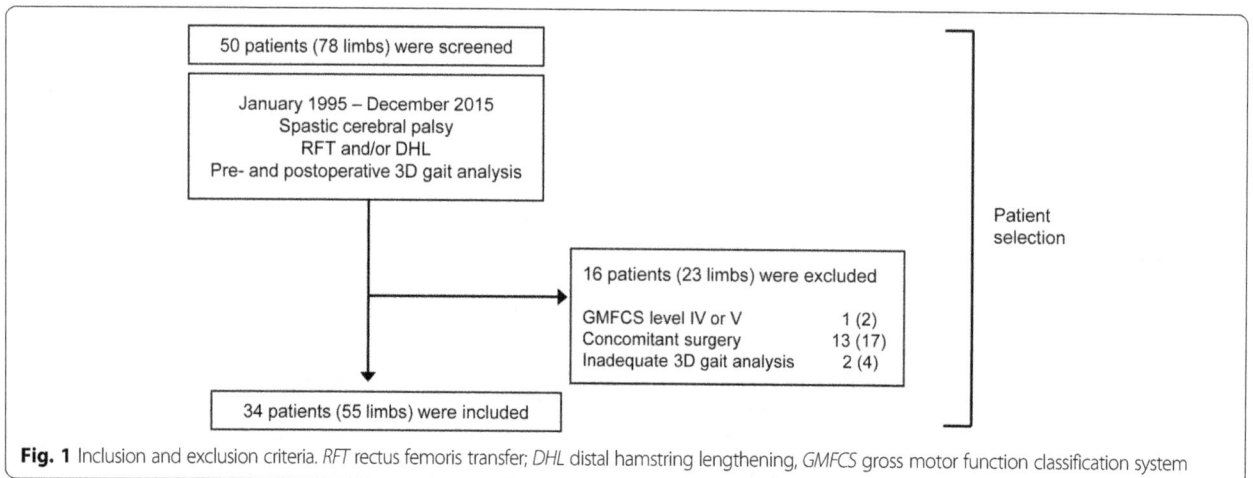

Fig. 1 Inclusion and exclusion criteria. *RFT* rectus femoris transfer; *DHL* distal hamstring lengthening, *GMFCS* gross motor function classification system

Table 2 Changes in gait parameters after surgery involving tendons around the knee

	Kinematics	[a]Reference value in children [15, 16]	Preoperative value(°)	Postoperative value (°)	Changes in parameter after the surgery (°)		
					Mean value	CI	P value
Knee	Knee flexion at IC	3.4–14.4	31.9 (SD 12.7)	22.8 (SD 9.7)	−9.1 (SD 14.1)	−12.9 – −5.3	< 0.001
	Peak knee flexion during swing	55.6–61.6	55.4 (SD 14.3)	58.3 (SD 11.0)	2.9 (SD 16.1)	−1.5 – 7.2	0.194
	Total knee ROM	46.8–57.2	38.9 (SD 14.0)	50.2 (SD 11.4)	11.2 (SD 14.6)	7.3–15.2	< 0.001
	Minimum knee flexion in the stance	7.6	16.5 (SD 14.9)	5.1 (SD 1.5)	−8.4 (SD 16.8)	−12.9 – −3.8	0.001
Ankle	Ankle dorsiflexion at IC	4.2	4.8 (SD 19.8)	3.5 (SD 8.7)	−1.2 (SD 19.5)	−6.5 – 4.0	0.641
	Peak ankle dorsiflexion during stance	9.0–14.8	21.6 (SD 21.2)	18.6 (SD 8.2)	−3.0 (SD 20.3)	−8.5 – 2.5	0.277
	Peak ankle dorsiflexion during swing	2.1–5.6	17.2 (SD 9.8)	15.2 (SD 7.3)	−2.0 (SD 10.2)	−4.8 – 0.7	0.142
	Dynamic ROM of the ankle	26.6–31.7	14.9 (SD 25.2)	11.5 (SD 7.5)	−3.4 (SD 22.7)	−9.6 – 2.7	0.269

[a]Reference value in children is the range of mean values of previous studies

knee flexion in the swing phase. We also found that pre- and postoperative ankle dorsiflexion at initial contact, peak ankle dorsiflexion in stance, and dynamic ankle ROM were smaller in the DHL with RFT group than in the DHL only group (Table 3). However, age at the time of knee surgery did not significantly affect ankle kinematics.

Discussion

Our study is the first to describe how surgery involving the tendons around the knee joint affects ankle motion during gait in patients with CP [16]. We have shown that DHL- or DHL with RFT-induced improvement in total knee ROM results in an improvement in ankle kinematics in the sagittal plane during gait.

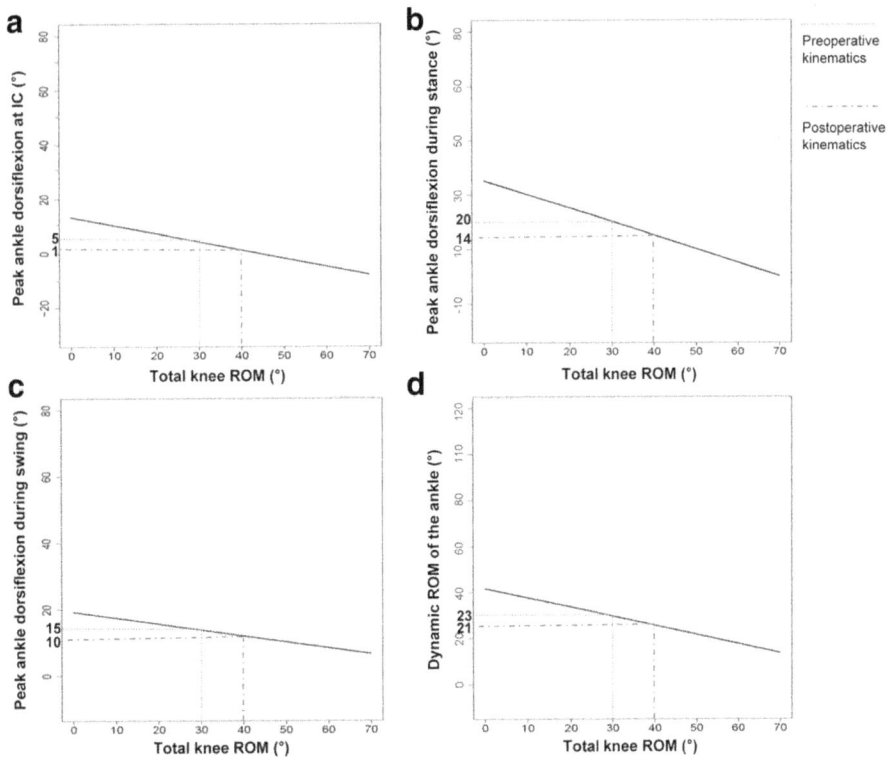

Fig. 2 Linear mixed model describing changes in ankle kinematics associated with postoperative improvement in total knee range of motion (ROM). The sloping lines indicate estimated changes in ankle kinematics according to the improvement of total knee ROM. For instance, one patient demonstrated 30° total knee ROM, 5° ankle dorsiflexion at initial contact (**a**), 20° peak ankle dorsiflexion in the stance phase (**b**), 15° peak ankle dorsiflexion in the swing phase (**c**), and 23° dynamic ROM of the ankle (**d**). If total knee ROM increased to 40° after the knee surgery, estimated ankle dorsiflexion at initial contact, peak ankle dorsiflexion in the stance and swing phases, and dynamic ankle ROM will be 1° (**a**), 14° (**b**), 10° (**c**), and 21° (**d**)

Table 3 Linear mixed model describing estimated and fixed effects on ankle kinematics after surgery involving tendons around the knee

Effect	Peak ankle dorsiflexion at IC			Peak ankle dorsiflexion during stance			Peak ankle dorsiflexion during swing			Dynamic ankle ROM		
	Estimate	CI	P-value	Estimate	CI	P-value	Estimate	CI	P-value	Estimate	CI	P-value
Intercept	13.8	−2.4– 30.1	0.091	25.6	8.4–42.7	0.005	8.0	−1.4–17.5	0.094	31.7	11.8–51.6	0.003
Age	−0.3	−0.9 – 0.3	0.314	−0.1	−0.7 – 0.5	0.749	− 0.3	− 0.6 – 0.1	0.119	− 0.2	− 0.9 – 0.5	0.583
Laterality (Right)	1.5	−4.0 – 6.9	0.594	1.2	−4.5 – 7.0	0.669	−1.0	−4.2 – 2.1	0.519	0.6	−6.1 – 7.3	0.862
DHL only	6.2	0.5–11.8	0.032	6.8	0.9–12.7	0.025	−1.0	−4.3 – 2.3	0.540	8.2	1.3–15.1	0.020
[a]Knee flexion at IC	0.2	−0.6 – 1.1	0.603	−0.5	−1.4 – 0.4	0.287	−0.7	−1.8 – 0.3	0.179	−0.4	−0.9 – 0.1	0.152
[a]Peak knee flexion during swing	0.0	−0.4 – 0.4	0.906	0.3	−0.1 – 0.7	0.132	0.0	−0.5 – 0.5	0.952	0.4	0.2–0.6	< 0.001
[a]Total knee ROM	−0.4	− 0.7 – − 0.1	0.016	−0.6	−1.0 – − 0.3	< 0.001	−0.5	− 1.0 – − 0.2	0.006	-0.2	−0.4 – 0.0	0.038
[a]Knee flexion in terminal swing	−0.2	−1.0 – 0.6	0.618	0.3	−0.6 – 1.1	0.515	0.6	−0.4 – 1.5	0.230	0.2	−0.2 – 0.7	0.289

CI 95% confidence interval, IC initial contact, ROM range of motion
[a]Each degree of increase in kinematics

Most sports and activities of daily living require the concomitant movement of various joints. The coordination of this joint movement is essential in human gait, which is the result of a combination of forces that allow maximum efficiency to be achieved at minimum cost [17]. The gastrocnemius muscle plays a role in this coordination, crossing the knee and ankle to act as both a knee flexor and an ankle plantar flexor in the sagittal plane. The resultant coupling of plantar flexion and knee extension is thought to underlie the knee and ankle kinematics that regulate the direction and modulus of ground reaction force to optimize gait [8]. Therefore, physicians should be aware of potential changes in ankle kinematics after knee surgery.

The present study found that improvement in total knee ROM resulted in decreased (i.e. improved) motion of the ankle joint in terms of peak ankle dorsiflexion at initial contact and during the stance and swing phases, as well as dynamic ankle ROM. Specifically, we estimated that peak ankle dorsiflexion at initial contact, peak ankle dorsiflexion in the stance phase, peak ankle dorsiflexion in the swing phase, and dynamic ankle ROM decreased by 0.4°, 0.6°, 0.2°, and 0.5°, respectively. Although these improvements seem small, they must be considered in terms of degree increase in total knee ROM. Because the ankle ROM is smaller than that of the knee during walking [15], these improvements in ankle kinematics actually represent substantial changes.

Furthermore, although these findings do not intuitively represent an improvement, they should be understood in the context of our patients undergoing surgery for tightness or shortness in the hamstring or rectus femoris. As such, the average preoperative total knee ROM was lower in our patients than in healthy children of a similar age (our patients, 38.9° vs. healthy children, 46.8°-57.2°), as was dynamic ankle ROM during walking [15, 18]. In contrast, peak ankle dorsiflexion parameters during walking were larger in our cohort than in healthy children, which might be related to weakness of the triceps surae. However, we found that improvement in knee kinematics after knee surgery was associated with a decrease in peak ankle dorsiflexion during gait. This suggests that increased preoperative ankle dorsiflexion represents a means of secondary compensation, triceps surae weakness, for decreased knee ROM. This is consistent with what is known about loss of knee ROM. Such loss of knee function is associated with gait problems including foot clearance and heel strike [13], which can be compensated for by increasing ankle dorsiflexion through the gait cycle. Thus, the decreased ankle dorsiflexion we found after surgery indicates less need for compensation and improved function. In addition, peak knee flexion during the swing phase showed a positive correlation with dynamic ankle ROM, but no correlation with ankle dorsiflexion at initial contact and during the stance and swing phases. We therefore suggest that improvement in peak knee flexion might allow effective push-off of the foot during the initial swing phase.

We also found that postoperative dynamic ROM of ankle and as well as peak ankle dorsiflexion at initial contact and in the stance phase, were larger in the DHL only group than in the DHL with RFT group. Since total knee ROM was negatively correlated with peak ankle dorsiflexion and dynamic ankle ROM during walking in our study, patients who underwent DHL with RFT also had larger improvements in total knee ROM than those who underwent only DHL. This is indicative of poorer results in the

DHL only group in terms of reducing the need for secondary compensation and enabling a larger decrease in ankle kinematics during gait to be achieved. This is unsurprising given that patients with stiff-knee gait generally required both DHL and RFT, the latter of which has been suggested to restore knee motion during the swing phase [3, 13]. Another possible reason for greater dynamic ankle ROM in the DHL only group involves patient selection. Patients who underwent DHL only exhibited hamstring tightness and shortness, which can contribute to jump-knee gait or crouch gait [19–21]. Since patients with jump-knee gait who required surgery for heel cord tightness (not hamstring tightness) were excluded, characteristics specific to patients with crouch gait might have contributed to the increased dynamic ankle ROM and as well as the increased ankle dorsiflexion at initial contact and in the stance phase, seen in the DHL only group.

Regarding other disadvantages of DHL, there are concerns that DHL may aggravate anterior pelvic tilt and lumbar lordosis, as well as induce crouch gait [11, 23, 24], despite its effectiveness at reducing knee flexion and improving knee motion [25]. Recent studies have also found that preservation of hip extension power and hip extension are better with than without the hamstring transfer procedure [5, 12, 26]. In our study, total knee ROM improved after knee surgery, and was correlated with a decrease in peak ankle dorsiflexion and dynamic ankle ROM during gait. These results suggest that in patients with crouch gait, excessive dorsiflexion of the ankle during gait may improve after DHL. Thus, we believe that in patients with CP, the effect of DHL on ankle motion might lead to an overall improvement in gait.

Despite the insights provided by this study, there are some limitations that should be addressed. First, because of the retrospective nature of this study, it was not possible to ensure consistency in the timeline of our evaluations. Therefore, the interval between pre- and postoperative 3D gait analyses varied with each case considered. To overcome the heterogeneity of this data set and adjust the interval between examinations, we used an LMM. This model quantifies the relationships between a continuous dependent variable and various predictor variables in a set of longitudinal data, thereby allowing within- and between-subject variations to be incorporated [26]. Therefore, we believe that our results are representative despite the limitations associated with the retrospective nature of our present study. Second, the ankle kinematics parameters measured using 3D gait analysis were considered to be the dependent variables in our study. However, the ankle kinematics assessed did not reflect motion in the coronal or transverse planes. Despite this limitation, we believe that our data are nevertheless very helpful in understanding changes in ankle kinematics after knee surgery.

Conclusions

We conclude that improvement in total knee ROM is correlated with improvement in ankle kinematics after DHL and DHL with RFT. Knee surgery might influence ankle kinematics during gait to the extent that additional surgical interventions involving the ankle joint become unnecessary. Furthermore, because motion of the knee and ankle joints is cross-linked, surgeons should be aware of potential changes in the ankle joint after knee surgery.

Abbreviations

3D: three-dimensional; AIC: Akaike information criterion; BIC: Bayesian information criterion; CI: Confidence intervals; CP: Cerebral palsy; DHL: Distal hamstring lengthening; GMFCS: Gross motor function classification system; LMM: Linear mixed model; RFT: Rectus femoris transfer; ROM: Range of motion; SEMLS: Single-event multilevel surgery

Acknowledgements

Not applicable.

Funding

This research was supported by the Basic Science Research Program through the National Research Foundation of Korea (NRF) funded by the Ministry of Science and ICT (NRF-2016R1C1B2008557), and was partly supported by the Technology Innovation Program funded By the Ministry of Trade, Industry and Energy (MOTIE) of Korea (10049785) and SNUBH research fund (grant no. 02-2012-018).

No benefits in any form have been received or will be received from a commercial party related directly or indirectly to the subject of this article.

Authors' contributions

All authors on this manuscript (SYL, S-SK, CYC, KHS, KML, SK, and MSP) made significant contributions to the study design. SK, KML, KHS, and SYL were involved in acquisition of data. SYL, S-SK, CYC, KML, and MSP were involved in the analysis and interpretation of data, as well as drafting the manuscript. All authors gave final approval of the version to be published.

Consent for publication

Not applicable.

Competing interests

The authors declare that they have no competing interests.

Author details

[1]Department of Orthopaedic Surgery, Ewha Womans University Mokdong Hospital, Seoul, South Korea. [2]Department of Mathematics, College of Natural Science, Ajou University, Suwon, Gyeonggi, South Korea. [3]Department of Orthopaedic Surgery, Seoul National University Bundang Hospital, 300 Gumi-Dong, Bundang-Gu, Seoungnam, Gyeonggi 463-707, South Korea. [4]Department of Orthopaedic Surgery, Seoul National University College of Medicine, Seoul, South Korea.

References

1. Wren TA, Rethlefsen S, Kay RM. Prevalence of specific gait abnormalities in children with cerebral palsy: influence of cerebral palsy subtype, age, and previous surgery. J Pediatr Orthop. 2005;25(1):79–83.
2. Rethlefsen SA, Blumstein G, Kay RM, Dorey F, Wren TA. Prevalence of specific gait abnormalities in children with cerebral palsy revisited: influence of age, prior surgery, and gross motor function classification system level. Dev Med Child Neurol. 2017;59(1):79–88.
3. Chung C, Stout J, Gage J. Rectus femoris transfer-Gracilis versus Sartorius. Gait Posture. 1997;6:137–46.
4. Khamis S, Martikaro R, Wientroub S, Hemo Y, Hayek S. A functional electrical

stimulation system improves knee control in crouch gait. J Child Orthop. 2015;9(2):137–43.

5.   Sung KH, Lee J, Chung CY, Lee KM, Cho BC, Moon SJ, Kim J, Park MS. Factors influencing outcomes after medial hamstring lengthening with semitendinosus transfer in patients with cerebral palsy. J Neuroeng Rehabil. 2017;14(1):83.

6.   Sossai R, Vavken P, Brunner R, Camathias C, Graham HK, Rutz E. Patellar tendon shortening for flexed knee gait in spastic diplegia. Gait Posture. 2015;41(2):658–65.

7.   Suzuki T, Chino K, Fukashiro S. Gastrocnemius and soleus are selectively activated when adding knee extensor activity to plantar flexion. Hum Mov Sci. 2014;36:35–45.

8.   Gage JR. Treatment principles for crouch gait. In: Gage JR, editor. The treatment of gait problems in cerebral palsy. 2nd edn. London: Mac Keith Press; 2004. p. 382–97.

9.   Koca K, Yildiz C, Yurttas Y, Bilgic S, Ozkan H, Kurklu M, Balaban B, Hazneci B, Basbozkurt M. Outcomes of combined hamstring release and rectus transfer in children with crouch gait. Ortop Traumatol Rehabil. 2009;11(4):333–8.

10. Rodda JM, Graham HK, Nattrass GR, Galea MP, Baker R, Wolfe R. Correction of severe crouch gait in patients with spastic diplegia with use of multilevel orthopaedic surgery. J Bone Joint Surg Am. 2006;88(12):2653–64.

11. Chang WN, Tsirikos AI, Miller F, Lennon N, Schuyler J, Kerstetter L, Glutting J. Distal hamstring lengthening in ambulatory children with cerebral palsy: primary versus revision procedures. Gait Posture. 2004;19(3):298–304.

12. De Mattos C, Patrick Do K, Pierce R, Feng J, Aiona M, Sussman M. Comparison of hamstring transfer with hamstring lengthening in ambulatory children with cerebral palsy: further follow-up. J Child Orthop. 2014;8(6):513–20.

13. Lee SY, Kwon SS, Chung CY, Lee KM, Choi Y, Kim TG, Shin WC, Choi IH, Cho TJ, Yoo WJ, et al. Rectus femoris transfer in cerebral palsy patients with stiff knee gait. Gait Posture. 2014;40(1):76–81.

14. Gage JR. Surgical treatment of knee dysfunction in cerebral palsy. Clin Orthop Relat Res. 1990;(253):45-54.

15. Calhoun M, Longworth M, Chester VL. Gait patterns in children with autism. Clin Biomech (Bristol, Avon). 2011;26(2):200–6.

16. Lee S, Lee K, Chun S. Influence of surgery involving tendons around the knee joint on ankle motion during gait in patients with cerebral palsy. In: Abstracts from the 6th IFFAS triennial meeting. Foot Ankle Sug. 2017;23(S1): 129. https://doi.org/10.1016/j.fas.2017.07.483.

17. Ralston HJ. Energy-speed relation and optimal speed during level walking. Int Z Angew Physiol. 1958;17(4):277–83.

18. Chung CY, Park MS, choi IH, Cho TJ, yoo WJ, kim JY. Three dimensional gait analysis in normal Korean: a preliminary report. J Korean Orthop Assoc. 2005;40:83–8.

19. Sutherland DH, Davids JR. Common gait abnormalities of the knee in cerebral palsy. Clin Orthop Relat Res. 1993;(288):139-147.

19. Carney BT, Oeffinger D, Meo AM. Sagittal knee kinematics after hamstring lengthening. J Pediatr Orthop B. 2006;15(5):348–50.

20. Laracca E, Stewart C, Postans N, Roberts A. The effects of surgical lengthening of hamstring muscles in children with cerebral palsy–the consequences of pre-operative muscle length measurement. Gait Posture. 2014;39(3):847–51.

21. Saraph V, Zwick EB, Zwick G, Steinwender C, Steinwender G, Linhart W. Multilevel surgery in spastic diplegia: evaluation by physical examination and gait analysis in 25 children. J Pediatr Orthop. 2002;22(2):150–7.

22. Zwick EB, Saraph V, Linhart WE, Steinwender G. Propulsive function during gait in diplegic children: evaluation after surgery for gait improvement. J Pediatr Orthop B. 2001;10(3):226–33.

23. Sung KH, Chung CY, Lee KM, Akhmedov B, Lee SY, Choi IH, Cho TJ, Yoo WJ, Park MS. Long term outcome of single event multilevel surgery in spastic diplegia with flexed knee gait. Gait Posture. 2013;37(4):536–41.

24. Feng L, Patrick Do K, Aiona M, Feng J, Pierce R, Sussman M. Comparison of hamstring lengthening with hamstring lengthening plus transfer for the treatment of flexed knee gait in ambulatory patients with cerebral palsy. J Child Orthop. 2012;6(3):229–35.

25. Nguyen DV, Senturk D, Carroll RJ. Covariate-adjusted linear mixed effects model with an application to longitudinal data. J Nonparametr Stat. 2008; 20(6):459–81.

22

Cartilage calcification of the ankle joint is associated with osteoarthritis in the general population

Jan Hubert[1*], Lukas Weiser[1], Sandra Hischke[2], Annemarie Uhlig[3], Tim Rolvien[4], Tobias Schmidt[4], Sebastian Karl Butscheidt[4], Klaus Püschel[5], Wolfgang Lehmann[1], Frank Timo Beil[1] and Thelonius Hawellek[1*]

Abstract

Background: Cartilage calcification (CC) is associated with osteoarthritis (OA) in weight-bearing joints, such as the hip and the knee. However, little is known about the impact of CC and degeneration on other weight-bearing joints, especially as it relates to the occurrence of OA in the ankles. The goal of this study is to analyse the prevalence of ankle joint cartilage calcification (AJ CC) and to determine its correlation with factors such as histological OA grade, age and BMI in the general population.

Methods: CC of the distal tibia and talus in 160 ankle joints obtained from 80 donors (mean age 62.4 years, 34 females, 46 males) was qualitatively and quantitatively analysed using high-resolution digital contact radiography (DCR). Correlations with factors, such as the joint's histological OA grade (OARSI score), donor's age and BMI, were investigated.

Results: The prevalence of AJ CC was 51.3% (95% CI [0.40, 0.63]), independent of gender ($p = 0.18$) and/or the joint's side ($p = 0.82$). CC of the distal tibia was detected in 35.0% (28/80) (95% CI [0.25, 0.47]) and talar CC in 47.5% (38/80) (95% CI [0.36, 0.59]) of all cases. Significant correlations were noted between the mean amount of tibial and talar CC ($r = 0.59$, $p = 0.002$), as well as between the mean amount of CC observed in one ankle joint with that of the contralateral side ($r = 0.52$, $p = 0.02$). Furthermore, although the amount of AJ CC observed in the distal tibia and talus correlated with the histological OA-grade of the joint ($r = 0.70$, $p < 0.001$ and $r = 0.72$, $p < 0.001$, respectively), no such correlation was seen in the general population with relation to age ($p = 0.32$ and $p = 0.49$) or BMI ($p = 0.51$ and $p = 0.87$).

Conclusion: The prevalence of AJ CC in the general population is much higher than expected. The relationship between the amount of AJ CC and OA, independent of the donors' age and BMI, indicates that CC may play a causative role in the development of OA in ankles.

Keywords: Cartilage calcification, Calcium crystals, Chondrocalcinosis, Ankle joint, Osteoarthritis, Cartilage

Background

Osteoarthritis (OA) is a major health problem that affects about 15% of the global population [1]. While OA in weight-bearing hip and knee joints is relatively common, in the ankle joint (AJ) it affects only 1% of the population [2]. It is often hypothesized that the development of AJ OA is mostly related to previous trauma [3, 4]. Valderrabano et al. reported a high prevalence of post-traumatic AJ OA (in 78% of cases) [4], while, other studies have shown a considerably lower prevalence (only 14%) [5]. The real impact of trauma on the development of AJ OA is yet to be fully understood, and the ability to accurately predict which patients will develop AJ OA in the future requires further investigations.

It is likely that the variations in individuals' articular cartilage composition will play a role in the development of AJ OA. Eckstein et al. reported surprisingly high variability in the quantitative distribution of cartilage in the ankles of patients [6], whereas Quinn et al. found intraindividual variations in the cartilage cells and matrix morphologies of knees and ankle joints [7].

* Correspondence: jan.hubert@med.uni-goettingen.de;
thelonius.hawellek@med.uni-goettingen.de
[1]Department of Trauma Surgery, Orthopaedics and Plastic Surgery, University Medical Center Göttingen, Robert-Koch-Straße 40, 37075 Göttingen, Germany
Full list of author information is available at the end of the article

Another possible explanation for the development of AJ OA could be the occurrence of calcification within the hyaline articular cartilage, also known as chondrocalcinosis [8]. A high prevalence of cartilage calcification (CC) as well as a significant correlation between CC and OA has been reported in both weight-bearing hip and knee joints as well as in the first metatarsophalangeal joint (MTP-I joint) [9–13]. Furthermore, in vitro studies have shown that calcium phosphate crystals can alter cartilage tissue via biomechanical [14, 15] and pro-inflammatory biochemical processes [16–19], all of which can lead to degeneration of the affected joint.

The prevalence of ankle joint cartilage calcification (AJ CC) in the general population is reported at around 4.7%, and is based on only one cross-sectional study in which the occurrence of calcification on the talar surface was analysed macroscopically [20] and an association between CC and OA of the talus was reported. However, early signs of CC are only measurable in the nano- to micrometre ranges, thus raising the possibility of underestimation with conventional imaging techniques. In order to detect the onset of CC, high-resolution imaging techniques like digital contact radiography (DCR) are required [21]. Taking this into account, the precision of the previously reported cross-sectional study might be called into question [20].

Therefore, the primary goal of this study was to evaluate and quantify the prevalence of AJ CC using high-resolution DCR. Secondly, we examined the correlations between the observed CC with age, BMI and the histological grade of osteoarthritis.

Methods

Both ankle joints ($n = 160$) of 80 donors were obtained from an unselected cohort who underwent autopsy at the Department for Legal Medicine, University Medical Center Hamburg-Eppendorf [22]. Only donors with bilaterally intact ankle joints with no signs of any other diseases (except for OA) were included in this study. Donors with a history of previous ankle surgery, tumours, infections and/or rheumatic diseases were excluded. The study was approved by the local Ethics Committee (PV 4570) and is in compliance with the Helsinki Declaration.

Sample preparation

Firstly, the whole ankle joint of the right and left limbs were extracted. Next, the soft tissue was carefully removed from the talus and the distal tibia along with the corresponding tibiofibular joint. For the calcification analysis, standardized 4 mm cartilage-bone specimens were cut in the coronal plane of the talus and

the distal tibia along with the corresponding tibiofibular joint (Fig. 1).

Digital contact radiography (DCR)

The prepared cartilage-bone specimens were then washed with physiological saline solution to remove residual bone debris before being subjected to standardized radiography (25 kV, 3.8 mAs, film focus distance of 8 cm) using a high-resolution digital radiography device (Faxitron X-Ray, Illinois, USA). Calcifications were detected as radiopaque spots within the cartilage matrix. Subsequently, the radiographs were qualitatively and quantitatively analysed using standard software (ImageJ 1.46, National Institutes of Health, Bethesda, USA) [9, 23]. The amount of calcification was determined as the percentage of the total area of the hyaline cartilage.

Histology

The histological OA grade was evaluated for the talar and distal tibial cartilage (central load-bearing zone) of all ankle joints. Therefore, a sample of full thickness hyaline cartilage of the previously extracted cartilage-bone-specimen was cut to the subchondral bone plate. All cartilage samples were fixed in 4% PFA for 24 h before being dehydrated using 80% alcohol and embedded in paraffin. Four-μm sections of all samples were stained with 1% Safranin-O (Fig. 2) in order to evaluate the samples' histological degeneration grade as it relates to the OARSI osteoarthritis cartilage histopathology assessment system (Grades 0 to 6) [24]. To confirm the occurrence of calcium phosphate deposition, von Kossa staining was performed.

Statistical analysis

The biometric characteristics of donors are reported as mean values ±standard deviations. For descriptive analysis, mean CC values for each joint were used. Logarithmic transformation was performed for further

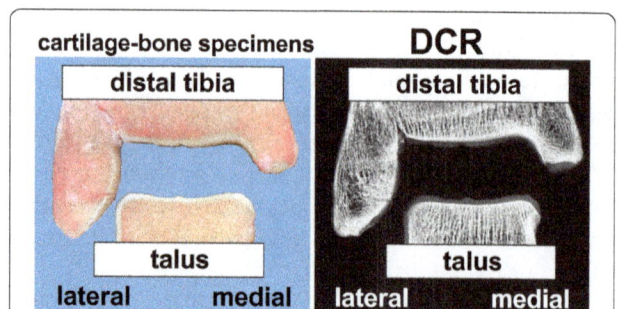

Fig. 1 Examplary samples of the ankle joint showing standardized, 4 mm cartilage-bone specimens (cut along the coronal plane) of the distal tibia and talus, as well as the corresponding digital contact radiographs. Calcification was detectable as radiopaque spots in the cartilage's matrix

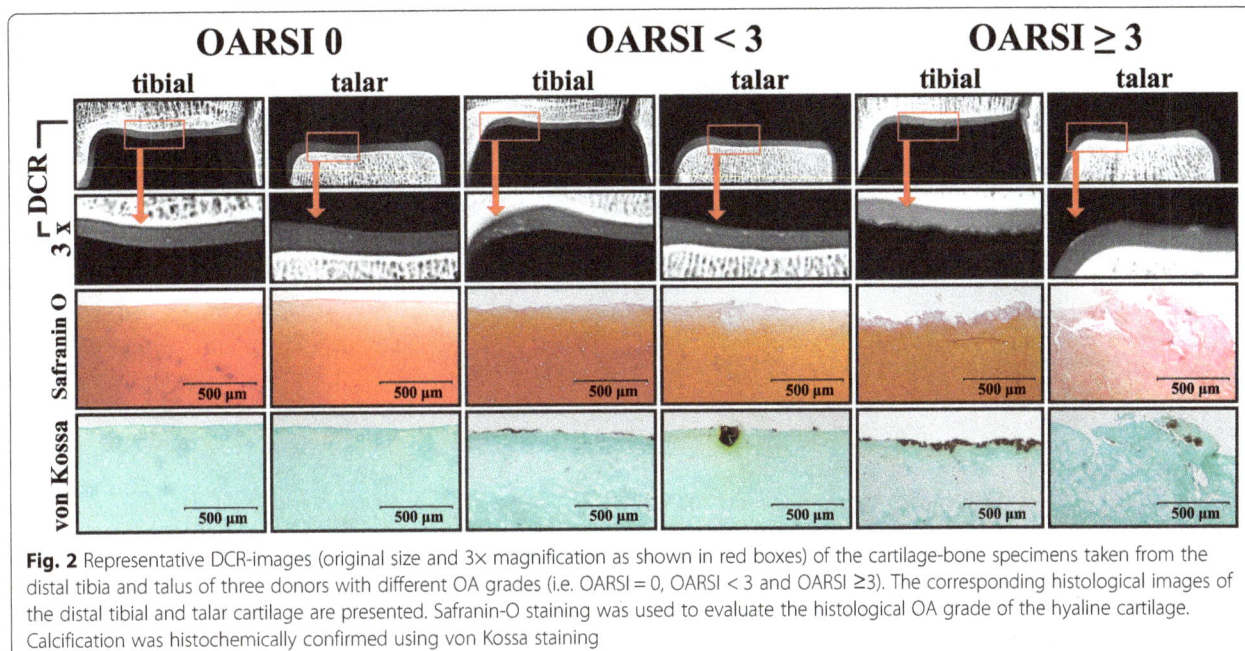

Fig. 2 Representative DCR-images (original size and 3× magnification as shown in red boxes) of the cartilage-bone specimens taken from the distal tibia and talus of three donors with different OA grades (i.e. OARSI = 0, OARSI < 3 and OARSI ≥3). The corresponding histological images of the distal tibial and talar cartilage are presented. Safranin-O staining was used to evaluate the histological OA grade of the hyaline cartilage. Calcification was histochemically confirmed using von Kossa staining

evaluation. Fisher's test was conducted to obtain categorical data, whereas side comparisons were evaluated using McNemar's Exact test. Differences between the mean amount of distal tibial and talar CC were analysed using a linear mixed model. The model takes into account the values of a donor's left and right ankle joints and uses them as random effects with compound symmetry covariance structure (as opposed to using the joint as a fixed effect). In addition, assumptions for the mixed model were checked using residual plots. To determine the association between continuous variables Pearson's (r) or Spearman's (r_s) rank correlation coefficient was calculated. Partial correlation calculations were carried out using the respective parameters (CC, histological degeneration grade and age) adjusted to avoid spurious correlations. All statistical analyses were performed with Software R, Version 3.1.1. [25]. P-values of less than 0.05 were considered statistically significant.

Results
The mean age of the study population was 62.4 years (SD ±17.7, range 23–95 years). Thirty-four of the donors were female, whereas 46 were male. Biometric characteristics of the study population are presented in Table 1.

Prevalence of cartilage calcification
In our study population, the prevalence of AJ CC was 51.3% (41/80) (95% CI [0.40, 0.63]). The left joint was affected in 37.5% (30/80) (95% CI [0.27, 0.49]) while the right joint in 40.0% (32/80) (95% CI [0.29, 0.52]) of all cases. No side showed signs of higher susceptibility to CC ($p = 0.82$). Bilateral CC was detected in 26.3% of donors (21/80). The prevalence of talar CC was 47.5% (38/80) (95% CI [0.36, 0.59]), whereas CC of the distal tibia was 35.0% (28/80) (95% CI [0.25, 0.47]). Bilateral talar CC was noted in 17.5% (14/80), while bilateral CC of the distal tibia was seen in only 8.8% (7/80) of all cases (Table 2).

Gender
AJ CC was detected in 58.7% (27/46) (95% CI [0.43, 0.73]), talar CC in 52.2% (24/46) (95% CI [0.37, 0.67]) and distal tibial CC in 39.1% (18/46) (95% CI [0.25, 0.55]) of all male donors. In the female donor cohort AJ CC was observed in 41.2% (14/34) (95% CI [0.25, 0.59]), talar CC in 41.2% (14/34) (95% CI [0.25, 0.59]) and distal tibial CC in 29.4% (10/34) (95% CI [0.15, 0.47]) (Table 2). There were no significant differences regarding the prevalence of AJ CC ($p = 0.18$), talar CC ($p = 0.37$) or distal tibial CC ($p = 0.48$) for gender.

Table 1 Biometric characteristics of the study population ($n = 80$)

Age [years]	62.4 ± 17.7
Male	59.2 ± 17.9
Female	66.6 ± 16.7
Height [cm]	
Male	177.5 ± 7.1
Female	161.7 ± 7.9
Body weight [kg]	
Male	81.9 ± 17.9
Female	72.3 ± 11.5
Body Mass Index [kg/m²]	25.4 ± 4.9

Table 2 Prevalence of DCR-detectable cartilage calcification (n = 80)

	Ankle		Talus		Distal tibia	
	n	%	n	%	n	%
Total CC	41/80	51.3	38/80	47.5	28/80	35.0
Bilateral CC	21/80	26.3	14/80	17.5	7/80	8.8
Unilateral	20/80	25.0	24/80	30.0	21/80	26.3
Left CC	30/80	37.5	26/80	32.5	15/80	18.8
Right CC	32/80	40.0	26/80	32.5	20/80	25.0
Male	27/46	58.7	24/46	52.2	18/46	39.1
Female	14/34	41.2	14/34	41.2	10/34	29.4

Quantitative analysis of cartilage calcification

The mean amount of AJ CC was quantitated at 0.17% (SD ± 0.52, range: 0.00–3.55); left AJ CC 0.22% (SD ± 0.77, range: 0.00–5.97) and right AJ CC 0.13% (SD ± 0.41, range: 0.00–3.03). Significant correlations were noted between the two joints ($r = 0.52$, $p = 0.02$) (Fig. 3a).

The mean amount of talar CC was quantified at 0.15% (SD ± 0.43, range: 0.00–3.04) and distal tibia CC at 0.39% (SD ± 1.53, range: 0.00–11.53). Significant correlations were found between the mean amount of CC noted in the talar and distal tibial cartilage ($r = 0.59$, $p = 0.002$) (Fig. 3b), however, no quantitative differences could be detected ($p = 0.06$) (Fig. 3c).

Cartilage degeneration (OARSI score)

The mean histological degeneration grade of the left/right distal tibia was 1.5 (SD ± 1.0, range: 0–5)/1.5 (SD ± 1.0, range: 0–6) and of the left/right talus 1.3 (SD ±1.1, range: 0–6)/1.6 (SD ± 1.1, range: 0–5). The distribution of the histological OA grade according to the OARSI score system (Grade 0–6) is presented in Table 3.

Cartilage calcification and histological degeneration
Distal tibial cartilage

Distal tibial CC was detected in only 11.9% (17/143) of the cases that were classified as 'mild cartilage damage' (OARSI < 3). However, distal tibial CC was reported in 82.4% (14/17) of the cases with 'severe cartilage degeneration' (OARSI ≥3), (Table 4). Quantitative analysis revealed significant correlations between the mean amount of distal tibial CC and the histological degeneration, both without ($r = 0.70$, $p < 0.001$, 95% CI [0.44, 0.85]) and after an adjustment for age ($r = 0.68$, $p < 0.001$) (Fig. 4a). Conversely, there was no significant correlation between the amount of distal tibial CC and the histological degeneration of the talus ($r = 0.23$, $p = 0.25$).

Talar cartilage

Talar CC was detected in only 21.5% (29/135) of the cases with 'mild cartilage damage' (OARSI < 3) and in 92.0% (23/25) of the cases with 'severe cartilage degeneration' (OARSI ≥3) (Table 4). Overall, a significant correlation was observed between the amount of talar CC and the histological degeneration grade of the talus, both without ($r = 0.72$, $p < 0.001$, 95% CI [0.52, 0.85]) and after an adjustment for age was conducted ($r = 0.72$, $p < 0.001$) (Fig. 4b). Additionally, significant correlations were noted between the amount of talar CC and distal tibial degeneration ($r = 0.61$, $p < 0.001$, 95% CI [0.36, 0.78]).

Cartilage calcification and age
Distal tibial cartilage

No correlation was observed between the amount of distal tibial CC and age without ($p = 0.32$) and after an adjustment for histological degeneration grade ($p = 0.75$) (Fig. 4c).

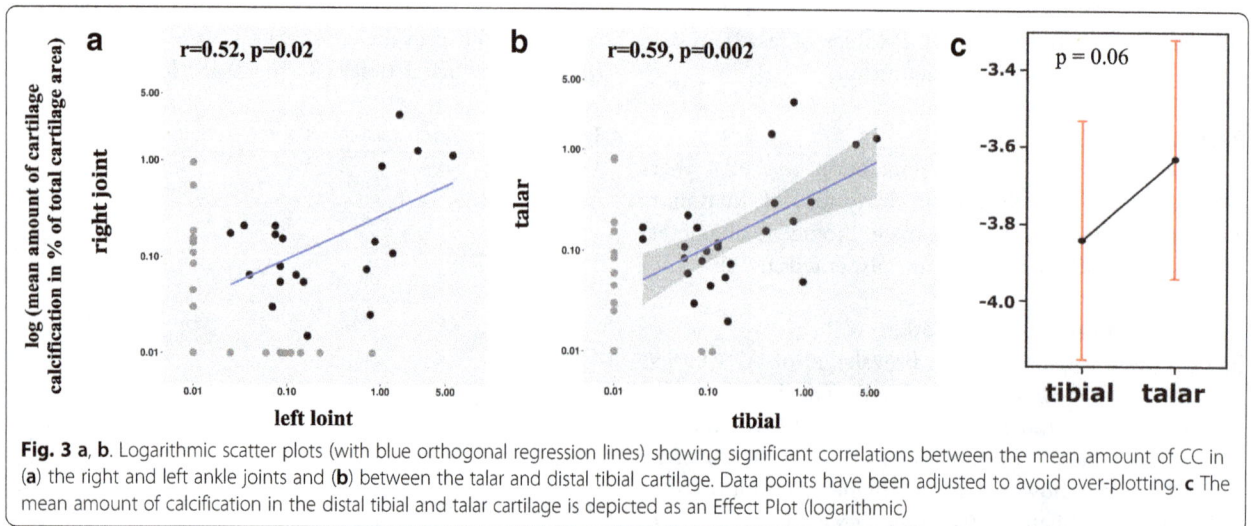

Fig. 3 a, b. Logarithmic scatter plots (with blue orthogonal regression lines) showing significant correlations between the mean amount of CC in (**a**) the right and left ankle joints and (**b**) between the talar and distal tibial cartilage. Data points have been adjusted to avoid over-plotting. **c** The mean amount of calcification in the distal tibial and talar cartilage is depicted as an Effect Plot (logarithmic)

Table 3 Distribution of the histological OA-grade by OARSI (n = 80)

OARSI	Distal tibia				Talus			
	Left		Right		Left		Right	
	n	%	n	%	n	%	n	%
0	9	11.3	12	15.0	18	22.5	12	15.0
1	37	46.3	33	41.3	35	43.8	32	40.0
2	26	32.5	26	32.5	17	21.3	21	26.3
3	5	6.3	7	8.8	6	7.5	11	13.8
4	1	1.3	1	1.3	3	3.8	3	3.8
5	2	2.5	0	0.0	0	0.0	1	1.3
6	0	0.0	1	1.3	1	1.3	0	0.0

Talar cartilage

There was no correlation between the amount of talar CC and age without ($p = 0.49$) and after an adjustment for histological degeneration grade ($p = 0.30$) (Fig. 4d).

Cartilage calcification and BMI

No correlation was detected between the amount of CC and the BMI of the donor for both the distal tibial ($p = 0.51$) and the talar cartilages ($p = 0.87$).

Histological degeneration grade and age

Correlations were noted between the histological degeneration grade of the distal tibial/talar hyaline cartilage and age (($r = 0.28$, $p = 0.01$, 95% CI [0.06, 0.47])/($r = 0.40$, $p < 0.001$, 95% CI [0.20, 0.57])).

Discussion

Independent of the donor's gender and side, an unexpectedly high prevalence of AJ CC (51.3%) was found in this study. Intraindividual correlations existed between the amount of CC of the left with that of the right AJ, as well as between the distal tibial and the talar cartilage. These findings underline the systemic appearance of ankle-related CC. Furthermore, since calcification has already been found in intact AJ cartilage and the amount of CC correlated with the histological OA grade, we hypothesize that CC may play a causative role in the pathogenesis of AJ OA.

So far, the prevalence of ankle-related CC has been reported in only one cross-sectional study [20]. However, since calcium phosphate deposition is known to begin in

Table 4 Distribution of joints with mild (OARSI < 3) and severe (OARSI ≥3) OA-grade with positive CC (n = 160)

OARSI	Distal tibia		Talus	
	n	%	n	%
< 3	17/143	11.9	29/135	21.5
≥ 3	14/17	82.4	23/25	92.0

the nano- to micrometre range, it is almost impossible to detect the early stages of calcification through macroscopic analysis or even using standard radiographic techniques. High-resolution imaging techniques such as Digital Contact Radiography (DCR) are therefore necessary for detection of the onset of CC [21]. Using DCR, we were able to establish that CC was prevalent in 51.3% of all cases; this was in stark contrast to previously published studies in which the prevalence of CC was a mere 4.7% [20]. Despite this, DCR has shown that AJ CC is relatively rare when compared to the prevalence of CC in other joints, such as the shoulder (98.9%) [26], the hip (96.6%) [11] or the knee (94.3–100%) [11, 23]. Nonetheless, the reason for the difference remains elusive. Interestingly, calcification is comparably prevalent in both the AJ and the MTP-I joint (48.1%) [12]. It has been theorized that weight-loading promotes pro-mineralization of the joints [27, 28], however, the results of our study contradict this point. Since the ankle generally bears enormous loads (many times greater than body weight), it stands to reason that the degree of calcification should be higher. Moreover, other studies have reported that calcification is more prevalent in non-weight bearing joints such as the shoulder [26] and has even been observed in non-weight-bearing parts of the knee cartilage [29]. Another factor to investigate is the impact of the donor's BMI on CC (additional mechanical stress induced by increasing BMI). We could not find any association between the donor's BMI and the mean amount of AJ CC. Given this, it can be assumed that mechanical load is not the predominant factor.

Our study highlighted significant correlations between the mean amount of CC in the left and right AJ, between the left and right distal tibia and talus, as well as correlations between the mean amount of calcification in the distal tibial and talar cartilage. These results underline the theory that the development of calcification is systemic [11, 26, 30].

Another interesting observation was the correlation between CC and the donor's histological OA grade. CC was detected in donors with histologically intact or almost intact hyaline cartilage (i.e. an OARSI grade < 3) in 12% and in 22% of the distal tibial and talar cartilage respectively. Given this, it can be indicated that CC is already present in the joint before the histological OA is even measurable, and might occur before the OA process initiates. Similar observations of spontaneous OA development have been found in two animal models [31, 32], wherein calcification was detectable before cartilage degeneration occurred.

In comparison with other joints [9–13, 26, 30, 33], there is also a clear association between CC and OA in the ankle. In our study, CC in the distal tibia was detectable in 82% of the donors with severe OA (i.e. an OARSI

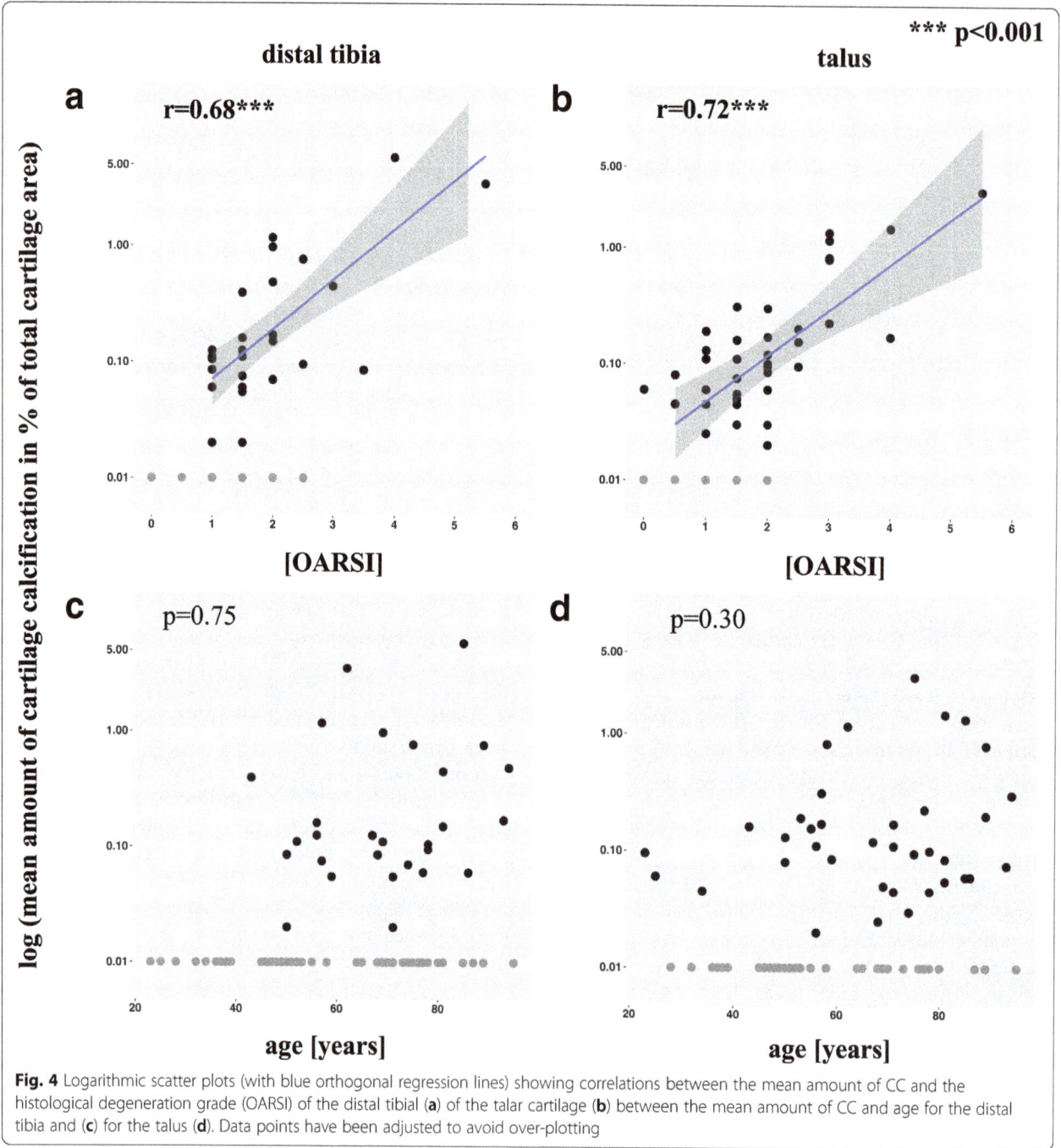

Fig. 4 Logarithmic scatter plots (with blue orthogonal regression lines) showing correlations between the mean amount of CC and the histological degeneration grade (OARSI) of the distal tibial (**a**) of the talar cartilage (**b**) between the mean amount of CC and age for the distal tibia and (**c**) for the talus (**d**). Data points have been adjusted to avoid over-plotting

grade ≥ 3), whereas talar CC was detected in 92%. Moreover, our quantitative analysis demonstrated that the mean amount of calcification in the distal tibial, as well as in the talar cartilage correlated with the histological degeneration grade. Muehlemann et al. also described an association between the prevalence of CC and macroscopic talar degeneration, even though no quantitative analysis was conducted for their study [20]. Taken together, there seems to be evidence that CC plays a crucial role in the development of AJ OA.

No correlation was found between the mean amount of AJ CC and the donors' age. This is in line with previously published results for other joints, including the shoulder [26], the hip/knee [11] and the MTP-I joint [12]. In contrast, Mitsuyama et al. [23] observed significant correlations between the mean amount of CC in the knee and age of the general population. However, since no adjustment for the donor's OA grade was conducted, it is conceivable that this association between CC and donor age might have been a spurious correlation, which would disappear once an adjustment for OA grade would be performed.

Certainly, there are some limitations to this study. There were no information about the donor lifestyle, activity and medical history, in particular ankle complaints. Even though the standardized cartilage-bone specimens of the distal tibia and talus used in this study were representative, they reflected only a small proportion of the ankle articulating surface. Lastly, the calcium-phosphate composition of DCR-detected CC was not thoroughly characterized in our study since such analyses require the use of specific diagnostic methods, e.g. FTIR spectroscopy [34] or X-Ray diffractometry [35], and were not specifically in the scope of our study. Nevertheless, none of these limitations is likely to influence the study's findings and conclusions.

Conclusion

DCR analysis revealed that the prevalence of ankle-related cartilage calcification is much higher than previously considered in general population. Even though it is independent of the donor's age and/or BMI, calcification seems to occur in histologically intact ankle cartilage and is linked with the joint's histological OA grade. These insights indicate that hyaline CC is an early, age-independent element and a possible causative factor in the development of ankle-related osteoarthritis. However, the exact pathophysiological role of CC in osteoarthritis and its subsequent importance in the disease's molecular mechanisms are yet to be identified and investigated.

Abbreviations

AJ: Ankle joint; CC: Cartilage calcification; DCR: Digital-contact radiography; OA: Osteoarthritis; OARSI: Osteoarthritis cartilage histopathology assessment system

Acknowledgements

We would like to thank Shahed Taheri for proofreading the manuscript and Elke Leicht of the Department of Osteology and Biomechanics, University Medical Centre Hamburg-Eppendorf for providing expert technical assistance throughout this project.

Authors' contributions

JH and TH contributed equally to the conception and design of the study, the acquisition analysis and interpretation of data, as well as to the creation and revision of the manuscript. SH and AU was responsible for conducting statistical analysis and interpreting the data. LW, TR, TS, and SKB conducted both DCR and histological analysis; they also contributed equally to the interpretation of the data. KP was responsible for data acquisition. WL and FTB conducted data interpretation and contributed equally to drafting and revising the manuscript. All authors have read and approved the final manuscript. All authors included on this paper have made substantial contributions to this work and have fulfilled the criteria for authorship. Both Jan Hubert (jan.hubert@med.uni-goettingen.de) and Thelonius Hawellek (thelonius.hawellek@med.uni-goettingen.de) take full responsibility for the integrity of this study from inception to completion.

Competing interests

All authors have disclosed all financial and personal relationships that could potentially and inappropriately influence this work. The authors declare that they have no competing interests.

Author details

[1]Department of Trauma Surgery, Orthopaedics and Plastic Surgery, University Medical Center Göttingen, Robert-Koch-Straße 40, 37075 Göttingen, Germany. [2]Department of Medical Biometry and Epidemiology, University Medical Center Hamburg-Eppendorf, Hamburg, Germany. [3]Department of Urology, University Medical Center Göttingen, Göttingen, Germany. [4]Department of Osteology and Biomechanics, University Medical Center Hamburg-Eppendorf, Hamburg, Germany. [5]Department of Legal Medicine, University Medical Center Hamburg-Eppendorf, Hamburg, Germany.

References

1. Felson DT. The epidemiology of osteoarthritis: prevalence and risk factors. In: Kuettner KE, Goldberg VM, editors. Osteoarthritis Disorders. Rosemont, IL: American Academy Orthopedic Surgeons; 1995. p. 13e24.
2. Peyron JG. The epidemiology of osteoarthritis. In: Moskowitz RW, Howell DS, Goldberg VM, Mankin HJ, editors. Osteoarthritis. Diagnosis and Treatment. Philadelphia, PA: WB Saunders; 1984. p. 9–27.
3. Saltzman CL, Salamon ML, Blanchard GM, et al. Epidemiology of ankle arthritis: report of a consecutive series of 639 patients from a tertiary orthopaedic center. Iowa Orthop J. 2005;25:44–6.
4. Valderrabano V, Horisberger M, Russell I, et al. Etiology of ankle osteoarthritis. Clin Orthop Relat Res. 2009;467(7):1800–6.
5. Lindsjö U. Operative treatment of ankle fracture-dislocations: a follow-up study of 306/321 consecutive cases. Clin Orthop Relat Res. 1985;199:28–38.
6. Eckstein F, Winzheimer M, Hohe J, et al. Interindividual variability and correlation among morphological parameters of knee joint cartilage plates: analysis with three-dimensional MR imaging. Osteoarthr Cartil. 2001;9(2):101–11.
7. Quinn TM, Häuselmann HJ, Shintani N, Hunziker EB. Cell and matrix morphology in articular cartilage from adult human knee and ankle joints suggests depth-associated adaptations to biomechanical and anatomical roles. Osteoarthr Cartil. 2013;21(12):1904–12.
8. Zhang W, Doherty M, Bardin T, et al. European league against rheumatism recommendations for calcium pyrophosphate deposition. Part I: terminology and diagnosis. Ann Rheum Dis. 2011;70(4):563–70.
9. Fuerst M, Bertrand J, Lammers L, et al. Calcification of articular cartilage in human osteoarthritis. Arthritis Rheum. 2009;60(9):2694–703.
10. Fuerst M, Niggemeyer O, Lammers L, et al. Articular cartilage mineralization in osteoarthritis of the hip. BMC Musculoskelet Disord. 2009;10:166. https://doi.org/10.1186/1471-2474-10-166.
11. Hawellek T, Hubert J, Hischke S, et al. Articular cartilage calcification of the hip and knee is highly prevalent, independent of age but associated with histological osteoarthritis: evidence for a systemic disorder. Osteoarthr Cartil. 2016;24(12):2092–9. https://doi.org/10.1016/j.joca.2016.06.020. Epub 2016 Jul 5
12. Hubert J, Hawellek T, Hischke S, et al. Hyaline cartilage calcification of the first metatarsophalangeal joint is associated with osteoarthritis but independent of age and BMI. BMC Musculoskelet Disord. 2016;17(1):474.
13. Neame RL, Carr AJ, Muir K, et al. UK community prevalence of knee chondrocalcinosis: evidence that correlation with osteoarthritis is through a shared association with osteophyte. Ann Rheum Dis. 2003;62(6):513–8.
14. Roemhildt ML, Beynnon BD, Gardner-Morse M. Mineralization of articular cartilage in the Sprague-Dawley rat: characterization and mechanical analysis. Osteoarthr Cartil. 2012;20(7):796–800.
15. Roemhildt ML, Gardner-Morse MG, Morgan CF, et al. Calcium phosphate particulates increase friction in the rat knee joint. Osteoarthr Cartil. 2014; 22(5):706–9.
16. McCarthy GM, Westfall PR, Masuda I, Christopherson PA, Cheung HS, Mitchell PG. Basic calcium phosphate crystals activate human osteoarthritic synovial fibroblasts and induce matrix metalloproteinase-13 (collagenase-3) in adult porcine articular chondrocytes. Ann Rheum Dis. 2001;60(4):399–406.
17. Morgan MP, Whelan LC, Sallis JD, et al. Basic calcium phosphate crystal-induced prostaglandin E2 production in human fibroblasts: role of cyclooxygenase 1, cyclooxygenase 2, and interleukin-1beta. Arthritis Rheum. 2004;50(5):1642–9.

18. Ea HK, Uzan B, Rey C, Lioté F. Octacalcium phosphate crystals directly stimulate expression of inducible nitric oxide synthase through p38 and JNK mitogen-activated protein kinases in articular chondrocytes. Arthritis Res Ther. 2005;7(5):R915–26.

19. Nasi S, So A, Combes C, et al. Interleukin-6 and chondrocyte mineralisation act in tandem to promote experimental osteoarthritis. Ann Rheum Dis. 2015. pii: annrheumdis-2015-207487. doi: https://doi.org/10.1136/annrheumdis-2015-207487. [Epub ahead of print].

20. Muehleman C, Li J, Aigner T, et al. Association between crystals and cartilage degeneration in the ankle. J Rheumatol. 2008;35(6):1108–17. Epub 2008 Apr 15

21. Abreu M, Johnson K, Chung CB, et al. Calcification in calcium pyrophosphate dihydrate (CPPD) crystalline deposits in the knee: anatomic, radiographic, MR imaging, and histologic study in cadavers. Skelet Radiol. 2004;33(7):392–8. Epub 2004 May 11

22. Püschel K. Teaching and research on corpses. Mortui vivos docent. Rechtsmedizin. 2016;26(2):115–9.

23. Mitsuyama H, Healey RM, Terkeltaub RA, et al. Calcification of human articular knee cartilage is primarily an effect of aging rather than osteoarthritis. Osteoarthr Cartil. 2007;15(5):559–65.

24. Pritzker KP, Gay S, Jimenez SA, et al. Osteoarthritis cartilage histopathology: grading and staging. Osteoarthr Cartil. 2006;14(1):13–29.

25. Team RC. R: A language and environment for statistical computing. Vienna: R Foundation for Statistical Computing; 2014. URL http://www.R-project.org

26. Hawellek T, Hubert J, Hischke S, et al. Articular cartilage calcification of the humeral head is highly prevalent and associated with osteoarthritis in the general population. J Orthop Res. 2016;34(11):1984–90. https://doi.org/10.1002/jor.23227. Epub 2016 Apr 6

27. Carlson AK, McCutchen CN, June RK. Mechanobiological implications of articular cartilage crystals. Curr Opin Rheumatol. 2017;29(2):157–62.

28. Taylor AM. Metabolic and endocrine diseases, cartilage calcification and arthritis. Curr Opin Rheumatol. 2013;25(2):198–203.

29. Nguyen C, Bazin D, Daudon M, et al. Revisiting spatial distribution and biochemical composition of calcium-containing crystals in human osteoarthritic articular cartilage. Arthritis Res Ther. 2013;15(5):R103.

30. Abhishek A, Doherty S, Maciewicz R, et al. Evidence of a systemic predisposition to chondrocalcinosis and association between chondrocalcinosis and osteoarthritis at distant joints: a cross-sectional study. Arthritis Care Res (Hoboken). 2013;65(7):1052e8.

31. Bendele AM, White SL. Early histopathologic and ultrastructural alterations in femorotibial joints of partial medial meniscectomized Guinea pigs. Vet Pathol. 1987;24(5):436–43.

32. Evans RG, Collins C, Miller P, et al. Radiological scoring of osteoarthritis progression in STR/ORT mice. Osteoarthr Cartil. 1994;2(2):103–9.

33. Hawellek T, Hubert J, Hischke S, et al. Microcalcification of lumbar spine intervertebral discs and facet joints is associated with cartilage degeneration, but differs in prevalence and its relation to age. J Orthop Res. 2017;35(12):2692–9.

34. Dessombz A, Nguyen C, Ea HK, et al. Combining μX-ray fluorescence, μXANES and μXRD to shed light on Zn2+ cations in cartilage and meniscus calcifications. J Trace Elem Med Biol. 2013;27(4):326–33.

35. Nguyen C, Ea HK, Thiaudiere D, et al. Calcifications in human osteoarthritic articular cartilage: ex vivo assessment of calcium compounds using XANES spectroscopy. J Synchrotron Radiat. 2011;18(Pt 3):475–80.

23

Locking plate for treating traumatic sternoclavicular joint dislocation

Rongguang Ao[†], Yalong Zhu[†], Jianhua Zhou[†], Zhen Jian, Jifei Shi, Cheng Li, Wankun Hu and Baoqing Yu[*]

Abstract

Background: Traumatic sternoclavicular joint dislocations are rare; closed reduction is the primary treatment. The failure of closed reduction or a prominent insult to the skin may require surgery to ensure the best possible outcome.

Methods: The records of 5 patients operated at our institution for sternoclavicular joint dislocation were reviewed. All patients were treated with open reduction and single 3.5-mm locking plate was used for fixation. Outcomes were evaluated with the Constant Shoulder Score (CSS) and Disability of the Arm, Shoulder, and Hand (DASH) questionnaire. Intraoperative and postoperative complications were recorded.

Results: All the patients had an average follow-up of 14 months (range, 11–16 months). At the final follow-up, the mean CSS score was 89.5 (range, 78–98) and the mean DASH score was 9.0 (range, 4–16). There were no early complications, including wound infection or neurologic or vascular deficits; there were also no broken or loosened screws or plates. No case of redislocation or arthrosis was observed.

Conclusion: Our study indicates that open reduction and fixation with a single locking plate for the treatment of traumatic sternoclavicular joint dislocation is a safe, relatively simple surgical procedure that can lead to satisfactory outcomes.

Keywords: Sternoclavicular joint, Dislocation, Open reduction and internal fixation

Background

Sternoclavicular joint dislocations (SCJ) are rare, accounting for approximately 3% of injuries to the shoulder girdle [1]. Some 90% to of 95% SCJ dislocations are anterior [2], and most can be treated with closed reduction. Once recurrence or instability of the anterior SCJ dislocation is noted, the prominence of the medial clavicle may cause discomfort, and operative management may become necessary [3]. Posterior SCJ dislocations are life-threatening injuries because of their potential for causing mediastinal compression, compression of the brachial plexus, pneumothorax, respiratory distress, as well as vascular injuries [4]. Prompt closed reduction is recommended for posterior dislocations of the SCJ. If

closed reduction fails, operative management is recommended [3].

Many surgical techniques have been used to treat unstable or chronic SCL dislocations, including osteosynthesis with pins [5] and K-wires [6], plate fixation [7–9], and ligament reconstruction [10–13]. But only three papers have reported on plate fixation for the treatment of SCJ dislocations, using three different types of implants: Balser plates [7], standard 3.5-mm LC/DCP with a ledge-plating technique [8], and a dual locking plate [9]. Good results were achieved with these techniques, but plate fixation has not been widely used.

In this paper, we report on the operative technique and outcomes of using a single locking plate to treat traumatic SCJ dislocation.

* Correspondence: 13131310044@fudan.edu.cn
[†]Equal contributors
Department of Orthopedics, Shanghai Pudong Hospital, Fudan University Pudong Medical Center, 2800 Gongwei Road, Huinan Town, Pudong, Shanghai 201399, People's Republic of China

Table 1 General conditions

Identifier	Gender/Age (y)	Affected side	Cause	Dislocation type	Associated injury	Follow-up (months)	DASH score/ Constant score
Patient 1	F/29	L	Traffic accident	Anterior	No	16	4/98
Patient 2	M/31	R	Sport injury	Posterior	No	11	6/96
Patient 3	F/43	R	Traffic accident	Anterior	Ipsilateral acromioclavicular joint dislocation (Rockwood type IV), left proximal humeral fracture	15	16/78
Patient 4	M/37	L	Traffic accident	Posterior	No	15	10/87.5
Patient 5	F/41	R	Traffic accident	Anterior	No	13	9/88

Methods

General data

Institutional review board approval for the study was obtained. A retrospective study that included all 8 cases of SCJ dislocation treated between October 2008 and December 2015 was performed. The primary management is closed reduction according to recommended reduction methods [3]. The indications for proceeding to surgery were as follows: (1) dislocations that could not be reduced by conservative management and (2) dislocations that appeared vulnerable to recurrence with movement of the shoulder joint, and cases in which there was a prominent insult to the skin. Five patients who met the criteria for surgery were treated with open reduction and internal fixation using a single 3.5-mm locking plate; these cases included three anterior and two posterior

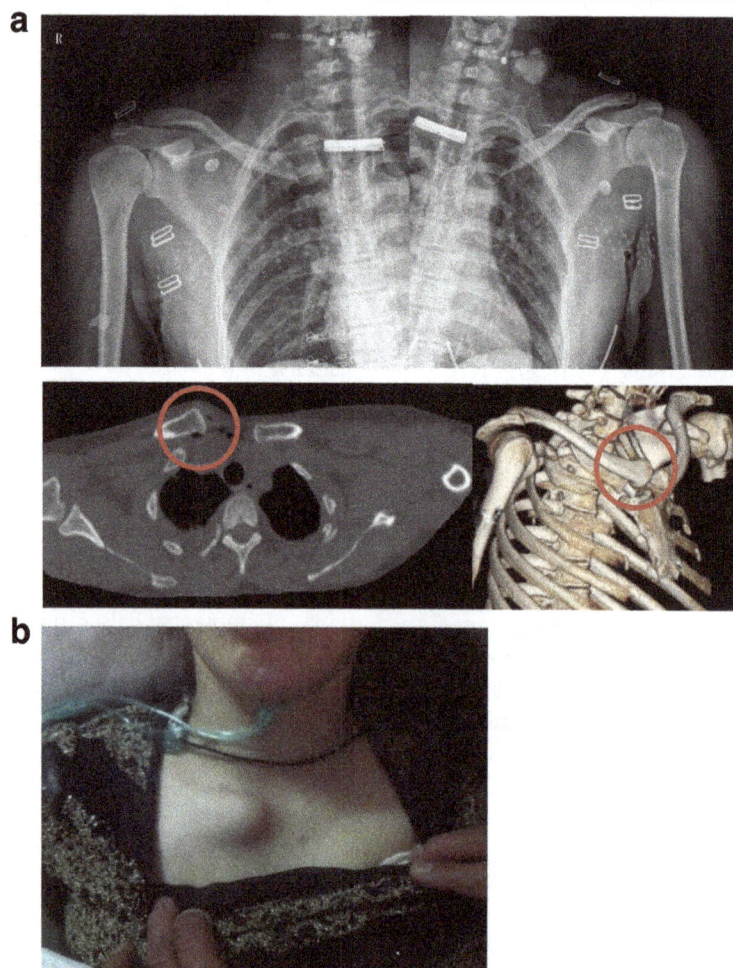

Fig. 1 In patient 3, a 43-year-old female, the preoperative x-ray and computed tomography scan (**a**) show a right anterior dislocation of the sternoclavicular joint and a left proximal humeral fracture. A preoperative photograph (**b**) showing an obvious prominence at the medial end of the clavicle

dislocations. The age, gender distribution, affected side, cause of the injuries, dislocation type, associated injuries, and duration of follow-up are listed in Table 1.

Surgical technique and rehabilitation

Surgery took place with the patient under general anesthesia and in the supine position. A transverse incision was made over the medial clavicle and sternum. The skin and subcutaneous tissues were dissected and, if possible, the platysma was incised and elevated as a separate layer. The periosteum of the medial clavicle was reflected superiorly and inferiorly, at which point the injured ligaments of the SCJ could be identified.

In the case of the anterior dislocations (Fig. 1), we found that the anterior capsule and ligaments were torn (Fig. 2a). After manual reduction of the SCJ, the medial end of clavicle would move anteriorly, indicating instability. Therefore we maintained reduction of the SCJ and used nonabsorbable suture to repair the torn ligaments and capsule (Fig. 2b), finally applying the locking plate for fixation. The plate was placed on the anterior part of the sternum and medial clavicle. First fixation at the medial clavicle was performed, using a short drill to protect the vascular structures (subclavian artery and vein). Bicrotic locking screws were used to maintain reduction of the SCJ. Then the anterior cortex of the sternum was carefully drilled and unicortical locking screws placed (Fig. 2c).

For posterior dislocations (Fig. 3a), we dissected the anterior ligament and capsule to expose the articular surface of the clavicle from the sternum side. Because the position of the medial clavicle was not visible (Fig. 3b), we identified the clavicle from the lateral side and then moved to the medial end of the clavicle. The injured upper limb was retracted with shoulder abduction to about 90 degrees. Reduction was then carefully held with forceps (Fig. 3c). A locking plate was used for fixation in the same manner as with the anterior dislocation (Figs. 3d and 4). Nonabsorbable suture was used to repair the ligament and capsule before plating.

After surgery, the injured extremity was immobilized in a sling for 3 weeks, during which active range-of-motion exercises for the elbow and shoulder were encouraged. Three weeks after operation, passive mobilization of the shoulder was increased while gradually transitioning to active exercises.

All patients were asked to follow up monthly for 3 months after their operations, and then every 3 to 6 months after implant removal. Functional evaluation was implemented using the Constant Shoulder Score (CSS) and Disability of the Arm, Shoulder, and Hand (DASH) questionnaire. Documented postsurgical complications included infection, implant failure, and

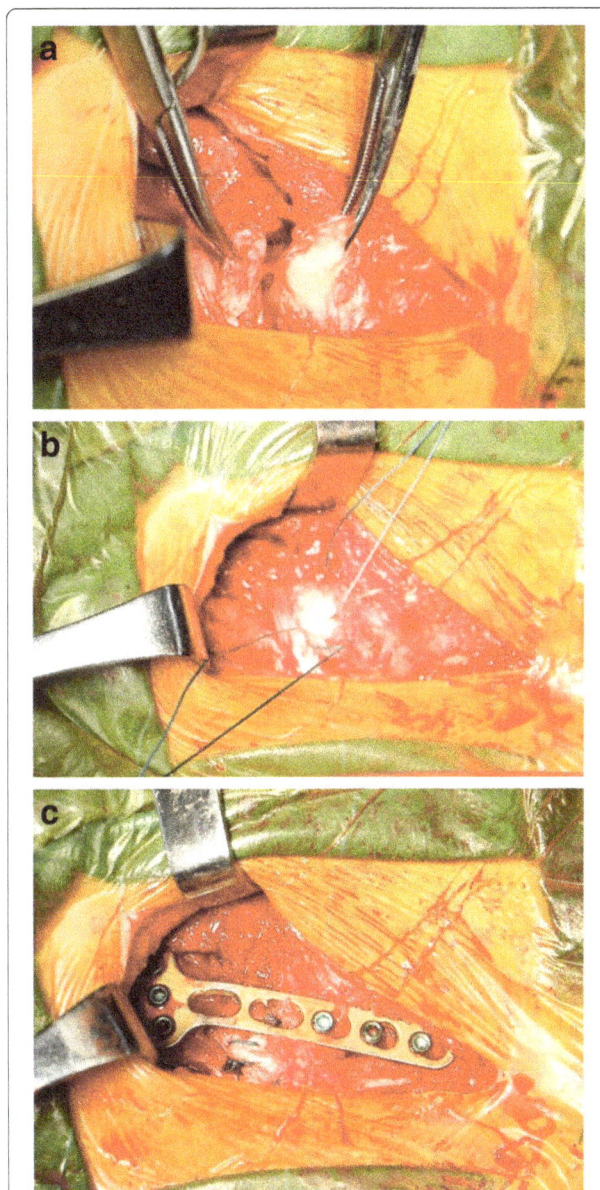

Fig. 2 Intraoperative **a** the anterior ligament was torn. **b** nonabsorbable suture was used to repair the torn ligament and **c** the 3.5-mm locking plate placed anteriorly with three screws in the manubrium and three in the clavicle

recurrent dislocation. All plates were removed after 6 months to avoid breakage or loosening of the plate and screws.

Results

The average follow-up was 14 months (range, 11–16 months). The mean age, gender distribution, dislocation type, and associated injuries are shown in Table 1. All patients had secondary operations for plate removal 6 months postoperatively. At the final follow-up, the mean CSS and DASH scores were 89.5 (range, 78–98) and 9.0 (range, 4–16), respectively (Table 1).

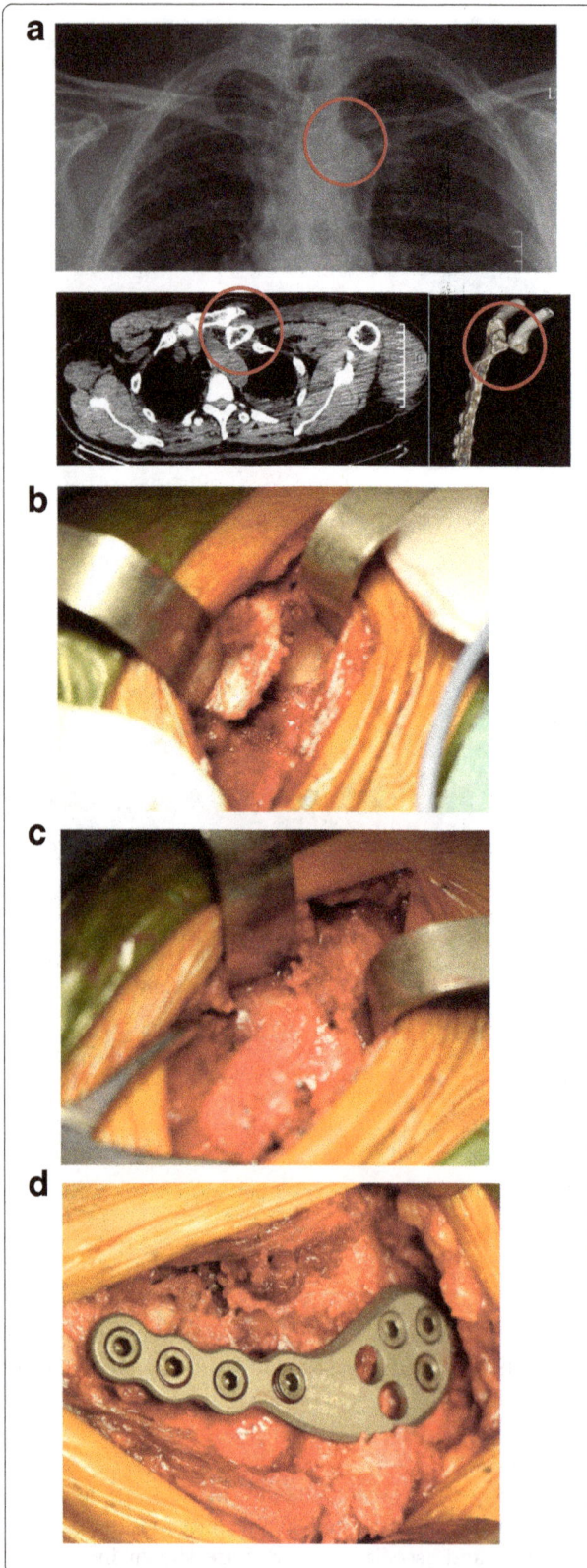

Fig. 3 In patient 2, a 31-year-old male, the preoperative x-ray and computed tomography scan **a** show a posterior dislocation of the sternoclavicular joint. Intraoperative **b** showing the exposed articular surface of the clavicle from the sternum side; and the position of the medial clavicle was not visible, **c** showing the medial end of the clavicle being reduced with forceps, and **d** showing the 3.5-mm locking plate placed anteriorly with three screws in the manubrium and four in the clavicle

There were no early complications, including wound infection or neurologic or vascular deficit; also, no screws or plates were broken or loosened. No case of redislocation or arthrosis was observed. Four patients were satisfied with the outcomes. All patients were able to return to their previous activities.

Only patient 3 had an unsatisfactory outcome. She had a right floating clavicular injury and a left proximal humeral fracture. She was initially diagnosed with a right anterior SCJ dislocation and left proximal humeral fracture (Fig. 1). Closed reduction for the anterior SCJ dislocation failed and open reduction and internal fixation for the two injuries were performed on the following day. The postoperative x-ray showed that the right acromioclavicular joint (ACJ) was dislocated—that is, the Rockwood type V (Fig. 5). After reviewing the initial CT scan again, we found that posterior ACJ dislocation was actually a Rockwood type IV (Fig. 6a). We therefore performed a second operation to treat the floating clavicle (Fig. 6b). The screws previously placed in the clavicle were removed and simultaneously reduction of the ACJ and SCJ dislocations was implemented (Fig. 6c). A hook plate was used to treat the ACJ dislocation. Three months after the second operation, the two implants for treating the floating clavicle were removed. At the last follow-up, although there was no pain or redislocation, abduction of the injured shoulder was limited to 110 degrees.

Disscussion

The SCJ is a saddle-type joint that represents less than half of the medial clavicle as it articulates with the upper angle of the sternum [1]. When the shoulder girdle moves, the SCJ has some range motion in three planes [1]. Despite its intrinsic instability owing to its bony anatomy, strong soft tissues stabilize the structures—including the ligaments, subclavius muscle, articular disc, and capsule—such that the SCJ is one of most rarely dislocated joints in the body [1].

Indirect force from shoulder girdle is the common mechanism of SCJ dislocation [3]. Occasionally, a direct force applied to the medial clavicle will lead to a posterior dislocation [3]. When the prominence of the medial clavicle is inspected after trauma, the anterior SCJ dislocation should be taken into account; a palpable defect

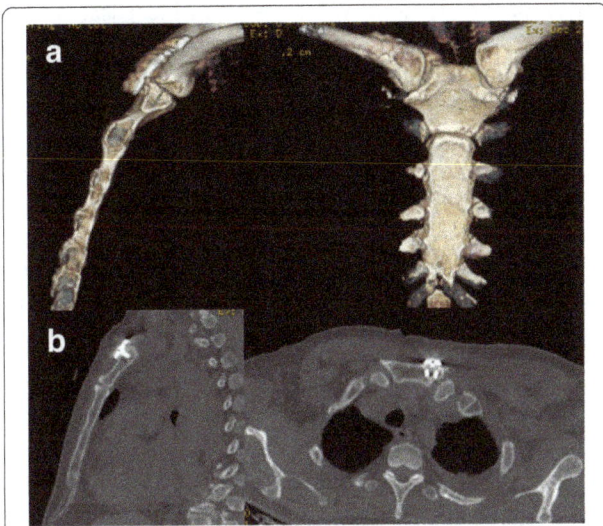

Fig. 4 Postoperative A postoperative three-dimensional computed tomography scan **a** showing good reduction and fixation with the locking plate, sagittal and transverse computed tomography **b** scans showing unicortical screw fixation in the sternum

of the medial end of the clavicle is the obvious sign of a posterior dislocation of the SJC [3]. After such a diagnosis, it is important that the entire clavicle and AC joint be examined. Especially for the anterior SCJ dislocation, the ACJ should be checked carefully to determine whether or not there is a posterior dislocation [14]. In the case of patient 3, we neglected to examine the ipsilateral ACJ and diagnosis of the floating clavicle was delayed.

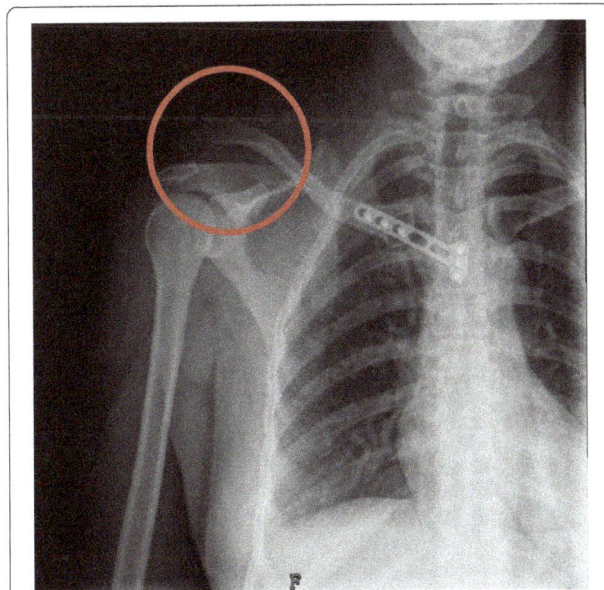

Fig. 5 A postoperative x-ray showing right acromioclavicular joint dislocation

Because it may be blocked by artifacts or neighboring structures, dislocation of the SJC can easily be missed on x-ray. A CT scan is the best diagnostic imaging method and can serve to distinguish between medial clavicular fractures, physeal separations, and SCJ dislocations. Careful scrutiny of a three-dimensional CT scan can serve to determine whether there is displacement of the SCJ and whether or not there is also a posterior AC dislocation.

Closed reduction is the primary choice for the treatment of an SCJ dislocation [15, 16]. For traumatic anterior SCJ dislocations, although there is a risk of recurrent instability, functional deficits after closed reduction have rarely occurred [3]. However, if the medial end of the clavicle clavicle is prominent, surgical correction may be preferred [3]. For traumatic posterior SCJ dislocations, there may be more potential complications; therefore such injuries should immediately be treated with closed reduction. When the posterior SCJ dislocation cannot be reduced in this way, an open reduction should be performed urgently to minimize the risk of cardiovascular compromise [3].

The objective of surgery is to restore the bony anatomy of the SCJ and restore stability to the joint. The risk in the intraoperative process is that of damaging the neighboring structures in the course of drilling holes in the sternum and the medial clavicle and also that of causing loose or unstable implants to migrate postoperatively. The optimal surgical process should minimize these risks as far as possible.

There are many operative methods to treat SCJ dislocation, including ligament repair with reconstruction [10–13], Kirschner wire or pin fixation [5, 6], as well as plate fixation [7–9]. The best choice among the various procedures is also controversial. Ligament repair with reconstruction is the most common method according to the literature [10–13]. These procedures require relatively complex operative manipulation, greater soft tissue dissection, and an extended time of postoperative immobilization. Kirschner wire or pin fixation is contraindicated owing to the associated high risk with their migration into vital structures [5, 6].

Up to now, three studies of plate fixation for the treatment of SCJ dislocation have been reported, including that of Franck et al., who utilized Balser plates for treating three posterior SCJ dislocation [7]. Shuler and Pappas used dual perpendicular locking plates to fix two posterior dialocations [8], and Hecox et al. used a ledge plating technique to treat two posterior dislocation [9]. The Balser plate requires a hook insert into the sternum, which appears to put vital structures at risk. Dual locking plates can achieve rigid fixation for the SCJ, but owing to additional soft tissue manipulation, medical cost will be greater. The ledge plating technique, which does not require the use of a drill or screws into the

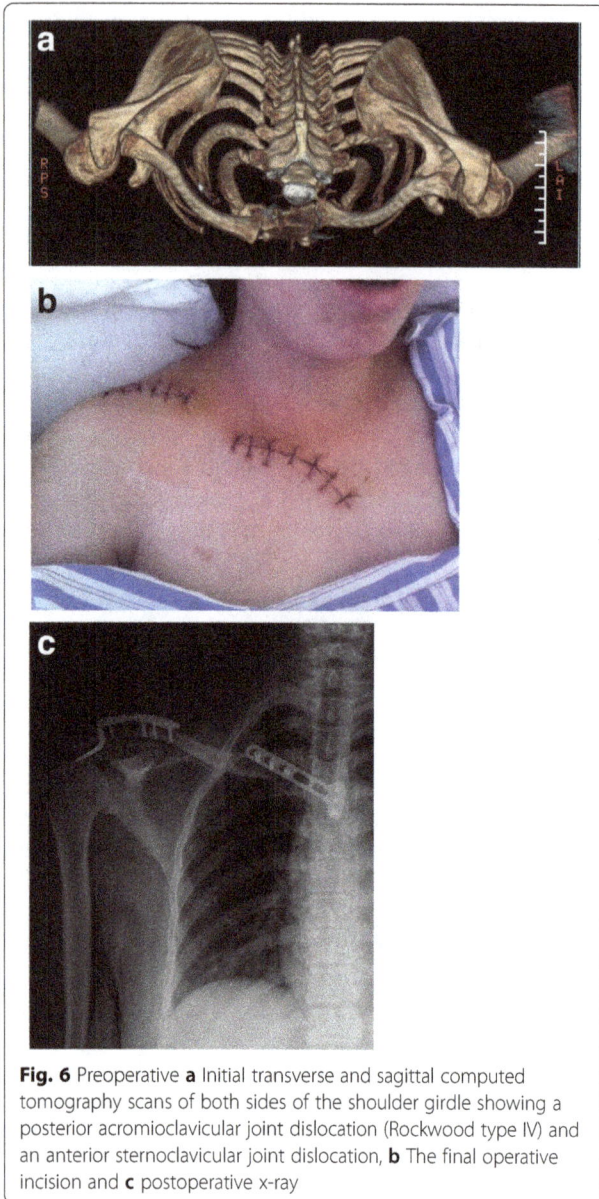

Fig. 6 Preoperative **a** Initial transverse and sagittal computed tomography scans of both sides of the shoulder girdle showing a posterior acromioclavicular joint dislocation (Rockwood type IV) and an anterior sternoclavicular joint dislocation, **b** The final operative incision and **c** postoperative x-ray

cortex of the sternum was drilled and bicortical screws were used for fixation. Finally, the locking plate allows relatively stable fixation as well as a certain degree of movement around the fracture fragment. Thus, in utilizing a single locking plate to treat the SCJ dislocation, we can also ensure a certain degree of joint movement, which facilitates healing and the recovery of shoulder function.

We believe that single locking plate fixation combined with repair of the ligament and capsul is easier to manipulate, minimizes the manipulation of soft tissues, and protects the periosteal blood supply. Unicortical drill and screw fixation in the sternum is a relatively safe operative process in terms of protecting the vital structures. Most of these patients have good function without recurrent dislocation or subluxation.

To avoid the migration of loose or broken implants, the locking plates must be removed about 3 months after surgery; that is the disadvantage of this technique.

Furthermore, this study has some limitations. It is a retrospective study involving a small number of patients with a short-term follow-up. A long-term follow-up would be needed to determine whether postoperative arthritis developed in these patients.

Conclusion

Fixation using a single locking plate combined with repair of the ligament and capsule is relatively easy to do; it decreases the risk of the soft tissues injury and protects the periosteal blood supply. Our study indicates that open reduction and single-locking-plate fixation for the treatment of traumatic sternoclavicular joint dislocations is a safe, relatively straightforward surgical procedure that can lead to satisfactory outcomes.

Abbreviations
ACJ: Acromioclavicular joint; CSS: Constant Shoulder Score; DASH: Disability of the Arm, Shoulder, and Hand; SCJ: Sternoclavicular joint

Acknowledgments
We thank LetPub (www.letpub.com) for providing linguistic assistance during the preparation of this manuscript.

Funding
Research Grant for Health Science and Technology of Pudong Municipal Commission of Health and family Planning of Shanghai (Grant No. PW2015A-15), Program for Outstanding Medical Academic Leader of Shanghai, Program for Medical Key Department of Shanghai (Grant No. ZK 2015B17) and Research Grant for Shanghai Municipal Commission of Health and family Planning (Grant No. 201440063).

Authors' contributions
RA, YZ, JZ, and BY conceived and designed the experiments. CL, WH, ZJ and JS analyzed the data. RA, and ZJ wrote the paper. All authors read and approved the final manuscript.

sternum, can obviously avoid damage to the vital structures, but the stability of fixation of the SCJ may be insufficient. The biomechanics involved in this innovative method requires further research.

Use of a single locking plate may be a preferable alternative for treating SCJ dislocations. The purpose of the locking plate is to maintain the SCJ reduction and allow the soft tissues around the joint to heal. In the surgical process, unicortical screws in the sternum and bicortical screws in the medial clavicle were used to maintain the stability of the SCJ. Meanwhile, we sutured the injured ligaments and capsules to provide preliminary stability to the joint. After stable fixation of the locking plate, the soft tissues can heal and the SCJ will be stable. In order to avoid iatrogenic injury, only the anterior

Consent for publication
Written consent to publish the content of this report along with the accompanying images was obtained from all patients.

Competing interests
The authors declare that they have no competing interests.

References
1. Renfree KJ, Wright TW. Anatomy and biomechanics of the acromioclavicular and sternoclavicular joints. Clinics in sports medicine. 2003;22(2):219–37.
2. Nettles JL, Linscheid RL. Sternoclavicular dislocations. The Journal of trauma. 1968;8(2):158–64.
3. Robinson CM, Jenkins PJ, Markham PE, Beggs I. Disorders of the sternoclavicular joint. The Journal of bone and joint surgery British volume. 2008;90(6):685–96.
4. Worman LW, Leagus C. Intrathoracic injury following retrosternal dislocation of the clavicle. The Journal of trauma. 1967;7(3):416–23.
5. Lyons FA, Rockwood CA Jr. Migration of pins used in operations on the shoulder. The Journal of bone and joint surgery American. 1990;72(8):1262–7.
6. Liu HP, Chang CH, Lin PJ, Chu JJ, Hsieh HC, Chang JP, Hsieh MC. Pulmonary artery perforation after Kirschner wire migration: case report and review of the literature. The Journal of trauma. 1993;34(1):154–6.
7. Franck WM, Jannasch O, Siassi M, Hennig FF. Balser plate stabilization: an alternate therapy for traumatic sternoclavicular instability. Journal of shoulder and elbow surgery. 2003;12(3):276–81.
8. Hecox SE, Wood GW 2nd. Ledge plating technique for unstable posterior sternoclavicular dislocation. Journal of orthopaedic trauma. 2010;24(4):255–7.
9. Shuler FD, Pappas N. Treatment of posterior sternoclavicular dislocation with locking plate osteosynthesis. Orthopedics. 2008;31(3):273.
10. Spencer EE, Kuhn JE, Huston LJ, Carpenter JE, Hughes RE. Ligamentous restraints to anterior and posterior translation of the sternoclavicular joint. Journal of shoulder and elbow surgery. 2002;11(1):43–7.
11. Armstrong AL, Dias JJ. Reconstruction for instability of the sternoclavicular joint using the tendon of the sternocleidomastoid muscle. The Journal of bone and joint surgery British volume. 2008;90(5):610–3.
12. Guan JJ, Wolf BR. Reconstruction for anterior sternoclavicular joint dislocation and instability. Journal of shoulder and elbow surgery. 2013;22(6):775–81.
13. Uri O, Barmpagiannis K, Higgs D, Falworth M, Alexander S, Lambert SM. Clinical outcome after reconstruction for sternoclavicular joint instability using a sternocleidomastoid tendon graft. The Journal of bone and joint surgery American. 2014;96(5):417–22.
14. Scapinelli R. Bipolar dislocation of the clavicle: 3D CT imaging and delayed surgical correction of a case. Archives of orthopaedic and trauma surgery. 2004;124(6):421–4.
15. Bicos J, Nicholson GP. Treatment and results of sternoclavicular joint injuries. Clinics in sports medicine. 2003;22(2):359–70.
16. Groh GI, Wirth MA, Rockwood CA Jr. Treatment of traumatic posterior sternoclavicular dislocations. Journal of shoulder and elbow surgery. 2011;20(1):107–13.

Permissions

All chapters in this book were first published in MD, by BioMed Central; hereby published with permission under the Creative Commons Attribution License or equivalent. Every chapter published in this book has been scrutinized by our experts. Their significance has been extensively debated. The topics covered herein carry significant findings which will fuel the growth of the discipline. They may even be implemented as practical applications or may be referred to as a beginning point for another development.

The contributors of this book come from diverse backgrounds, making this book a truly international effort. This book will bring forth new frontiers with its revolutionizing research information and detailed analysis of the nascent developments around the world.

We would like to thank all the contributing authors for lending their expertise to make the book truly unique. They have played a crucial role in the development of this book. Without their invaluable contributions this book wouldn't have been possible. They have made vital efforts to compile up to date information on the varied aspects of this subject to make this book a valuable addition to the collection of many professionals and students.

This book was conceptualized with the vision of imparting up-to-date information and advanced data in this field. To ensure the same, a matchless editorial board was set up. Every individual on the board went through rigorous rounds of assessment to prove their worth. After which they invested a large part of their time researching and compiling the most relevant data for our readers.

The editorial board has been involved in producing this book since its inception. They have spent rigorous hours researching and exploring the diverse topics which have resulted in the successful publishing of this book. They have passed on their knowledge of decades through this book. To expedite this challenging task, the publisher supported the team at every step. A small team of assistant editors was also appointed to further simplify the editing procedure and attain best results for the readers.

Apart from the editorial board, the designing team has also invested a significant amount of their time in understanding the subject and creating the most relevant covers. They scrutinized every image to scout for the most suitable representation of the subject and create an appropriate cover for the book.

The publishing team has been an ardent support to the editorial, designing and production team. Their endless efforts to recruit the best for this project, has resulted in the accomplishment of this book. They are a veteran in the field of academics and their pool of knowledge is as vast as their experience in printing. Their expertise and guidance has proved useful at every step. Their uncompromising quality standards have made this book an exceptional effort. Their encouragement from time to time has been an inspiration for everyone.

The publisher and the editorial board hope that this book will prove to be a valuable piece of knowledge for researchers, students, practitioners and scholars across the globe.

List of Contributors

Emma Olsson
Medical Radiation Physics, Department of Translational Medicine, Lund University, Inga Marie Nilssons gata 49, SE-205 02 Malmö, Sweden

Pernilla Peterson and Lars E. Olsson
Medical Radiation Physics, Department of Translational Medicine, Lund University, Inga Marie Nilssons gata 49, SE-205 02 Malmö, Sweden
Department of Oncology and Radiation Physics, Skåne University Hospital, Inga Marie Nilssons gata 49, SE-205 02 Malmö, Sweden

Carl Johan Tiderius
Department of Clinical Sciences, Lund University, Skåne University Hospital, SE-221 85 Lund, Sweden

Björn Lundin
Department of Medical Imaging and Physiology, Skåne University Hospital, SE-221 85 Lund, Sweden

Annemarie Uhlig
Department of Urology, University Medical Center Göttingen, Göttingen, Germany

Tim Rolvien, Tobias Schmidt and Sebastian Karl Butscheidt
Department of Osteology and Biomechanics, University Medical Center Hamburg-Eppendorf, Hamburg, Germany

Klaus Püschel
Department of Legal Medicine, University Medical Center Hamburg-Eppendorf, Hamburg, Germany

Seung Yeol Lee and Sangwoo Kim
Department of Orthopaedic Surgery, Ewha Womans University Mokdong Hospital, Seoul, South Korea

Soon-Sun Kwon
Department of Mathematics, College of Natural Science, Ajou University, Suwon, Gyeonggi, South Korea

Kyoung Min Lee Moon Seok Park and Ki Hyuk Sung
Department of Orthopaedic Surgery, Seoul National University Bundang Hospital, 300 Gumi-Dong, Bundang-Gu, Seoungnam, Gyeonggi 463-707, South Korea

Chin Youb Chung
Department of Orthopaedic Surgery, Seoul National University Bundang Hospital, 300 Gumi-Dong, Bundang-Gu, Seoungnam, Gyeonggi 463-707, South Korea
Department of Orthopaedic Surgery, Seoul National University College of Medicine, Seoul, South Korea

Ricky Watari
Faculty of Kinesiology, University of Calgary, Calgary, Alberta, Canada
Coordination for the Improvement of Higher Education Personnel (CAPES), Brasilia, Brazil

Sean T. Osis
Faculty of Kinesiology, University of Calgary, Calgary, Alberta, Canada
Running Injury Clinic, University of Calgary, 2500 University Drive NW, Calgary, Alberta T2N 1N4, Canada

Angkoon Phinyomark
Institute of Biomedical Engineering, University of New Brunswick, Fredericton, New Brunswick, Canada
Reed Ferber Faculty of Kinesiology, University of Calgary, Calgary, Alberta, Canada
Coordination for the Improvement of Higher Education Personnel (CAPES), Brasilia, Brazil
Running Injury Clinic, University of Calgary, 2500 University
Drive NW, Calgary, Alberta T2N 1N4, Canada
Faculty of Nursing, University of Calgary, Calgary, Alberta, Canada

Keiji Yoshioka, Tomochika Kisukeda, Ryoji Zuinen, Yosuke Yasuda and Kenji Miyamoto
Central Research Lab., Research & Development Div., Seikagaku Corporation, 1253, Tateno 3-chome, Higashiyamato-shi, Tokyo 207-0021, Japan

Sarah Drew and Christopher Lavy
Oxford NIHR Musculoskeletal Biomedical Research Unit, Nuffield Department of Orthopaedics, Rheumatology and Musculoskeletal Sciences, University of Oxford, Windmill Road, Headington, Oxford OX3 7LD, UK

Rachael Gooberman-Hill
School of Clinical Sciences, University of Bristol, Learning and Research Building, Level 1, Southmead Hospital, Bristol BS10 5NB, UK
National Institute for Health Research Bristol Biomedical Research Centre, University of Bristol, Bristol, UK

M. E. van Eck, C. M. Lameijer and M. El Moumni
University of Groningen, University Medical Center Groningen, Department of Surgery, Groningen, The Netherlands

Jan Hubert, Lukas Weiser, Wolfgang Lehmann, Frank Timo Beil and Thelonius Hawellek
Department of Trauma Surgery, Orthopaedics and Plastic Surgery, University Medical Center Göttingen, Robert-Koch-Straße 40, 37075 Göttingen, Germany

Sandra Hischke
Department of Medical Biometry and Epidemiology, University Medical Center Hamburg-Eppendorf, Hamburg, Germany

Linda C. Li and Lynne M. Feehan
Faculty of Medicine, Arthritis Research Canada, University of British Columbia, Vancouver, Canada

Angela Schlager, Kerstin Ahlqvist, Ronnie Pingel and Per Kristiansson
Department of Public Health and Caring Sciences, Uppsala University, Husargatan 3, 752 37 Uppsala, Sweden

Jonas Svensson
Medical Radiation Physics, Department of Translational Medicine, Lund
University, Inga Marie Nilssons gata 49, SE-205 02 Malmö, Sweden Orthopedics, Department of Medical Imaging and Physiology, Skåne University Hospital, SE-221 85 Lund, Sweden

N. Berger, M. Salzmann and P. M. Prodinger
Klinikum rechts der Isar der Technischen Universität München, Munich, Germany

D. Lewens and L. Döderlein
Behandlungszentrum Aschau im Chiemgau, Aschau, Germany

A. Hapfelmeier
Klinikum rechts der Isar der Technischen Universität München, Munich, Germany
Institute of Medical Informatics, Statistics and Epidemiology, Technical University Munich, Munich, Germany

Jeremy S. Somerson
University of Texas Medical Branch, 301 University Blvd, Galveston, TX 77555, USA

Aaron J. Bois
Sport Medicine Centre, University of Calgary, 2500 University Drive NW, Calgary, AB T2N 1N4, Canada

Jeffrey Jeng
University of California Los Angeles, Los Angeles, USA

Kamal I. Bohsali
Jacksonville Orthopaedic Institute-Beaches Division, 6100 Kennerly Road Suite 101, Jacksonville, FL 32216, USA

John W. Hinchey and Michael A. Wirth
Department of Orthopaedics, The University of Texas Health Science Center San Antonio, 7703 Floyd Curl Drive – MC 7774, San Antonio, TX 78229, USA

Juan Wu, Jianhua Xu, Qicui Zhu, Jingyu Cai and Jiale Ren
Department of Rheumatology and Immunology, Arthritis Research Institute, the First Affiliated Hospital of Anhui Medical University, 218 Jixi Street, Hefei, China

Shuang Zheng
Department of Rheumatology and Immunology, Arthritis Research Institute, the First Affiliated Hospital of Anhui Medical University, 218 Jixi Street, Hefei, China

Kang Wang
Department of Rheumatology and Immunology, Arthritis Research Institute, the First Affiliated Hospital of Anhui Medical University, 218 Jixi Street, Hefei, China
Menzies Institute for Medical Research, University of Tasmania, Hobart, TAS 7000, Australia

Changhai Ding
Department of Rheumatology and Immunology, Arthritis Research Institute, the First Affiliated Hospital of Anhui Medical University, 218 Jixi Street, Hefei, China
Menzies Institute for Medical Research, University of Tasmania, Hobart, TAS 7000, Australia
Institute of Bone & Joint Translational Research, Southern Medical University, Guangzhou, Guangdong, China

Emma Louise Healey, Ebenezer K. Afolabi, John J. Edwards, Clare Jinks, Elaine M. Hay and Krysia S. Dziedzic
Research Institute for Primary Care and Health Sciences, Keele University, Keele, Staffordshire ST5 5BG, UK

Martyn Lewis and Kelvin P. Jordan
Research Institute for Primary Care and Health Sciences, Keele University, Keele, Staffordshire ST5 5BG, UK
Keele Clinical Trials Unit, David Weatherall Building, Keele University, Staffordshire, UK

Andrew Finney
Research Institute for Primary Care and Health Sciences, Keele University, Keele, Staffordshire ST5 5BG, UK
School of Nursing and Midwifery, Keele University, Staffordshire, UK

Alison Hammond and Yeliz Prior
Centre for Health Sciences Research (OT), L701 Allerton, University of Salford, Frederick Road, Salford M6 6PU, UK

Sarah Tyson
Division of Nursing, Midwifery & Social Work, University of Manchester, Manchester, UK

Yuji Kohno, Mitsuru Mizuno, Nobutake Ozeki, Hisako Katano, Koji Otabe and Ichiro Sekiya
Center for Stem Cells and Regenerative Medicine, Tokyo Medical and Dental
University, 1-5-45 Yushima, Bunkyo-ku, Tokyo 113-8510, Japan

Hideyuki Koga
Department of Joint Surgery and Sports Medicine, Tokyo Medical and Dental University, 1-5-45 Yushima, Bunkyo-ku, Tokyo 113-8510, Japan

Mikio Matsumoto, Haruka Kaneko and Yuji Takazawa
Department of Orthopaedics, Juntendo University School of Medicine, 3-1-3 Hongo, Bunkyo-ku, Tokyo 113-8431, Japan

Matthias Aurich
Center for Orthopaedic and Trauma Surgery, Klinikum Mittleres Erzgebirge, Alte Marienberger, Str. 52, 09405 Zschopau, Germany
Department of Trauma, Hand and Reconstructive Surgery, Universitätsklinikum Jena, Erlanger Allee 101, 07747 Jena, Germany
Department of Biochemistry, Rush Medical College, 1735 W. Harrison St, Chicago, IL 60612, USA

Gunther O. Hofmann and Florian Gras
Department of Trauma, Hand and Reconstructive Surgery, Universitätsklinikum Jena, Erlanger Allee 101, 07747 Jena, Germany

Bernd Rolauffs
G.E.R.N. Tissue Replacement, Regeneration & Neogenesis, Department of Orthopedics and Trauma Surgery, Medical Center - Albert-Ludwigs-University of Freiburg, Faculty of Medicine, Albert-Ludwigs-University of Freiburg, Hugstetter Straße 55, 79106 Freiburg, Germany
Massachusetts Institute of Technology, Center for Biomedical Engineering, 500 Technology Sq, Cambridge, MA 02139, USA

Jong Jin Yoo
Department of Internal Medicine, Kangdong Sacred Heart Hospital, Seoul, South Korea

Dong Hyun Kim
Department of Social and Preventive Medicine, Hallym University College of Medicine, Chuncheon, South Korea

Hyun Ah Kim
Rheumatology Division, Department of Internal Medicine, Hallym University Sacred Heart Hospital, 896, Pyongchondong, Dongan-gu, Anyang, Kyunggi-do 431-070, South Korea

Cliodhna Farthing, Gernot Lang, Matthias J. Feucht, Norbert P. Südkamp and Kaywan Izadpanah
Department of Orthopedic and Trauma Surgery, Medical Center - Albert-Ludwigs-University of Freiburg, Faculty of Medicine, Freiburg im Breisgau, Germany

Jing Wu, Yuan Qu, Yu-Ping Zhang, Jia-Xin Deng and Qing-Hong Yu
Department of Rheumatology and Clinical Immunology, ZhuJiang Hospital, Southern Medical University, 253 Gongye Ave GuangZhou, Guang Dong 510282, China

Philipp Ahrens
Department of Orthopaedic Sports Medicine, Klinikum rechts der Isar, Technische Universitaet Muenchen, Germany, Ismanninger, Str. 22, D- 81675 Muenchen, Germany
Sportklinik Stuttgart, Taubenheimstraße 8, D-70372 Stuttgart, Germany

Dirk Mueller
Schön Klinik Harthausen, Dr.-Wilhelm-Knarr- Weg 1-3, D-83043 Bad Aibling, Germany

Sebastian Siebenlist
Department of Orthopaedic Sports Medicine, Klinikum rechts der Isar, Technische Universitaet Muenchen, Germany, Ismanninger, Str. 22, D- 81675 Muenchen, Germany

Andreas Lenich
Department of Orthopaedic Sports Medicine, Klinikum rechts der Isar, Technische Universitaet Muenchen, Germany, Ismanninger, Str. 22, D- 81675 Muenchen, Germany
Helios Klinikum München West, Steinerweg 5, D- 81241 Muenchen, Germany

Gunther H. Sandmann
BG Unfallklinik Tuebingen, Schnarrenbergstraße 95, 72076 Tuebingen, Germany
Sportklinik Ravensburg, Bachstraße 57, 88214 Ravensburg, Germany

Tracey Smythe and Allen Foster
International Centre for Evidence in Disability, London School of Hygiene & Tropical Medicine, Keppel Street, London WC1E7HT, UK

Ryan S. Falck Patrick C. Y. Chan, Teresa Liu-Ambrose and John R. Best
Faculty of Medicine, Aging, Mobility and Cognitive Neuroscience Laboratory, Djavad Mowafaghian Centre for Brain Health, Department of Physical Therapy, University of British Columbia, 212-2177 Wesbrook Mall, Vancouver, BC V6T 1Z3, Canada

Ulrich Stoeckle
BG Unfallklinik Tuebingen, Schnarrenbergstraße 95, 72076 Tuebingen, Germany

Eva Rasmussen-Barr
Karolinska Institutet, Department of Neurobiology, Care Sciences and Society, Division of Physiotherapy, Huddinge, Sweden

Elisabeth Krefting Bjelland
Department of Public Health and Caring Sciences, Uppsala University, Husargatan 3, 752 37 Uppsala, Sweden
Department of Obstetrics and Gynecology, Akershus University Hospital, Lørenskog, Norway

Christina Olsson and Lena Nilsson-Wikmar
Karolinska Institutet, Department of Neurobiology, Care Sciences and Society, Division of Physiotherapy, Huddinge, Sweden
Academic Primary Healthcare Centre, Stockholm County Council, Huddinge, Sweden

Haixia Cao, Qiuxiang Zhang, Ting Fu, Rulan Yin, Yunfei Xia and Zhifeng Gu
Department of Rheumatology, Affiliated Hospital of Nantong University, 20th Xisi Road, 226001 Nantong, People's Republic of China

Lijuan Zhang
Department of Rheumatology, Affiliated Hospital of Nantong University, 20th Xisi Road, 226001 Nantong, People's Republic of China
Department of Rheumatology, Ruijin Hospital, Shanghai Jiao Tong University School of Medicine, 197 Ruijin 2nd Road, Shanghai 200025, China

Liren Li
Department of Rheumatology, Affiliated Hospital of Nantong University, 20th Xisi Road, 226001 Nantong, People's Republic of China
School of Nursing, Nantong University, 19th Qixiu Road, 226001 Nantong, People's Republic of China

Rongguang Ao, Yalong Zhu, Jianhua Zhou, Zhen Jian, Jifei Shi, Cheng Li, Wankun Hu and Baoqing Yu
Department of Orthopedics, Shanghai Pudong Hospital, Fudan University
Pudong Medical Center, 2800 Gongwei Road, Huinan Town, Pudong, Shanghai 201399, People's Republic of China

Index

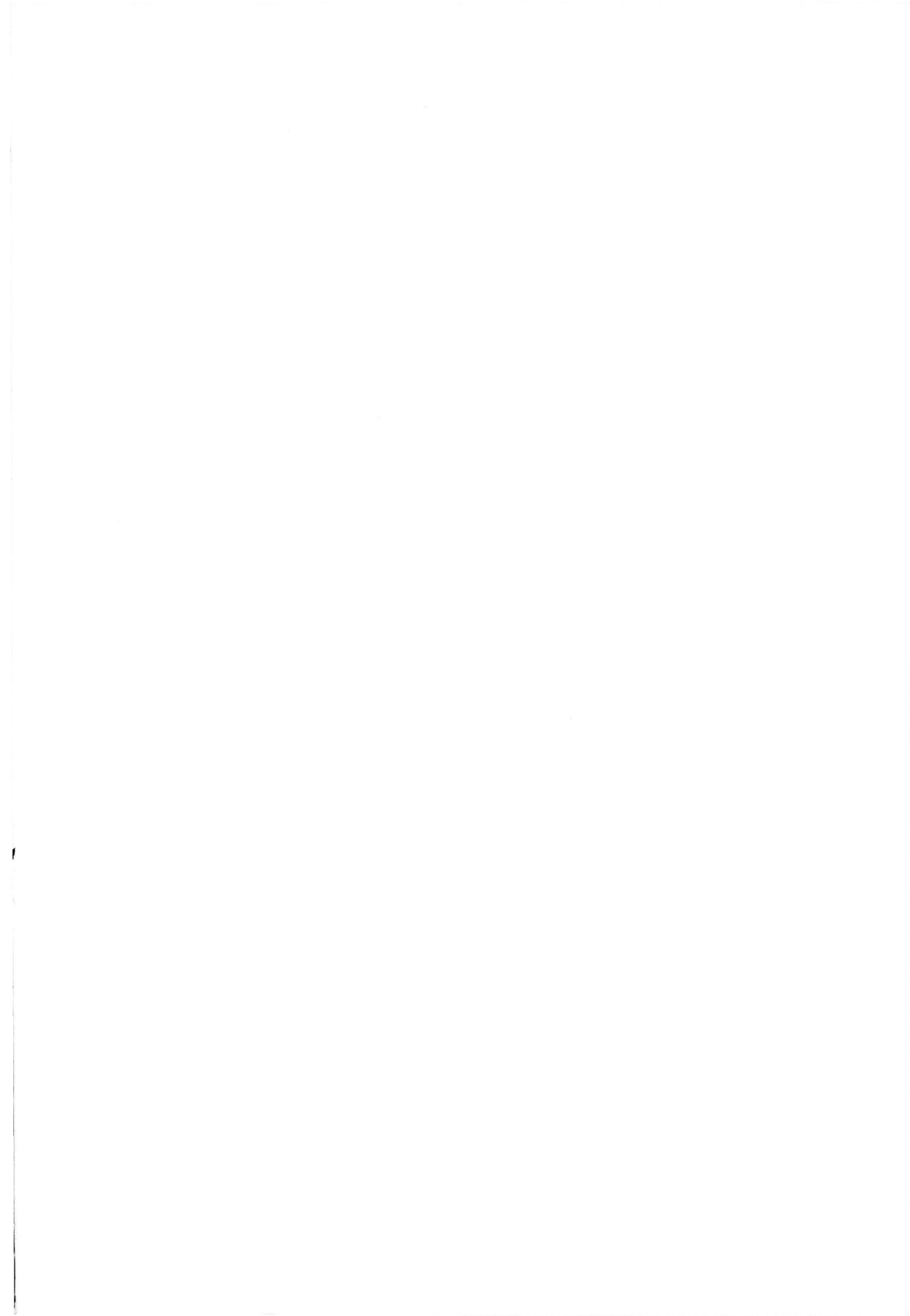